Patient Management with Stable Ischemic Heart Disease

Editors

ALEXANDER C. FANAROFF
JOHN W. HIRSHFELD JR

MEDICAL CLINICS OF NORTH AMERICA

www.medical.theclinics.com

Consulting Editor
JACK ENDE

May 2024 • Volume 108 • Number 3

ELSEVIER

1600 John F. Kennedy Boulevard • Suite 1800 • Philadelphia, Pennsylvania, 19103-2899

http://www.theclinics.com

MEDICAL CLINICS OF NORTH AMERICA Volume 108, Number 3
May 2024 ISSN 0025-7125, ISBN-13: 978-0-443-29368-9

Editor: Taylor Hayes
Developmental Editor: Malvika Shah

Medical Clinics of North America (ISSN 0025-7125) is published bimonthly by Elsevier Inc., 360 Park Avenue South, New York, NY 10010-1710. Months of publication are January, March, May, July, September, and November. Business and editorial offices: 1600 John F. Kennedy Boulevard, Suite 1800, Philadelphia, PA 19103-2899. Periodicals postage paid at New York, NY, and additional mailing offices. Subscription prices are USD $336.00 per year (US individuals), $100.00 per year (US Students), $433.00 per year (Canadian individuals), $200.00 per year for (foreign students), $100.00 per year for (Canadian students), $479.00 per year (foreign individuals). For institutional access pricing please contact Customer Service via the contact information below. To receive student/resident rate, orders must be accompanied by name of affiliated institution, date of term, and the signature of program/residency coordinator on institution letterhead. Orders will be billed at individual rate until proof of status is received. Foreign air speed delivery is included in all Clinics' subscription prices. All prices are subject to change without notice. **POSTMASTER:** Send address changes to *Medical Clinics of North America*, Elsevier Health Sciences Division, Subscription Customer Service, 3251 Riverport Lane, Maryland Heights, MO 63043. **Customer Service: Telephone: 1-800-654-2452** (U.S. and Canada); **1-314-447-8871** (outside U.S. and Canada). **Fax: 314-447-8029. E-mail: journalscustomerserviceusa@elsevier.com** (for print support); **journalsonlinesupport-usa@elsevier.com** (for online support).

Reprints. For copies of 100 or more of articles in this publication, please contact the Commercial Reprints Department, Elsevier Inc., 360 Park Avenue South, New York, NY 10010-1710. Tel.: 212-633-3874; Fax: 212-633-3820; E-mail: reprints@elsevier.com.

Medical Clinics of North America is also published in Spanish by McGraw-Hill Interamericana Editores S. A., P.O. Box 5-237, 06500 Mexico, D.F., Mexico.

Medical Clinics of North America is covered in *MEDLINE/PubMed (Index Medicus), Current Contents, ASCA, Excerpta Medica, Science Citation Index, and ISI/BIOMED.*

PROGRAM OBJECTIVE
The goal of the *Medical Clinics of North America* is to keep practicing physicians up to date with current clinical practice by providing timely articles reviewing the state of the art in patient care.

TARGET AUDIENCE
All practicing physicians and other healthcare professionals.

LEARNING OBJECTIVES
Upon completion of this activity, participants will be able to:
1. Review the diagnostic evaluation options for individuals presenting with stable ischemic heart disease symptoms.
2. Explain current modalities for enhancing the quality and equity of chronic coronary disease (CCD) management, concerning racial and ethnic disparities.
3. Discuss primary and secondary optimal medical therapies for preventing recurrent ischemic events in patients with chronic coronary disease.

ACCREDITATION
The Elsevier Office of Continuing Medical Education (EOCME) is accredited by the Accreditation Council for Continuing Medical Education (ACCME) to provide continuing medical education for physicians.

The EOCME designates this journal-based CME activity for a maximum of 13 *AMA PRA Category 1 Credit*(s)™. Physicians should claim only the credit commensurate with the extent of their participation in the activity.

All other healthcare professionals requesting continuing education credit for this enduring material will be issued a certificate of participation.

DISCLOSURE OF CONFLICTS OF INTEREST
The EOCME assesses conflict of interest with its instructors, faculty, planners, and other individuals who are in a position to control the content of CME activities. All relevant conflicts of interest that are identified are thoroughly vetted by EOCME for fair balance, scientific objectivity, and patient care recommendations. EOCME is committed to providing its learners with CME activities that promote improvements or quality in healthcare and not a specific proprietary business or a commercial interest.

The planning committee, staff, authors, and editors listed below have identified no financial relationships or relationships to products or devices they or their spouse/life partner have with commercial interest related to the content of this CME activity:
Timothy Abrahams, MBBS; Khawaja Hassan Akhtar, MD; Alexander P. Ambrosini, MD; Tanesha Beebe-Peat, MD; Alex J. Chang, MD; Andrew M. Cheng, MD; Abdulla A. Damluji, MD, PhD; Jacob A. Doll, MD; Emily S. Fishman, MD; Eleonore Grant, MD; Steven A. Hamilton, MD; John W. Hirshfeld Jr, MD; Rand Ibrahim, MD; Anita M. Kelsey, MD, MBA; Sherrie Khadanga, MD; Yilin Liang, MD, MPH; Michelle Littlejohn; Puja K. Mehta, MD; Brett M. Montelaro, MD; Nkiru Osude, MD, MS; Merlin Packiam; Parth P. Patel, MD; Monika Sanghavi, MD; Wilson Lay Tang, MD; Marc Thames, MD

The planning committee, staff, authors, and editors listed below have identified financial relationships to products or devices they or their spouse/life partner have with commercial interest related to the content of this CME activity:
Andrew P. Ambrosy, MD: Researcher: Abbott, Amarin, Edwards Lifesciences, Esperion Therapeutics, Novartis

Usman Baber, MD, MS: Consultant: Amgen, AstraZeneca, Boston Scientific, Abbott

Alexander C. Fanaroff, MD, MHS: Researcher: Abbott, Prolocor; Consultant: Abbott, Intercept Pharmaceuticals, Areteia Therapeutics, Anthos Therapeutics

Michelle D. Kelsey, MD: Consultant/Advisor: Bayer, HeartFlow

Michael G. Nanna, MD, MHS: Consultant: HeartFlow, Merck

Adam J. Nelson, MBBS, MBA, MPH, PhD: Researcher: Amgen, Lilly, Novartis, Boehringer Ingelheim; Consultant: Amgen, AstraZeneca, Boehringer Ingelheim, Lilly, Merck, Sanofi, Novo Nordisk, CSL Seqirus, Vaxxinity

Stephen J. Nicholls, MBBS, PhD: Researcher: AstraZeneca, Amgen, Anthera Pharmaceuticals, CSL Behring, Cerenis Therapeutics, Lilly, Esperion, Resverlogix, Novartis, InfraReDx, Sanofi-Regeneron;

Consultant: Amgen, Akcea, AstraZeneca, Boehringer Ingelheim, CSL Behring, Lilly, Esperion, Kowa, Merck, Takeda, Pfizer, Sanofi-Regeneron, Novo Nordisk, CSL Seqirus, Vaxxinity

Neha Pagidipati, MD, MPH: Researcher: Alnylam, Amgen, Boehringer Ingelheim, Eggland's Best, Lilly, Novartis, Novo Nordisk, Verily Life Sciences; Consultant/Advisor: Bayer, Boehringer Ingelheim, CRISPR Therapeutics, Eli Lilly, Esperion, AstraZeneca, Merck, Novartis, Novo Nordisk, Johnson & Johnson, Miga Health

Fatima Rodriguez, MD, MPH: Consultant: Health Pals, Novartis, Amgen, NovoNordisk, Movano Health, Kento Health

UNAPPROVED/OFF-LABEL USE DISCLOSURE
The EOCME requires CME faculty to disclose to the participants;
1. When products or procedures being discussed are off-label, unlabelled, experimental, and/or investigational (not US Food and Drug Administration [FDA] approved); and
2. Any limitations on the information presented, such as data that are preliminary or that represent ongoing research, interim analyses, and/or unsupported opinions. Faculty may discuss information about pharmaceutical agents that is outside of FDA-approved labelling. This information is intended solely for CME and is not intended to promote off-label use of these medications. If you have any questions, contact the medical affairs department of the manufacturer for the most recent prescribing information.

TO ENROLL
To enroll in the *Medical Clinics of North America* Continuing Medical Education program, call customer service at 1-800-654-2452 or sign up online at http://www.theclinics.com/home/cme. The CME program is available to subscribers for an additional annual fee of USD 319.00.

METHOD OF PARTICIPATION
In order to claim credit, participants must complete the following;
1. Complete enrolment as indicated above.
2. Read the activity.
3. Complete the CME Test and Evaluation. Participants must achieve a score of 70% on the test. All CME Tests and Evaluations must be completed online.

CME INQUIRIES/SPECIAL NEEDS
For all CME inquiries or special needs, please contact elsevierCME@elsevier.com.

MEDICAL CLINICS OF NORTH AMERICA

Contributors

CONSULTING EDITOR

JACK ENDE, MD, MACP
The Schaeffer Professor of Medicine, Perelman School of Medicine of the University of Pennsylvania, Philadelphia, Pennsylvania, USA

EDITORS

ALEXANDER C. FANAROFF, MD, MHS
Assistant Professor of Medicine, Division of Cardiovascular Medicine, University of Pennsylvania Perelman School of Medicine, Philadelphia, Pennsylvania, USA

JOHN W. HIRSHFELD Jr, MD
Emeritus Professor of Medicine, Division of Cardiovascular Medicine, University of Pennsylvania Perelman School of Medicine, Philadelphia, Pennsylvania, USA

AUTHORS

TIMOTHY ABRAHAMS, MBBS
Cardiology Registrar, Victorian Heart Institute, Monash University, Melbourne, Victoria, Australia

KHAWAJA HASSAN AKHTAR, MD
Cardiology Fellow, Department of Medicine, Section of Cardiovascular Medicine, University of Oklahoma Health Sciences Center, Oklahoma City, Oklahoma, USA

ALEXANDER P. AMBROSINI, MD
Resident, Department of Internal Medicine, Yale School of Medicine, New Haven, Connecticut, USA

ANDREW P. AMBROSY, MD
Department of Cardiology, Kaiser Permanente San Francisco Medical Center, San Francisco, California, USA; Assistant Medical Director, Clinical Trials Program, Division of Research, Kaiser Permanente Northern California, Oakland, California, USA

USMAN BABER, MD, MS
Chief, Cardiovascular Section, Associate Professor of Medicine, University of Oklahoma Health Sciences Center, Oklahoma City, OK, USA

TANESHA BEEBE-PEAT, MD
Chief Internal Medicine Resident, Department of Medicine, University of Vermont Medical Center, Burlington, Vermont, USA

ALEX J. CHANG, MD
Resident, Department of Medicine, Kaiser Permanente San Francisco Medical Center, San Francisco, California, USA

ANDREW M. CHENG, MD
Assistant Professor, Division of Cardiology, Department of Medicine, University of Washington, Seattle, Washington, USA

ABDULLA A. DAMLUJI, MD, PhD
Director, Inova Center of Outcomes Research, Inova Heart and Vascular Institute, Falls Church, Virginia, USA; Associate Professor, Johns Hopkins University School of Medicine, Baltimore, Maryland, USA

JACOB A. DOLL, MD
Assistant Professor, Division of Cardiology, Department of Medicine, University of Washington, Seattle, Washington, USA

ALEXANDER C. FANAROFF, MD, MHS
Assistant Professor of Medicine, Division of Cardiovascular Medicine, University of Pennsylvania Perelman School of Medicine, Philadelphia, Pennsylvania, USA

EMILY S. FISHMAN, MD
Resident, Department of Internal Medicine, Yale School of Medicine, New Haven, Connecticut, USA

ELEONORE GRANT, MD
Resident Physician, Department of Internal Medicine, University of Pennsylvania, Philadelphia, Pennsylvania, USA

STEVEN A. HAMILTON, MD
Fellow, Department of Cardiology, Kaiser Permanente San Francisco Medical Center, San Francisco, California, USA

JOHN W. HIRSHFELD Jr, MD
Emeritus Professor of Medicine, Division of Cardiovascular Medicine, University of Pennsylvania Perelman School of Medicine, Philadelphia, Pennsylvania, USA

RAND IBRAHIM, MD
Resident Physician, Division of Cardiology, Department of Medicine, J. Willis Hurst Internal Medicine Residency Training Program, Emory University School of Medicine, Atlanta, Georgia, USA

ANITA M. KELSEY, MD, MBA
Professor, Division of Cardiology, Department of Medicine, Duke University, Durham, North Carolina, USA

MICHELLE D. KELSEY, MD
Assistant Professor, Division of Cardiology, Department of Medicine, Duke University, Duke Clinical Research Institute, Durham, North Carolina, USA

SHERRIE KHADANGA, MD
Assistant Professor, Division of Cardiology, Department of Medicine, Vermont Center on Behavior and Health, University of Vermont, Burlington, Vermont, USA

YILIN LIANG, MD, MPH
Resident, Department of Medicine, Kaiser Permanente San Francisco Medical Center, San Francisco, California, USA

PUJA K. MEHTA, MD
Associate Professor, Division of Cardiology, Department of Medicine, Emory University, Director, Women's Translational Cardiovascular Research, Emory Women's Heart Center, Emory Clinical Cardiovascular Research Institute, Atlanta, Georgia, USA

BRETT M. MONTELARO, MD
Resident Physician, Division of Cardiology, Department of Medicine, J. Willis Hurst
Internal Medicine Residency Training Program, Emory University School of Medicine,
Atlanta, Georgia, USA

MICHAEL G. NANNA, MD, MHS
Assistant Professor, Section of Cardiovascular Medicine, Yale School of Medicine, New
Haven, Connecticut, USA

ADAM J. NELSON, MBBS, MBA, MPH, PhD
Cardiologist, Victorian Heart Institute, Monash University, Melbourne, Victoria, Australia;
Associate Professor, Adelaide Medical School, University of Adelaide, Adelaide, South
Australia

STEPHEN J. NICHOLLS, MBBS, PhD
Director, Victorian Heart Institute, Monash University, Melbourne, Victoria, Australia

NKIRU OSUDE, MD, MS
Cardiovascular Fellow, Cardiovascular Division, Duke University, Durham, North Carolina,
USA

NEHA J. PAGIDIPATI, MD, MPH
Associate Professor, Cardiovascular Division, Duke University School of Medicine,
Durham, North Carolina, USA

PARTH P. PATEL, MD
Physician, Department of Medicine, University of Pennsylvania, Philadelphia,
Pennsylvania, USA

FATIMA RODRIGUEZ, MD, MPH
Associate Professor, Center for Academic Medicine, Division of Cardiovascular Medicine,
Cardiovascular Institute, Department of Medicine, Stanford University School of
Medicine, Stanford, California, USA

MONIKA SANGHAVI, MD
Associate Professor, Division of Cardiology, University of Pennsylvania, Philadelphia,
Pennsylvania, USA

WILSON LAY TANG, MD
IM Resident, Department of Medicine, Stanford University, Stanford, California, USA

MARC THAMES, MD
Division of Cardiology, Assistant Professor, Department of Medicine, Emory University,
Atlanta, Georgia, USA

Contents

Chronic coronary heart disease encompasses a broad spectrum of disorders that range in severity from trivial to imminently life-threatening. The primary care physician encounters coronary disease at all stages. The number of available diagnostic and therapeutic options for evaluating and treating coronary disease is vast, presenting a complex selection strategy challenge when making choices for the individual patient. The primary care physician is responsible to tailor evaluation and management strategies to each individual patient based on his/her particular disease characteristics. There are many categories of diagnostic studies and therapeutic interventions that have been shown at the population level in clinical trials to improve patient outcomes. Blindly applying the findings of all demonstrated studies and therapies to a patient with coronary disease would saddle him/her with an unsustainable burden of diagnostic tests and therapies. The core principle of the approach outlined in this article is to tailor diagnostic and therapeutic choices to the operative pathophysiology that drives a particular patient's disorder. This introductory article is intended to provide a conceptual framework for studying and applying the specialized topics discussed in the articles that follow.

There are unique advantages and disadvantages to functional versus anatomic testing in the work-up of patients who present with symptoms suggestive of obstructive coronary artery disease. Evaluation of these individuals starts with an assessment of pre-test probability, which guides subsequent testing decisions. The choice between anatomic and functional testing depends on this pre-test probability. In general, anatomic testing has particular utility among younger individuals and women; while functional testing can be helpful to rule-in ischemia and guide revascularization decisions. Ultimately, selection of the most appropriate test should be individualized to the patient and clinical scenario.

Hypertension and dyslipidemia are 2 highly prevalent and modifiable risk factors in patients with stable ischemic heart disease. Multiple lines of evidence demonstrate that lowering blood pressure and low-density lipoprotein cholesterol improves clinical outcomes in patients with ischemic heart disease. Accordingly, clinical guidelines recommend intensive treatment targets for these high-risk patients. This article summarizes the pathophysiology, supporting evidence, and treatment recommendations for management of hypertension and dyslipidemia among patients with manifest ischemic heart disease and points to future research and unmet clinical needs.

Chronic coronary disease (CCD) is a major cause of morbidity and mortality worldwide. The most common symptom of CCD is exertional angina pectoris, a discomfort in the chest that commonly occurs during activities of daily life. Patients are dismayed by recurring episodes of angina and seek medical help in preventing or minimizing episodes. Angina occurs when the coronary arteries are unable to supply sufficient blood flow to the cardiac muscle to meet the metabolic needs of the left ventricular myocardium. While lifestyle changes and aggressive risk factor modification play a critical role in the management of CCD, management of angina usually requires pharmacologic therapy. Medications such as beta-blockers, calcium channel blockers, nitrates, ranolazine, and others ultimately work to improve the mismatch between myocardial blood flow and metabolic demand. This manuscript briefly describes the pathophysiologic basis for symptoms of angina, and how currently available anti-anginal therapies contribute to preventing or minimize the occurrence of angina.

Patients with type 2 diabetes and/or obesity and established cardiovascular disease are at increased risk for recurrent cardiovascular events. The indications of glucagon-like peptide-1 receptor agonists (GLP-1RAs) and sodium–glucose cotransporter-2 inhibitors have been expanded in the last decade due to benefit in cardiovascular outcome trials and are now considered guideline-recommended therapy for patients with type 2 diabetes and cardiovascular disease. Emerging data have begun to suggest that GLP-1RAs can decrease major adverse cardiovascular events among patients with obesity without diabetes. Overall, prescription of these agents remains low, despite being key to improve disparities in recurrent cardiovascular events. In this review, we discuss optimal medical therapy for secondary prevention for stable ischemic heart disease.

Antiplatelet therapy is the cornerstone of the secondary prevention of cardiovascular disease. Aspirin is indicated for all patients with chronic coronary disease to prevent recurrent ischemic events. A more potent antithrombotic therapy—including P2Y12 inhibitor monotherapy, dual antiplatelet therapy, or vascular dose anticoagulation—reduces the risk of ischemic events but also increases bleeding risk. Clinicians must weigh both ischemic risks and bleeding risks when determining an optimal antithrombotic therapy for patients with chronic coronary disease, and soliciting patient involvement in shared decision-making is critical.

Given the prevalence of chronic coronary disease, efforts should be made toward risk factor modification. Cardiac rehabilitation is a secondary prevention program consisting of tailored exercise and lifestyle counseling and has been shown to not only reduce cardiovascular morbidity and mortality but also improve quality of life and exercise capacity. Despite the benefits, it remains underutilized. Efforts should be made to increase referral for patients with chronic coronary disease to aid in symptom management and reduction of cardiovascular risk factors.

Revascularization is an effective adjunct to medical therapy for some patients with chronic coronary disease. Despite numerous randomized trials, there remains significant uncertainty regarding if and how to revascularize many patients. Coronary artery bypass grafting is a class I indication for patients with significant left main stenosis or multivessel disease with ejection fraction $\leq$ 35%. For other patients, clinicians must carefully consider the potential benefits of symptom improvement and reduction of future myocardial infarction or CV death against the risk and cost of revascularization. Although guidelines provide a framework for these decisions, each individual patient will have distinct coronary anatomy, clinical factors, and preferences.

Dual antiplatelet therapy (DAPT) with aspirin and a $P2Y_{12}$ inhibitor is recommended for at least 6 and 12 months following percutaneous coronary intervention with drug-eluting stents among patients with stable ischemic heart disease and acute coronary syndrome, respectively. Additional exposure to antiplatelet therapy reduces ischemic events but also increases bleeding risk. Conversely, shorter durations of DAPT are preferred among those at high bleeding risk. Hence, decisions surrounding duration of DAPT after revascularization should include clinical judgment, assessment of the risk of bleeding and ischemic events, and time after revascularization.

Ischemic cardiomyopathy (ICM) is the most common underlying etiology of heart failure in the United States and is a significant contributor to deaths due to cardiovascular disease worldwide. The diagnosis and management of ICM has advanced significantly over the past few decades, and the evidence for medical therapy in ICM is both compelling and robust. This contrasts with evidence for coronary revascularization, which is more controversial and favors surgical approaches. This review will examine landmark clinical trial results in detail as well as provide a comprehensive overview of the current epidemiology, diagnostic approaches, and management strategies of ICM.

This review synthesizes the current understanding of ischemic heart disease in women, briefly discussing differences in risk factors, presentation, and treatment. We have underscored the unique clinical phenotype of IHD in women with a higher prevalence of ischemia with non-obstructive coronary arteries. Further research is needed to elucidate the complexities of ischemic heart disease in women, understand the discordance between ischemic burden and clinical symptoms, and optimize treatment strategies.

The number of older adults age ≥ 75 with chronic coronary disease (CCD) continues to rise. CCD is a major contributor to morbidity, mortality, and disability in older adults. Older adults are underrepresented in randomized controlled trials of CCD, which limits generalizability to older adults living with multiple chronic conditions and geriatric syndromes. This review discusses the presentation of CCD in older adults, reviews the guideline-directed medical and invasive therapies, and recommends a patient-centric approach to making treatment decisions.

Chronic coronary disease (CCD) comprises a continuum of conditions that include obstructive and non-obstructive coronary artery disease with or without prior acute coronary syndrome. Racial and ethnic representation disparities are pervasive in CCD guideline-informing clinical trials and evidence-based management. These disparities manifest across the entire spectrum of CCD management, spanning from non-pharmacological lifestyle changes to guideline-directed medical therapy, and cardiac rehabilitation to invasive procedures. Recognizing and addressing the historical factors underlying these disparities is crucial for enhancing the quality and equity of CCD management within an increasingly diverse population.

Foreword
Collaborative Care

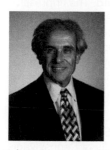

Jack Ende, MD, MACP
Consulting Editor

Writing recently for *Harrison's Textbook of Medicine (21st edition)*,[1] my colleague, Jeff Berns, and I explored the science and art of medical consultation. We emphasized several points, including the importance of the consultant collecting his or her own database; the execution of the consultation in a timely manner, in keeping with the urgency of the clinical situation; the necessary engagement of the patient to insure he or she agrees that the consultation is appropriate and understands the intended outcomes; and, of course, the importance of communication, that is, communication between the primary care clinician and the consultant.

Effective communication between referring clinicians and cardiologists in the care of chronic coronary disease underlies the most important aspect of this joint clinical effort, which is collaboration. Note that we are discussing here the care of the patient whose coronary disease is chronic. The patient may already have experienced angina or myocardial infarction, or already been diagnosed with ischemic cardiomyopathy. Now the terms change from acute care to chronic care, and the focus changes from urgent care to prevention and management, from the coronary care unit to the office. It is time to collaborate.

The word itself, collaboration, comes from the Latin *collaborer* or *collaboratio*, meaning "work together." Not sequentially, not separately, and definitely not at cross-purposes. How can effective collaboration be achieved?

I see three key ingredients to this. First is shared goals; that is, the primary care clinician and the consulting cardiologist need to understand the patient's goals and work together to achieve them. Second is communication. Here, the two (or more) clinicians must be in-sync, in a fashion that ensures they are working together. Finally, there must be coordination so that appointments mesh, the clinical plan is carried out smoothly, and the patient's care for chronic coronary disease fits within their overall health care, including comorbidities and socioeconomic factors.

Med Clin N Am 108 (2024) xv–xvi
https://doi.org/10.1016/j.mcna.2024.01.001
0025-7125/24/© 2024 Published by Elsevier Inc.

medical.theclinics.com

Embedded in all this is that just as the cardiologist needs to understand, or at least be familiar with, the patient's noncardiologic issues, so too, the referring primary care physician needs to be familiar with the cardiologic advances in diagnosis and treatment if they are to remain central to the patient's overall care. That is why this issue of *Medical Clinics of North America* is so important and so timely. Care of the patient with chronic coronary disease is ever-changing and moving forward. The impressive decline in coronary mortality referenced by our two Guest Editors, Alexander Fanaroff, MD, and John Hirshfeld, MD, reflects this. But we can and should do better. Drs Fanaroff and Hirshfeld have provided a well-organized and comprehensive update of this important area of internal medicine with articles written by experts who not only are at the forefront of their fields but also know what referring clinicians need to know. They have set the stage for more effective collaboration.

Jack Ende, MD, MACP
Perelman School of Medicine
of the University of Pennsylvania
Philadelphia, PA, USA

E-mail address:
jack.ende@pennmedicine.upenn.edu

REFERENCE

1. Berns J, Ende J. Chapter 478: Approach to medical consultation. In: Loscalzo J, Fauci AS, Kasper DL, et al, editors. Harrison's principles of internal medicine. 21st edition. New York: McGraw-Hill; 2022.

Preface

Chronic Coronary Disease

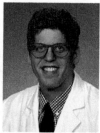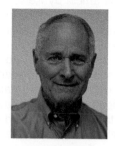

Alexander C. Fanaroff, MD, MHS   John W. Hirshfeld Jr, MD
Editors

Chronic coronary disease (CCD), a disease state characterized by the development of atherosclerosis in the coronary arteries, affects over 20 million people in the United States and approximately 200 million people worldwide.[1–3] CCD includes people with previous myocardial infarction and/or revascularization, those with chronic stable angina pectoris, and those diagnosed with atherosclerotic coronary artery disease only on invasive or noninvasive testing. Over the past decade, deaths from CCD have declined by 25%; however, CCD remains the leading cause of death in the United States and worldwide, responsible for nearly 1 million deaths in the United States and 9 million worldwide.[2,3]

The primary care physician often provides the first patient encounter upon the initial presentation of CCD and initiates evaluation and management. In addition, because the number of people living with CCD in the United States and worldwide far exceeds the number of patients able to be cared for by cardiovascular specialists, the primary care provider has an important responsibility to manage atherosclerosis and CCD. This issue's purpose is to aggregate the knowledge base that informs current evaluation and management practices.

The main risk factors for CCD—hypertension, hyperlipidemia, diabetes mellitus, tobacco use, and sedentary lifestyle—have been well known since the middle of the twentieth century,[4] and many treatments for CCD—such as antihypertensive agents, antiplatelet agents, lipid-lowering therapies, exercise, and revascularization—have been established for nearly as long.[5] However, over several years, there have been a number of important advances in the epidemiology and management of CCD, and this issue seeks to present these updates in a clinically relevant format for the practicing primary care provider or general internist.

The article in this issue by Hirshfeld, "The pathophysiologic basis of managing chronic atherosclerotic cardiovascular disease," serves as a broad overview of

Med Clin N Am 108 (2024) xvii–xx
https://doi.org/10.1016/j.mcna.2023.12.007
0025-7125/24/© 2023 Published by Elsevier Inc.

the management of CCD, providing a pathophysiologic basis for understanding the strategies and therapies discussed further in the remainder of the issue. In the realm of diagnosis of CCD, several randomized clinical trials have established the efficacy of coronary computed tomographic angiography (CCTA),[6,7] and we provide an updated, patient-centered approach to deciding between CCTA and traditional stress testing in the article by Kelsey and Kelsey entitled, "Diagnosing coronary artery disease in the patient presenting with stable ischemic heart disease: the role of anatomic versus functional testing." There have also been multiple advances in secondary prevention, with novel lipid-lowering agents and therapies for hypertension covered in the article by Abrahams and colleagues entitled, "Optimal medical therapy for stable ischemic heart disease in 2024: focus on blood pressure and lipids," and novel therapies for diabetes and obesity covered in the article by Osude and Pagidipati entitled, "A new age for secondary prevention: optimal medical therapy for stable ischemic heart disease among patients with diabetes and/or obesity." In addition, though antiplatelet therapy has been the cornerstone of secondary prevention of cardiovascular events since the 1970s, multiple novel antithrombotic therapies have been introduced in the past 15 years, and a dizzying number of randomized clinical trials have attempted to define the optimal antithrombotic regimen to balance bleeding and ischemic events in various patient subgroups. The article, "Optimal medical therapy for chronic coronary disease in 2024: focus on antithrombotic therapy" by Patel and Fanaroff, provides an evidence-based approach to antithrombotic therapy for patients with CCD, and "Antiplatelet therapy for patients that have undergone revascularization within the past year: which agents and for how long" by Hassan Akhtar and Baber focuses specifically on patients with recent revascularization. Among patients with more severe or symptomatic CCD, the role of revascularization has been clarified by several recent randomized clinical trials,[8,9] and we provide an updated approach to selecting patients for revascularization in the article, "When to consider coronary revascularization for stable coronary artery disease," by Cheng and Doll. These trials have also demonstrated the similarity of outcomes with medical antianginal therapy and revascularization in many patients with CCD, and we cover available antianginal therapies in the article by Montelaro and colleagues entitled, "Optimal medical therapy for stable ischemic heart disease: focus on anti-anginal therapy." Improving diet and increasing exercise is important for all patients with CCD, and the efficacy of cardiac rehabilitation in improving these measures of a healthy lifestyle has been established for decades. However, cardiac rehabilitation remains underused, and the article by Khadanga and Beebe-Peat entitled, "Optimal medical therapy for stable ischemic heart disease in 2024: focus on exercise and cardiac rehabilitation," provides an overview targeted toward the general internist who might refer patients.

Finally, we focus on epidemiology and management considerations of CCD in specific patient populations, including patients with ischemic cardiomyopathy ("Medical decision making and revascularization in ischemic cardiomyopathy" by Chang and colleagues), women ("Ischemic heart disease in women" by Grant and Sanghavi), older adults ("Chronic coronary disease in older adults" by Ambrosini and colleagues), and racial and ethnic minorities ("Racial and ethnic disparities in the management of chronic coronary disease" by Tang and Rodriguez). CCD is often undertreated in these groups, due to complexity or social determinants of health, and these articles are intended to build general internists' confidence in managing or comanaging these patients.

DISCLOSURE

A.C. Fanaroff discloses research funds to the institution from Abbott and Prolocor; consulting fees from Abbott Laboratories, Intercept Pharmaceuticals, Areteia Therapeutics, and Anthos Therapeutics; consulting (unpaid) for Centers for Medicare and Medicaid Services. J.W. Hirshfeld has nothing to disclose.

Alexander C. Fanaroff, MD, MHS
Division of Cardiovascular Medicine
University of Pennsylvania
Perelman School of Medicine
Perelman Center for Advanced Medicine
11-103 South Pavilion
3400 Civic Center Boulevard
Philadelphia, PA 19104, USA

John W. Hirshfeld Jr, MD
Division of Cardiovascular Medicine
University of Pennsylvania
Perelman School of Medicine
Perelman Center for Advanced Medicine
11-109 South Pavilion
3400 Civic Center Boulevard
Philadelphia, PA 19104, USA

E-mail addresses:
alexander.fanaroff@pennmedicine.upenn.edu (A.C. Fanaroff)
hirshfel@pennmedicine.upenn.edu (J.W. Hirshfeld)

REFERENCES

1. Virani SS, Newby LK, Arnold SV, et al. 2023 AHA/ACC/ACCP/ASPC/NLA/PCNA guideline for the management of patients with chronic coronary disease: a report of the American Heart Association/American College of Cardiology Joint Committee on Clinical Practice Guidelines. Circulation 2023;148(9): e9–119.

2. Vos T, Lim SS, Abbafati C, et al. Global burden of 369 diseases and injuries in 204 countries and territories, 1990–2019: a systematic analysis for the Global Burden of Disease Study 2019. Lancet 2020;396(10258):1204–22.

3. Tsao CW, Aday AW, Almarzooq ZI, et al. Heart disease and stroke statistics—2023 update: a report from the American Heart Association. Circulation 2023;147(8): e93–621.

4. Mahmood SS, Levy D, Vasan RS, et al. The Framingham Heart Study and the epidemiology of cardiovascular disease: a historical perspective. Lancet 2014; 383(9921):999–1008.

5. Weintraub WS, Taggart DP, Mancini GBJ, et al. Historical milestones in the management of stable coronary artery disease over the last half century. Am J Med 2018;131(11):1285–92.

6. Douglas PS, Hoffmann U, Patel MR, et al. Outcomes of anatomical versus functional testing for coronary artery disease. N Engl J Med 2015 2;372(14): 1291–300.

7. SCOT-HEART Investigators, Newby DE, Adamson PD, et al. Coronary CT Angiography and 5-year risk of myocardial infarction. N Engl J Med 2018;379(10): 924–33.
8. Boden WE, O'Rourke RA, Teo KK, et al. Optimal medical therapy with or without PCI for stable coronary disease. N Engl J Med 2007;356(15):1503–16.
9. Maron DJ, Hochman JS, Reynolds HR, et al. Initial invasive or conservative strategy for stable coronary disease. N Engl J Med 2020;382(15):1395–407.

The Pathophysiologic Basis of Managing Chronic Atherosclerotic Cardiovascular Disease

John W. Hirshfeld Jr, MD

KEYWORDS

- Coronary artery disease • Atherosclerosis • Atherothrombosis
- Myocardial infarction • Myocardial ischemia • Prevention of atherosclerosis

KEY POINTS

- Coronary heart disease is a complex disorder with many different manifestations and degrees of severity.
- The diagnostic and therapeutic strategy for managing coronary disease is based on assessing the particular patient's disease status and applying the understanding of the multiple contributing pathophysiologic processes.
- A cornerstone of chronic coronary heart disease management involves attenuating atherosclerosis progression and preventing its complications.
- Appropriate management of coronary artery disease also includes a responsibility to undertake primary prevention initiatives when appropriate.

INTRODUCTION/BACKGROUND

The primary care physician encounters and participates in managing the entire spectrum of chronic coronary disease from presymptomatic coronary atherosclerosis to advanced heart failure due to ischemic cardiomyopathy. Management responsibilities encompass many topics (as covered in this monograph) ranging from primary and secondary prevention, to symptom management and advanced therapy selection.

The chronic coronary disease knowledge base is vast—a multimodality discipline that integrates multiple disciplines and knowledge bases. The 2023 American Heart Association/ American College of Cardiology /American College of Clinical Pharmacy/American Society For Preventive Cardiology/NLA/PCNA Guideline for the Management of Patients With Chronic Coronary Disease is 83 printed pages long with hundreds of references.[1]

Cardiovascular Division, Perelman University of Pennsylvania School of Medicine, 11-109 South Pavilion, 3400 Civic Center Boulevard, Philadelphia, PA 19104, USA
E-mail address: hirshfel@pennmedicine.upenn.edu

Med Clin N Am 108 (2024) 419–425
https://doi.org/10.1016/j.mcna.2023.12.002
0025-7125/24/© 2023 Elsevier Inc. All rights reserved.

How does the primary care physician master and apply this knowledge base to optimize care of the individual patient? The totality of available diagnostic and therapeutic options is large requiring informed choices among them.

This article describes a conceptual framework that applies a mechanistic understanding of coronary disease to navigate the totality of the coronary disease knowledge bases and management guidelines.

The principles of coronary disease evaluation and management are rooted in its pathogenesis and pathophysiology. Accordingly understanding the operative disease processes informs evaluation and management strategy. Individual patitent-specific management choices should be driven by the particular pathophysiologic processes involved.

The strategies that underpin this approach may be summarized as follows.

- Atherosclerosis prevention/attenuation
- Recognition of coronary disease and severity assessment ("Staging")
- Management of symptoms caused by coronary disease
- Prevention of atherothrombosis.
- Prevention and management of end-organ complications.

ATHEROSCLEROSIS PREVENTION/ATTENUATION

Arterial atherosclerosis, a generalized chronic progressive disorder, is the underlying cause of virtually all chronic coronary disease and, additionally, can affect virtually every organ system. Uncommon exceptions to this generality include spontaneous coronary artery dissection and arterial fibromuscular dysplasia. (See Eleonore Grant and Monika Sanghavi's article, "Ischemic Heart Disease in Women," in this issue). It is important to bear in mind that atherosclerosis occurs throughout the body. Consequently, a patient who has coronary artery atherosclerosis likely has significant atherosclerotic disease elsewhere and vice versa.

Most adverse cardiovascular events due to coronary heart disease are triggered by complications of atherosclerosis that are the consequence of ongoing disease progression. Thus, prevention and attenuation of the atherosclerotic process is foundational to coronary heart disease management. In particular, successful reduction of elevated low-density lipoprotein (LDL) cholesterol has major cardiovascular health benefits.[2]

Atherosclerosis is nearly universally prevalent in adults of all ages. Typically, it develops asymptomatically in early in life at which time early lesions are functionally unimportant. it progresses at variable rates, generally over many years, until it causes sufficient vascular obstruction to declare its presence. The patient's particular progression rate determines the age at first clinical presentation, and is modulated by a number of well-characterized genetic and behavioral characteristics.[3]

Prevention and/or attenuation of atherosclerosis progression is among the most important treatments that the primary care physician may institute. The aggressiveness and stage of an individual patient's atherosclerotic process determines the approach to this issue. (see article by Nelson and colleagues & Pagidipati and colleagues) The determinants of atherosclerotic risk are well characterized and include plasma LDL cholesterol, hypertension, diabetes mellitus, and cigarette smoking.[4] All patients who have clinically evident symptomatic atherosclerosis benefit from aggressive risk factor modification (secondary prevention). Completely asymptomatic patients may harbor advanced presymptomatic atherosclerotic disease and may benefit from preemptive preventative treatment (primary prevention) as may young people who have no evident atherosclerosis but have characteristics associated with particularly extreme risk.

Consequently, the primary care physician is responsible to treat atherosclerotic risk factors in patients who have clinically evident atherosclerotic disease as well as to identify asymptomatic patients who have genetic and behavioral markers of increased atherosclerotic risk who will benefit from preemptive primary preventative treatment (see article by Nelson and colleagues & Pagidipati and colleagues). Recently, diabetes and obesity, long recognized as coronary risk factors, have assumed greater prominence not only as risk factors but also, with the emergence of Glucagon-like peptide receptor 1 agonists (GLP-1RA) and Sodium-Glucose cotransporter 2 inhibitors (SGLT-2 inhibitors) have become independent therapeutic targets.

Thus, by careful attention to treatment of atherosclerotic risk factors, the primary care physician is in a position to have a strongly positive impact on coronary artery disease outcomes.

CORONARY DISEASE RECOGNITION, "STAGING" AND SEVERITY ASSESSMENT

Atherosclerosis by itself does not cause symptoms, but declares its presence by impairing arterial perfusion of the affected vascular bed causing either ischemia or infarction. Clinically evident coronary disease (symptomatic or asymptomatic) is a spectrum of conditions whose severity and prognosis ranges from a trivial nuisance to malignantly life-threatening.

As a generality, the prognosis associated with a given case of coronary disease is strongly related to the anatomic extent of the disease and the severity of cardiac ischemia that it causes. A therapeutic intervention's benefit potential is linked to the disease severity. Patients with the most severe coronary disease stand to benefit the most from therapeutic interventions whereas patients with less severe disease may have a favorable natural history without treatment.

There is a wealth of data relating coronary disease severity to prognosis and outcomes (see Michelle D. Kelsey and Anita M. Kelsey's article, "Diagnosing Coronary Artery Disease in the Patient Presenting with Stable Ischemic Heart Disease: the Role of Anatomic Versus Functional Testing," in this issue). Any clinical event that declares the definite or possible presence of coronary artery disease, such as the emergence of a chest pain syndrome or a myocardial infarction, demands an initial risk stratification evaluation to detect disease presence and assess its severity. The initial approach to coronary disease management involves assessing the anatomic (cofonary artery imaging) and functional (stress testing) disease severity. Anatomic and functional assessments provide complementary information and the best risk stratification combines both modalities.[5]

As the importance and value of therapies is linked to disease severity, diagnostic "staging" of coronary disease informs the understanding of a patient's prognosis enabling the physician to counsel the patient accurately with respect to the implications of his/her particular situation. It also informs therapeutic choices (see articles by Mehta and colleagues, Pagidipati and colleagues, Sherrie Khadanga and Tanesha Beebe-Peat's article, "Optimal Medical Therapy for Stable Ischemic Heart Disease in 2024: Focus on Exercise and Cardiac Rehabilitation"; Parth P. Patel and Alexander C. Fanaroff's article, "Optimal Medical Therapy for Chronic Coronary Disease in 2024: Focus on Antithrombotic Therapy"; Andrew M. Cheng and Jacob A. Doll's article, "When to Consider Coronary Revascularization for Stable Coronary Artery Disease," in this issue) such as the choice between medical and revascularization management.

MANAGEMENT OF SYMPTOMS CAUSED BY CORONARY ATHEROSCLEROSIS

As a generality, coronary disease causes symptoms in 1 of 2 ways.

- Symptom-producing myocardial ischemia
- Cardiac dysfunction secondary to either infarction, ischemia, or both.

Myocardial ischemia occurs when, because of epicardial coronary artery obstruction, there is a disparity between myocardial metabolic requirements and available coronary blood flow. The disparity may be ameliorated either by decreasing myocardial metabolic demand or by augmenting coronary blood supply. Most medical management strategies are based on attenuating myocardial metabolic requirements while coronary revascularization—by percutaneous intervention or coronary bypass surgery—is done to augment coronary blood supply.

Medical therapy for angina is a multidisciplinary process that utilizes different pharmacologic mechanisms to decrease myocardial metabolic requirements enabling satisfactory metabolism within a circumstance of constrained coronary supply (see article by Mehta and colleagues). Exercise training and conditioning can also alter this relationship favorably. (See Sherrie Khadanga and Tanesha Beebe-Peat's article, "Optimal Medical Therapy for Stable Ischemic Heart Disease in 2024: Focus on Exercise and Cardiac Rehabilitation," in this issue). The multiple pharmacologic approaches to attenuating metabolic demand include beta-blockers, calcium channel blockers and other vasodilators and myocardial metabolism modifiers.[6] As each of the agents works through a different mechanism, the choice of which agent(s) to employ, singly or in combination, is based on the assessment of the particular patient's characteristics.

It is noteworthy that successful medical therapy for symptomatic cardiac ischemia accomplishes more than just symptom attenuation. In particular, beta blockers exert their clinical effects by decreasing myocardial oxygen demand, improving ischemic threshold, and impeding maladaptive LV remodeling.[6]

Revascularization, either by percutaneous coronary intervention or by coronary bypass grafting, improves the myocardial supply-demand relationship by improving the coronary flow supply. In appropriately selected patients, successful revascularization can achieve gratifyingly greater symptomatic improvement, than can be achieved by medical therapy alone. Similarly, revascularization applied to properly selected patients with more severe coronary disease can lower the risk of cardiovascular death, myocardial infarction, and urgent revascularization.[7]

Selection of candidates for revascularization and of revascularization modalities is a complex process that involves weighing considerations of symptom and ischemia severity as well as anatomic suitability for successful revascularization. (See Andrew M. Cheng and Jacob A. Doll's article, "When to Consider Coronary Revascularization for Stable Coronary Artery Disease," in this issue).

Coronary artery disease also can cause cardiac dysfunction either because of loss of myocardium due to myocardial infarction or due to ischemic dysfunction or chronic myocardial fibrosis. Such patients fall at some point on the spectrum of chronic congestive heart failure. Consequently these patients, in addition to requiring therapy to ameliorate myocardial ischemia, also require failure for heart failure adjusted to the particular patient's heart failure stage (see Alex J. Chang and colleagues' article, "Medical Decision Making and Revascularization in Ischemic Cardiomyopathy," in this issue). There is some overlap between ischemia-specific and heart failure–specific therapy. For example, beta-blockers, blood pressure–lowering agents, and anti-diabetic agents have established roles in both conditions.

PREVENTION OF ATHEROTHROMBOSIS

Acute coronary syndromes constitute a spectrum ranging from unstable angina through non ST elevation myocardial infarction to ST elevation myocardial infarction. The vast majority of these scenarios are caused by intracoronary thrombi that generally form on a preexisting atherosclerotic plaque. A notable exception is spontaneous coronary artery dissection—a rare but clinically important event occurring predominantly in younger women with little or no accompanying coronary atherosclerosis. (See Eleonore Grant and Monika Sanghavi's article, "Ischemic Heart Disease in Women," in this issue). Consequently, preventing thrombus formation is a cornerstone of therapy of patients who harbor coronary atherosclerosis.

Because intracoronary thrombi are arterial rather than venous, the platelet is the therapeutic target. Consequently, therapeutic focus is on platelet inhibitors. Anticoagulants are of little, if any value. (See Khawaja Hassan Akhtar and Usman Baber's article, "Antiplatelet Therapy for Patients that Have Undergone Revascularization within the Past Year: Which Agents and for How Long," in this issue).

There are 2 categories of oral platelet-inhibiting drugs all of which act by inhibiting platelet actdivation. Aspirin acts on 1 of the 5 platelet activation mechanisms by permanently acetylating cyclooxygenase-1 (COX-1) in platelets, leading to the inhibition of thromboxane A_2 (TXA_2) synthesis. A second class of platelet inhibitors, including clopidogrel, prasugrel, and ticagrelor, act through a second platelet-activating mechanism by rendering the P2Y12 receptor unable to respond to adenosine diphosphate stimulation. Consequently, neither class of platelet inhibitors inactivates platelets completely and there is sufficient synergism between the 2 drug classes such that administering both classes concurrently produces greater platelet inhibition than either class by itself.

Low-dose (81 mg) aspirin has long been foundational therapy in patients with known coronary artery disease and is essential during acute coronary syndromes.[8] Numerous clinical trials have examined whether more aggressive platelet inhibition employing other platelet inhibiting drug clases–either in isolation or in combination with aspirin–can provide greater protection against future acute coronary events. In general, these trials show that increasingly aggressive platelet inhibition may modestly decrease acute coronary syndrome incidence, but at the price of increased bleeding.[9] Thus, the role of dual antiplatelet therapy in the management of chronic coronary disease is controversial whereas it is well accepted as temporary therapy for recently implanted coronary stents in most circumstances. It most likely should not be considered in patients who have any characteristic that increases bleeding risk including, in particular, patients who require oral anticoagulation for other reasons such as atrial fibrillation.

PREVENTION AND MANAGEMENT OF END-ORGAN COMPLICATIONS

Acute cardiac ischemic episodes and chronic myocardial ischemia can cause multiple detrimental effects on the heart impairing its contractile function and, thus, exposing the patient to the risk of congestive heart failure. The pathogenesis is multifactorial including loss of functioning myocardium secondary to an ST elevation myocardial infarction event or progressive loss due to multiple small ischemic injury events which are not individually recognizable. Chronically ischemic myocardium can reprogram its metabolism to decrease its contractile function in order to preserve cellular viability in the setting of jeopardized coronary flow supply. This process, termed "hibernation," is potentially reversible if coronary flow is restored. In addition, in response to chronically inadequate coronary blood flow and adverse neurohumoral input, myocardium can remodel both physically and metabolically. The end result of these processes leads to distortion of left ventricular size and geometry, development of myocardial fibrosis, and emergence of secondary functional mitral regurgitation.[10] (See Alex J. Chang and colleagues' article, "Medical Decision Making and Revascularization in Ischemic Cardiomyopathy," in this issue).

Once this process is established, it has the potential to become self-perpetuating leading to an ischemic cardiomyopathy with progressive chronic congestive heart failure. Naturally, should this clinical picture develop, a patient is on a very undesirable trajectory.

In addition to congestive heart failure, patients with severely decreased left ventricular contractile function are at risk of other problems including mitral regurgitation which can compound the effects of impaired ventricular contractility. It also creates the potential for ventricular thrombus formation with secondary risk of systemic embolization. In some patients a previous myocardial infarction can create an unstable electrophysiologic substrate that can cause ventriclar tachycardia. Finally, such patients can develop persistent atrial fibrillation with all of its adverse consequences.

Consequently, it is important to recognize the potential that ischemic cardiomyopathy may develop and to vigilantly monitor patients who have evident coronary artery disease for early harbingers of this adverse process.

SUMMARY AND CLINICS CARE POINTS

Coronary artery disease is a complex multifaceted disorder with a spectrum of severities and clinical manifestations. Its underlying pathogenetic mechanism is coronary artery atherosclerosis. Consequently, the primary care physician should always be focused on recognition of atherosclerotic risk and identification of its presence. Aggressive atherosclerosis preventative measures are important for any patient who has evident atherosclerosis and also for asymptomatic patients who have an adverse risk factor profile.

Once coronary disease is detected, its extent and severity should be assessed ("staged") by a combination of anatomic imaging and functional testing for cardiac ischemia. The therapeutic choices available for managing coronary artery disease are vast and include ischemia-modifying pharmacologic therapy and revascularization. Patients with known coronary disease should be systematically monitored for potential complicatations with a particular focus on preventing the development of ischemic cardiomyopathy.

REFERENCES

1. Virmani SS, Newby LC, Arnold SV, et al. 2023 AHA/ACC/ACCP/ASPC/NLA/PCNA guideline for the management of patients with chronic coronary disease: a report of the american heart association/american college of cardiology joint committee on clinical practice guidelines. Circulation 2023;148:e9–119.

2. Cholesterol Treatment Trialists' Collaboration. Efficacy and safety of statin therapy in older people: a meta-analysis of individual participant data from28 randomised controlled trials. Lancet 2019;393:407–15.

3. Arnett DK, Blumenthal RS, Albert MA, et al. 2019 ACC/AHA guideline on the primary prevention of cardiovascular disease: a report of the American College of Cardiology/American Heart Association Task Force on Clinical Practice Guidelines. J Am Coll Cardiol 2019;74:e177–232.

4. American College of Cardiology, AmericanHeart Association. ASCVD Risk Estimator. Available at: https://tools.acc.org/ldl/ascvd_risk_estimator/index.html#!/calulate/estimator.
5. Weintraub WS, Hartigan PM, Mancini GBJ, et al. Effect of coronary anatomy and myocardial ischemia on long-term survival in patients with stable ischemic heart disease. Circ Cardiovasc Qual Outcomes 2019;12:e005079.
6. Sorbets E, Steg PG, Young R, et al. Beta-blockers, calcium antagonists, and mortality in stable coronary artery disease: an international cohort study. Eur Heart J 2019;40:1399–407.
7. Navarese EP, Lansky AJ, Kereiakes DJ, et al. Cardiac mortality in patients randomised to elective coronary revascularisation plus medical therapy or medical therapy alone: a systematic review and meta-analysis. Eur Heart J 2021;42:4638–51.
8. Baigent C, Blackwell L, Collins R, et al. Aspirin in the primary and secondary prevention of vascular disease: collaborative meta-analysis of individual participant data from randomised trials. Lancet 2009;373:1849–60.
9. Udell JA, Bonaca MP, Collet JP, et al. Long-term dual antiplatelet therapy for secondary prevention of cardiovascular events in the subgroup of patients with previous myocardial infarction: a collaborative meta-analysis of randomized trials. Eur Heart J 2016;37:390–9.
10. Bhatt AS, Ambrosy AP, Velazquez EJ. Adverse remodeling and reverse remodeling after myocardial infarction. Curr Cardiol Rep 2017;19(8):71.

Diagnosing Coronary Artery Disease in the Patient Presenting with Stable Ischemic Heart Disease

The Role of Anatomic versus Functional Testing

Michelle D. Kelsey, MD[a,b,*], Anita M. Kelsey, MD, MBA[a]

KEYWORDS

- Stable ischemic heart disease • Stress testing
- Coronary computed tomographic angiography

KEY POINTS

- There are many options for diagnostic evaluation of individuals presenting with symptoms of stable ischemic heart disease.
- Both functional and anatomic diagnostic tests can be useful to identify ischemic or obstructive coronary artery disease and risk stratify patients.
- The choice between diagnostic testing modalities depends on individual patient characteristics.

INTRODUCTION/HISTORY/DEFINITIONS/BACKGROUND

The management of patients presenting with suspected stable coronary artery disease (CAD) can be challenging. The evaluation of such an individual includes assessment of his or her pretest probability, with a clinical history, followed by diagnostic testing where appropriate, to further risk stratify and define the extent of disease. This work-up requires identifying both the categorical classification of coronary disease (present vs absent) and, if coronary disease is present, the graded finding of functional disease severity. There are several options for evaluation, including functional stress testing with a variety of imaging modalities, or anatomic testing using diagnostic coronary angiography or coronary computed tomographic angiography (CCTA). In this article, we will

[a] Division of Cardiology, Department of Medicine, Duke University, 2301 Erwin Road, Durham, NC 27710, USA; [b] Duke Clinical Research Institute, 300 West Morgan Street, Durham, NC 27701, USA
* Corresponding author. 300 West Morgan Street, Durham, NC 27701.
E-mail address: Michelle.kelsey@duke.edu
Twitter: @MDKelseyMD (M.D.K.); @AnitaKelseyMD (A.M.K.)

Med Clin N Am 108 (2024) 427–439
https://doi.org/10.1016/j.mcna.2023.11.002
0025-7125/24/

review the characteristics of both functional and anatomic testing, the risks and benefits of both categories, and the principles of selecting the most appropriate test for the individual patient.

Clinical Presentation

The first essential step in the evaluation of a patient presenting with stable chest pain is a careful clinical history and a resting electrocardiogram (ECG).[1] This precedes all consideration of diagnostic evaluation, as a thoughtful clinical assessment with estimation of pre-test probability is the foundation of this work-up. There are several validated scores which use a variety of clinical information to predict pre-test probability of disease.[2–4] Some guidelines also recommend incorporating information on coronary artery calcium burden to enhance pre-test probability estimates.[1] Regardless of methodology used, this part of the work-up guides all further steps in the diagnosis—both the need for additional testing and the choice of that specific test.

Observation/Assessment/Evaluation

Once pre-test probability has been established, there are many diagnostic imaging modalities to choose from for the work-up of CAD. While each test has unique advantages and disadvantages, ultimately the optimal test depends on local availability and the ability to achieve high quality images with expert interpretation.[1]

Functional tests

Functional testing for CAD can be performed with or without imaging and uses exercise or pharmacologic agents to induce or mimic stress on the heart and vasculature. In general, functional tests are designed to detect myocardial ischemia as a surrogate marker for obstructive CAD. Exercise is typically preferred over use of pharmacologic agents in functional stress testing (in patients who do not otherwise have a contraindication).[5] Exercise ECG is recommended by the American College of Cardiology (ACC)/American Heart Association (AHA) as a first line test for low-risk individuals to exclude myocardial ischemia, and is considered reasonable for intermediate to high risk individuals with no known CAD.[1] Patients must have an interpretable ECG (without baseline ST-T wave abnormalities, pacing, left bundle branch block, or pre-excitation) and be able to exercise to a satisfactory workload.[6] Although the diagnostic accuracy of exercise ECG is lower than other forms of stress testing, the data gathered from this test provide useful prognostic information—as lower exercise capacity with earlier ECG changes suggests higher risk.[7,8] Exercise ECG may also be economically reasonable. When studied as a part of tiered testing with selective stress echocardiography, exercise ECG was shown to be cost-effective for the level of diagnostic accuracy offered.[9]

Functional testing with imaging has improved sensitivity and specificity compared with exercise ECG for the diagnosis of obstructive CAD. Stress testing with echocardiography, cardiac magnetic resonance imaging (CMR), single-photon emission computerized tomography (SPECT) or positron-emission tomography (PET) myocardial perfusion imaging (MPI) are all deemed effective for the diagnosis of myocardial ischemia in intermediate-high risk patients who present with stable angina.[1] The performance characteristics of these tests are relatively similar. In comparison to quantitative coronary angiography for the diagnosis of obstructive CAD (>50% stenosis), stress echocardiography has a sensitivity of 0.85 (0.80–0.89) and specificity of 0.82 (0.72–0.89); CMR has a sensitivity of 0.90 (0.83–0.94) and specificity of 0.80 (0.69–0.88); SPECT has a sensitivity of 0.87 (0.83–0.90) and specificity of 0.70 (0.63–0.76); and PET has a sensitivity of 0.90 (0.78–0.96) and specificity 0.85 (0.78–0.90).[10,11]

While these tests perform relatively equally in the diagnosis of obstructive CAD, there are some circumstances in which one is favored over another. In general, PET MPI (when available) is preferred over SPECT for those with and without known obstructive CAD presenting with stable chest pain.[1] PET has been shown to have better diagnostic accuracy than SPECT[12] and can also provide quantitative assessment of myocardial blood flow which adds prognostic information.[13] Stress echocardiography also provides useful prognostic data, and can lend insight into hemodynamic changes with stress (eg, changes in diastolic function or pulmonary artery pressure response).[14,15] CMR has shown to be as useful as MPI in the work-up of stable chest pain, and also provides highly accurate assessment of left ventricular function and other changes to myocardial tissue (eg, scarring, inflammation, etc.).[16,17] In terms of radiation exposure, neither stress echocardiography nor CMR use radiation. The average radiation exposure for SPECT and PET MPI depend on the imaging protocol and radio-tracer used. In general, the average dose for PET is 3 mSv when Rubidium-82 is used and the average dose for SPECT in 10 mSv when Technetium-99m is used.[18]

Beyond the binary diagnosis of obstructive CAD, each functional test modality offers important prognostic information that can help guide further management of the patient presenting with stable angina symptoms. Exercise ECG provides a wealth of data on exercise capacity and heart rate and blood pressure response to exercise, which have been associated with longer-term risk. In particular, individuals with reduced exercise capacity on exercise ECG testing have been shown to have increased all-cause mortality.[19,20] Similarly, abnormal heart rate response to exercise (ie, inability to achieve 85% of the age-predicted maximum heart rate with activity) and abnormal heart rate recovery after exercise (ie, a smaller fall in heart rate at 1 minute after stopping activity) have been associated with increased cardiovascular (CV) and all-cause mortality.[21–23] Other variables, such as a fall in systolic blood pressure with exercise,[24] ventricular ectopy during recovery,[25] or exercise-induced left bundle branch block,[26] have also been associated with increased risk. Some of these factors have been combined into risk scores, such as the Duke treadmill score (which combines exercise time, ST segment deviation with activity, and degree of angina), in order to predict both severity of obstructive CAD and downstream survival.[7,27]

Functional tests with imaging also offer important prognostic information, in addition the data derived from exercise parameters. On myocardial perfusion imaging, the extent of ischemia, presence of large fixed perfusion defect, reduced left ventricular function, and left ventricular cavity dilation have been associated with increased risk for CV events.[28–30] Similarly, on stress echocardiography, left ventricular size and function and the number and degree of left ventricular wall motion abnormality with stress, as well as ischemic ECG changes in the absence of regional wall motion abnormalities, have been associated with higher risk.[14,31–33] Finally, on stress CMR, stress-induced wall motion abnormality, extent of perfusion defects and degree of late gadolinium enhancement (suggestive of scarring), are associated with increased risk for major CV events.[34] While exercise stress testing is generally preferred over pharmacologic stress testing (when able), these tests can also provide prognostic information.[5,32]

It is critical to integrate these prognostic variables in the interpretation of stress testing results, beyond simply diagnosing obstructive CAD. The spectrum of findings from a stress test can help guide revascularization decisions, and should be used to tailor preventive care, to optimize CV risk factor control particularly among individuals with high risk features.

Anatomic tests

CCTA is used to visualize the coronary arteries and directly evaluate atherosclerotic plaque. CCTA is recommended for evaluation of intermediate-high risk individuals without known CAD who present with stable chest pain.[1] CCTA can also be used for individuals with known history of CAD who have already undergone revascularization, who present with stable chest pain, to assess stent or bypass graft patency.[1] CCTA not only offers percent stenosis of each coronary artery, but also can provide details on atherosclerotic plaque characteristics. Certain radiographic features (low attenuation plaque, positive remodeling) have been associated with higher risk plaque.[35,36] Fractional flow reserve (FFR-CT) can be calculated from CT angiographic data and can estimate ischemia or a specific stenotic lesion within the vessel or flow at the distal end of the vessels.[37] Individuals undergoing CCTA are often pretreated with beta blockers to ensure heart rates are low and stable, and are given nitroglycerin to increase the size of the arteries for better visualization. Individuals with contraindications to either of these agents, or with heart rates that are variable due to arrhythmia, may not be appropriate for CCTA imaging.[38] Patients undergoing CCTA must also be able to cooperate during the scan (hold their breath at certain times) to optimize image acquisition.[38] Finally, significant calcification in the coronary arteries can impact the ability to see vessel details. Depending on the distribution of calcification, this can decrease diagnostic accuracy.[10] The average radiation dose from CCTA is 3 to5 mSv.[39]

Invasive coronary angiography has long been considered the gold standard for the diagnosis of CAD. Beyond visual assessment, there are many tools available to quantify stenosis and to characterize coronary atherosclerotic lesions. Intravascular ultrasound and optical coherence tomography can be used to visualize intraluminal coronary structure. Instantaneous wave-free ratio (iFR) and fractional flow reserve (FFR) can be used for intracoronary physiologic assessment, to understand the hemodynamic significance of a stenotic region.[40] These techniques are performed at the time of the procedure using specialized equipment. There are also methods of quantitative coronary angiography using software to analyze angiographic images to compute a more exact percent stenosis.[41] These technologies improve the accuracy of invasive coronary angiography and help to select the most appropriate patients for revascularization.[40]

Though invasive coronary angiography remains the gold standard for the diagnosis of CAD, there are risks associated with this procedure. Major complications are rare, occurring less than 2% of the time in modern practice. Other risks include the following: infection (<1%), contrast induced nephropathy (3.3%–16.5%), cholesterol emboli (<2%), local vascular injury (0.7%–11.7%), hematoma requiring blood transfusion (2.8%), retroperitoneal bleeding (0.3%), arrhythmia (1.3%–2.5%), or death (<1%).[42] Invasive coronary angiography also carries radiation exposure of approximately 8 to 10 mSv.[43]

Though invasive coronary angiography has been considered the gold standard for the diagnosis of obstructive CAD, it is no longer routinely recommended as a first test in the work-up of stable chest pain (unless very high clinical likelihood).[1] Multiple randomized trials suggest that CCTA or other functional stress testing can be used safely for first-line evaluation in the majority of individuals. This allows for appropriate triaging of patients, higher yield invasive coronary angiography, and lower rates of procedural complications.[44,45]

Similar to functional testing, anatomic tests also provide prognostic information, which should be integrated into the evaluation of patients presenting with stable angina. On CCTA, the presence of any stenosis, higher degree of stenosis, and proximal location of stenosis have been associated with increased CV risk.[46,47] Lower FFR-CT values have also been associated with higher risk of subsequent events including myocardial infarction or unplanned revascularization.[48] Similarly, invasive coronary artery flow measures, using iFR or FFR, have also demonstrate an association between positive (obstructive) values and increased risk for adverse CV events.[49,50] As with functional testing, these prognostic variables should be incorporated into the overall assessment of individuals presenting with stable angina, in order to guide revascularization decisions and optimize preventive care for individuals at high risk.

Current Evidence

The ACC/AHA guidelines offer slightly different recommendations for anatomic versus functional testing in the work-up of patients with stable chest pain (**Table 1**[51,52]).[1] Notably, among intermediate-high risk individuals without known CAD, anatomic evaluation with CCTA has a Class 1, level of evidence A indication, while other functional stress imaging has Class 1, but slightly lower level of evidence B-R.[1]

There is a growing body of evidence of head-to-head comparison studies between functional and anatomic testing in the evaluation of stable angina. The results of these comparisons are variable, depending on the outcome measure selected and the population studied (**Table 2**). Among the largest, were the Prospective Multicenter Imaging Study for Evaluation of Chest Pain (PROMISE) trial, published in 2015, and the Scottish Computed Tomography of the Heart (SCOT-HEART) trial, published in 2018. PROMISE randomized outpatients with stable symptoms suggestive of CAD to CCTA or functional testing with SPECT, stress echo or exercise ECG. After a median follow-up of 25 months, there were similar event rates (a composite of death, myocardial infarction, hospitalization for unstable angina, or major procedural complication) between the functional and anatomic testing arms.[53] SCOT-HEART randomized outpatients with stable symptoms suggestive of CAD to CCTA with standard of care (most commonly exercise ECG) or CCTA alone. At 5 years of follow-up, there were lower rates of CV death or myocardial infarction in the CCTA with standard of care arm.[54]

Anatomic testing with CCTA typically leads to more refined selection of patients for invasive coronary angiography. In both PROMISE and SCOT-HEART, when invasive coronary angiography was pursued, participants were more likely to have obstructive CAD at the time of catheterization.[53–55] This suggests a higher yield selection for invasive testing after anatomic evaluation. Similarly, in both PROMISE and in SCOT-HEART, there was increased coronary revascularization in the CCTA arms, likely a downstream consequence of increased catheterization with obstructive CAD.[53–55] Anatomic testing also leads to more changes in preventive medications than functional testing. In SCOT-HEART, there were increased prescriptions of anti-platelet agents and statins after anatomic evaluation.[55] As CCTA can diagnose both obstructive and non-obstructive CAD, it often prompts more changes in medical therapy.

Ultimately, one must consider individual patient characteristics to select the most appropriate diagnostic imaging modality for work-up of stable chest pain. CCTA is more often recommended in those at lower clinical risk, as it has higher diagnostic accuracy among patients with lower pre-test probability or disease.[56] Conversely, functional testing is often recommended for those at higher risk, as it can be more helpful to rule-in obstructive coronary disease, and guide subsequent revascularization decisions.[4] Along these lines, there is some evidence to suggest that functional testing may have more prognostic utility among older adults over 65 years of age; while anatomic testing with CCTA better risk stratified those under 65 years.[57] CCTA may have particular utility in women, as some evidence suggests that anatomic testing

Table 1
Selected randomized trials of anatomic vs. functional testing for stable coronary artery disease[51-54,61]

Randomized Trial (Year)	Patient Population (N)	Diagnostic Testing Modalities	Primary Endpoint	Result
Min et al,[51] 2012	Outpatients with stable CAD symptoms (N = 180)	CCTA vs SPECT	Angina-specific health status	Change in angina stability CCTA 30 ± 37.0 vs SPECT 22.9 ± 30.1, $P = .11$
CAPP,[52] 2014	Troponin-negative stable chest pain, without known CAD (N = 500)	CCTA vs ETT	Composite of all-cause mortality, STEMI/NSTEMI, HF admission, stroke	ETT: 1 death, 2 NSTEMI CCTA: 1 death, 1 NSTEMI
PROMISE,[53] 2015	Outpatients with stable CAD symptoms (N = 10,003)	CCTA vs Functional testing (SPECT, stress echo, ETT)	Composite of death, MI, unstable angina, major procedural complication	aHR 1.04 (95% CI: 0.83–1.29), $P = .75$
SCOT-HEART,[54] 2018	Outpatients with stable CAD symptoms (N = 4,146)	Standard of care and CCTA vs standard of care (ETT or SPECT)	Composite of CV death or MI	HR 0.59 (95% CI: 0.41–0.84), $P = .004$
PRECISE,[61] 2023	Outpatients with stable CAD symptoms (N = 2,103)	CCTA with FFR-CT vs Functional testing (SPECT, stress echo, ETT, MRI) or ICA	Composite of death, MI and catheterization without obstructive CAD	aHR 0.29 (95% CI: 0.20–0.31), $P < .001$

Abbreviations: aHR, adjusted hazard ratio; CAD, coronary artery disease; CCTA, coronary compute tomographic angiography; CI, confidence interval; Echo, echocardiography; ETT, exercise treadmill testing; FFR-CT, fractional flow reserve computed tomography; HF, heart failure; HR, hazard ratio; MI, myocardial infarction; ICA, invasive coronary angiography; NSTEMI, non-ST elevation myocardial infarction; SPECT, single-photon emission computerized tomography; STEMI, ST elevation myocardial infraction.

Table 2
American college of cardiology/american heart association guideline recommendations for anatomic vs. functional testing in patients with stable chest pain

	Anatomic Testing Recommendations	COR, LOE	Functional Testing Recommendations	COR, LOE
Low-risk Patients without known CAD	CAC testing is reasonable as first line to identify low risk patients	2a, B-R	Exercise testing without imaging is reasonable as first line	2a, B-R
Intermediate-High Risk without known CAD	CCTA is effective for diagnosis of CAD	1, A	Stress imaging (stress echo, PET/SPECT MPI or CMR) is effective for diagnosis of ischemia	1, B-R
Sequential Testing in Intermediate-High Risk	If CCTA is inconclusive, stress imaging is reasonable	2a, B-NR	After inconclusive or abnormal exercise ECG or stress imaging, CCTA is reasonable	2a, B-NR
	If coronary stenosis of 40%–90% in proximal or middle vessel segment on coronary CCTA, FFR-CT can be used	2a, B-NR		
Known non-obstructive CAD	CCTA is reasonable to determine plaque burden and progression to obstructive disease	2a, B-NR	Stress imaging (stress echo, PET/SPECT MPI or CMR) is reasonable for the diagnosis of ischemia	2a, C-LD
Known obstructive CAD	CCTA is reasonable to evaluate bypass graft anatomy or stent patency (for stents $\geq$ 3 mm)	2a, B-NR	For chest pain despite optimal medical therapy, stress testing (PET/SPECT MPI, CMR or stress echo) is recommended	1, B-NR
Prior CABG Surgery	If suspected myocardial ischemia, CCTA is reasonable	2a, C-LD	If suspected myocardial ischemia, stress testing is reasonable	2a, C-LD

Abbreviations: CABG, coronary artery bypass grafting; CAC, coronary artery calcium; CAD, coronary artery disease; CCTA, coronary computed tomographic angiography; CMR, cardiac magnetic resonance imaging; COR, class of recommendation; ECG, electrocardiogram; FFR-CT, fractional flow reserve computed tomography; LOE, level of evidence; MPI, myocardial perfusion imaging; PET, positron emission tomography; SPECT, single-photon emission computerized tomography.

may provide more prognostic information among this demographic.[58] Thus, individual patient characteristics and pre-test probability of disease must be considered in order to select the optimal test to evaluate for obstructive CAD.

Emerging Therapies/Emerging Treatment

While both functional and anatomic testing can be useful in the work-up of suspected CAD, there may be some individuals who do not require any such evaluation. Both the ESC guidelines on the diagnosis of chronic coronary syndromes,[4] and the ACC/AHA guideline on the evaluation and diagnosis of chest pain[1] suggest that testing can be deferred in individuals who have a low pretest probability for obstructive coronary disease and who have an overall favorable prognosis. The ESC guidelines specifically recommend deferring testing in those with a pre-test probability less than or equal to 5%, and it can also be considered in those with a pre-test probability of 5% to 15%. This is because clinical outcomes are favorable in this populations and testing may be low-yield unless there is some other compelling reason to pursue (eg, limiting symptoms or need for additional clarification).[59,60]

This strategy of deferred testing among low risk patients was tested prospectively in the Prospective Randomized Trial of the Optimal Evaluation of Cardiac Symptoms and Revascularization trial.[61] In this pragmatic randomized control trial, patients presenting with stable anginal symptoms were randomized to a precision strategy vs. usual testing for work-up of suspected CAD. Every participant was risk stratified using the PROMISE Minimal Risk Score (PMRS). The PMRS was derived from the PROMISE trial dataset and was designed to identify individuals at very low risk of obstructive CAD with likewise low risk of CV events. Participants in the precision strategy arm who were deemed low risk were not immediately offered testing, and instead offered reassurance and medical therapy. Low risk individuals randomized to usual care were offered functional testing or coronary angiography, based on their clinician preference. Importantly, in this study, individuals randomized to the precision strategy with deferred testing had no CV events at 1 year (no death, no myocardial infarction) and 64% never received subsequent testing.[62] There was similar improvement in angina symptoms between low risk precision strategy and low risk usual care arms. The results of this study support guideline recommendations and offer additional reassurance that testing may be safely deferred in low risk individuals.

DISCUSSION

The evaluation of individuals presenting with stable chest pain can be challenging. The first step in this work-up includes a careful clinical history in order to determine pre-test probability of disease. This clinical information and baseline risk are then used to guide the selection of an appropriate diagnostic test (if any). There are many diagnostic tests available to evaluate for the presence of obstructive CAD. There are both functional tests and anatomic tests, which have very different indications and contraindications and provide slightly different diagnostic and prognostic information. The choice of the optimal diagnostic test depends first on the local availability and expertise to accurately acquire and interpret the clinical data. Provided this is available, the decision between functional testing and anatomic testing depends on individual patient characteristics. Anatomic testing with CCTA can be useful in lower risk populations, to rule out obstructive CAD. This testing performs particularly well in younger individuals and in women, and leads to more downstream initiation of preventive therapies, which can have long term clinical benefit. Functional testing can be useful among higher risk individuals. When ischemia is detected, functional testing can help to guide revascularization decisions. Both anatomic and functional testing offer unique advantages and disadvantages, and the choice between the 2 depends heavily on the clinical scenario at hand.

SUMMARY

The evaluation of patients who presents with stable chest pain suspicious for obstructive CAD starts with an assessment of pre-test probability using clinical history. There are both functional and anatomic tests available for those that would benefit from additional diagnostic evaluation. The decision between these testing modalities depends on individual patient characteristics.

CLINICS CARE POINTS

- Assessment of pre-test probability is an essential first step in the evaluation of patients present with stable chest pain.
- Anatomic testing has particular utility among younger individuals and women
- Functional testing can be helpful to rule-in ischemia and guide revascularization decisions
- Low risk individuals presenting with stable angina may not require any further diagnostic testing, given low diagnostic yield of tests in this population and overall low clinical event rates.
- Selection of the most appropriate test (or deferred test) should be individualized to the patient and clinical scenario.

DISCLOSURE

M D. Kelsey reports consultation/advisory panels for Bayer, Heartflow. The remaining authors report nothing to disclose.

REFERENCES

1. Gulati M, Gulati M, Levy PD, et al. 2021 AHA/ACC/ASE/CHEST/SAEM/SCCT/ SCMR Guideline for the Evaluation and Diagnosis of Chest Pain. J Am Coll Cardiol 2021;78(22):e187–285.
2. Juarez-Orozco LE, Saraste A, Capodanno D, et al. Impact of a decreasing pre-test probability on the performance of diagnostic tests for coronary artery disease. European Heart Journal-Cardiovascular Imaging 2019;20(11):1198–207.
3. Fordyce CB, Douglas PS, Roberts RS, et al. Identification of Patients With Stable Chest Pain Deriving Minimal Value From Noninvasive Testing: The PROMISE Minimal-Risk Tool, A Secondary Analysis of a Randomized Clinical Trial. JAMA Cardiology 2017;2(4):400–8.
4. Knuuti J, Wijns W, Saraste A, et al. 2019 ESC Guidelines for the diagnosis and management of chronic coronary syndromes: The Task Force for the diagnosis and management of chronic coronary syndromes of the European Society of Cardiology (ESC). Eur Heart J 2019;41(3):407–77.
5. Navare SM, Mather JF, Shaw LJ, et al. Comparison of risk stratification with pharmacologic and exercise stress myocardial perfusion imaging: a meta-analysis. J Nucl Cardiol 2004;11(5):551–61.
6. Gibbons RJ, Balady GJ, Bricker JT, et al. ACC/AHA 2002 guideline update for exercise testing: summary article: a report of the American College of Cardiology/

American Heart Association Task Force on Practice Guidelines (Committee to Update the 1997 Exercise Testing Guidelines). Circulation 2002;106(14):1883–92.

7. Mark DB, Hlatky MA, Harrell FE, et al. Exercise treadmill score for predicting prognosis in coronary artery disease. Ann Intern Med 1987;106(6):793–800.

8. Shaw LJ, Mieres JH, Hendel RH, et al. Comparative effectiveness of exercise electrocardiography with or without myocardial perfusion single photon emission computed tomography in women with suspected coronary artery disease: results from the What Is the Optimal Method for Ischemia Evaluation in Women (WOMEN) trial. Circulation 2011;124(11):1239–49.

9. Genders TS, Petersen SE, Pugliese F, et al. The optimal imaging strategy for patients with stable chest pain: a cost-effectiveness analysis. Ann Intern Med 2015; 162(7):474–84.

10. Saraste A, Barbato E, Capodanno D, et al. Imaging in ESC clinical guidelines: chronic coronary syndromes. European Heart Journal - Cardiovascular Imaging 2019;20(11):1187–97.

11. Knuuti J, Ballo H, Juarez-Orozco LE, et al. The performance of non-invasive tests to rule-in and rule-out significant coronary artery stenosis in patients with stable angina: a meta-analysis focused on post-test disease probability. Eur Heart J 2018;39(35):3322–30.

12. Neglia D, Rovai D, Caselli C, et al. Detection of significant coronary artery disease by noninvasive anatomical and functional imaging. Circulation: Cardiovascular Imaging 2015;8(3):e002179.

13. Taqueti VR, Hachamovitch R, Murthy VL, et al. Global coronary flow reserve is associated with adverse cardiovascular events independently of luminal angiographic severity and modifies the effect of early revascularization. Circulation 2015;131(1):19–27.

14. Marwick TH, Case C, Vasey C, et al. Prediction of mortality by exercise echocardiography: a strategy for combination with the duke treadmill score. Circulation 2001;103(21):2566–71.

15. Metz LD, Beattie M, Hom R, et al. The prognostic value of normal exercise myocardial perfusion imaging and exercise echocardiography: a meta-analysis. J Am Coll Cardiol 2007;49(2):227–37.

16. Greenwood JP, Ripley DP, Berry C, et al. Effect of care guided by cardiovascular magnetic resonance, myocardial perfusion scintigraphy, or NICE guidelines on subsequent unnecessary angiography rates: the CE-MARC 2 randomized clinical trial. JAMA 2016;316(10):1051–60.

17. Kramer CM, Barkhausen J, Bucciarelli-Ducci C, et al. Standardized cardiovascular magnetic resonance imaging (CMR) protocols: 2020 update. J Cardiovasc Magn Reson 2020;22(1):1–18.

18. Einstein AJ, Berman DS, Min JK, et al. Patient-centered imaging: shared decision making for cardiac imaging procedures with exposure to ionizing radiation. J Am Coll Cardiol 2014;63(15):1480–9.

19. Myers J, Prakash M, Froelicher V, et al. Exercise capacity and mortality among men referred for exercise testing. N Engl J Med 2002;346(11):793–801.

20. Goraya TY, Jacobsen SJ, Pellikka PA, et al. Prognostic value of treadmill exercise testing in elderly persons. Ann Intern Med 2000;132(11):862–70.

21. Elhendy A, Mahoney DW, Khandheria BK, et al. Prognostic significance of impairment of heart rate response to exercise: impact of left ventricular function and myocardial ischemia. J Am Coll Cardiol 2003;42(5):823–30.

22. Lauer MS, Okin PM, Larson MG, et al. Impaired heart rate response to graded exercise. Prognostic implications of chronotropic incompetence in the Framingham Heart Study. Circulation 1996;93(8):1520–6.
23. Cole CR, Pashkow FJ, et al. Heart-rate recovery immediately after exercise as a predictor of mortality. N Engl J Med 1999;341(18):1351–7.
24. Dubach P, Froelicher VF, Klein J, et al. Exercise-induced hypotension in a male population. Criteria, causes, and prognosis. Circulation 1988;78(6):1380–7.
25. Lee V, Perera D, Lambiase P. Prognostic significance of exercise-induced premature ventricular complexes: a systematic review and meta-analysis of observational studies. Heart Asia 2017;9(1):14–24.
26. Grady TA, Chiu AC, Snader CE, et al. Prognostic significance of exercise-induced left bundle-branch block. JAMA 1998;279(2):153–6.
27. Shaw LJ, Peterson ED, Shaw LK, et al. Use of a prognostic treadmill score in identifying diagnostic coronary disease subgroups. Circulation 1998;98(16):1622–30.
28. Hachamovitch R, Berman DS, Shaw LJ, et al. Incremental prognostic value of myocardial perfusion single photon emission computed tomography for the prediction of cardiac death: differential stratification for risk of cardiac death and myocardial infarction. Circulation 1998;97(6):535–43.
29. McClellan JR, Travin MI, Herman SD, et al. Prognostic importance of scintigraphic left ventricular cavity dilation during intravenous dipyridamole technetium-99m sestamibi myocardial tomographic imaging in predicting coronary events. Am J Cardiol 1997;79(5):600–5.
30. Yao SS, Rozanski A. Principal uses of myocardial perfusion scintigraphy in the management of patients with known or suspected coronary artery disease. Prog Cardiovasc Dis 2001;43(4):281–302.
31. McCully RB, Roger VL, Mahoney DW, et al. Outcome after normal exercise echocardiography and predictors of subsequent cardiac events: follow-up of 1,325 patients. J Am Coll Cardiol 1998;31(1):144–9.
32. Sicari R, Pasanisi E, Venneri L, et al. Stress echo results predict mortality: a large-scale multicenter prospective international study. J Am Coll Cardiol 2003;41(4):589–95.
33. Daubert MA, Sivak J, Dunning A, et al. Implications of Abnormal Exercise Electrocardiography With Normal Stress Echocardiography. JAMA Intern Med 2020;180(4):494–502.
34. Lipinski MJ, McVey CM, Berger JS, et al. Prognostic value of stress cardiac magnetic resonance imaging in patients with known or suspected coronary artery disease: a systematic review and meta-analysis. J Am Coll Cardiol 2013;62(9):826–38.
35. Motoyama S, Ito H, Sarai M, et al. Plaque characterization by coronary computed tomography angiography and the likelihood of acute coronary events in mid-term follow-up. J Am Coll Cardiol 2015;66(4):337–46.
36. Ferencik M, Mayrhofer T, Bittner DO, et al. Use of high-risk coronary atherosclerotic plaque detection for risk stratification of patients with stable chest pain: a secondary analysis of the PROMISE randomized clinical trial. JAMA cardiology 2018;3(2):144–52.
37. Nørgaard BL, Fairbairn TA, Safian RD, et al. Coronary CT angiography-derived fractional flow reserve testing in patients with stable coronary artery disease: recommendations on interpretation and reporting. Radiology: Cardiothoracic Imaging 2019;1(5):e190050.
38. Narula J, Chandrashekhar Y, Ahmadi A, et al. SCCT 2021 expert consensus document on coronary computed tomographic angiography: a report of the

society of cardiovascular computed tomography. Journal of cardiovascular computed tomography 2021;15(3):192–217.

39. Stocker TJ, Deseive S, Leipsic J, et al. Reduction in radiation exposure in cardio-vascular computed tomography imaging: results from the PROspective multi-center registry on radiaTion dose Estimates of cardiac CT anglOgraphy iN daily practice in 2017 (PROTECTION VI). Eur Heart J 2018;39(41):3715–23.

40. Lotfi A, Davies JE, Fearon WF, et al. Focused update of expert consensus state-ment: Use of invasive assessments of coronary physiology and structure: A po-sition statement of the society of cardiac angiography and interventions. Cathet Cardiovasc Interv 2018;92(2):336–47.

41. Athanasiou LS, Fotiadis DI, Michalis LK. 3 - Quantitative Coronary Angiography Methods. In: Athanasiou LS, Fotiadis DI, Michalis LK, editors. Atherosclerotic pla-que characterization methods based on coronary imaging. Oxford: Academic Press; 2017. p. 49–69.

42. Tavakol M, Ashraf S, Brener SJ. Risks and complications of coronary angiog-raphy: a comprehensive review. Glob J Health Sci 2012;4(1):65–93.

43. Vijayalakshmi K, Kelly D, Chapple CL, et al. Cardiac catheterisation: radiation doses and lifetime risk of malignancy. Heart 2007;93(3):370–1.

44. Trial Group DISCHARGE, Maurovich-Horvat P, Bosserdt M, Kofoed KF, et al. CT or Invasive Coronary Angiography in Stable Chest Pain. N Engl J Med 2022; 386(17):1591–602.

45. Chang H-J, Lin FY, Gebow D, et al. Selective referral using CCTA versus direct referral for individuals referred to invasive coronary angiography for suspected CAD. JACC (J Am Coll Cardiol): Cardiovascular Imaging 2019;12(7_Part_2): 1303–12.

46. Carrigan TP, Nair D, Schoenhagen P, et al. Prognostic utility of 64-slice computed tomography in patients with suspected but no documented coronary artery dis-ease. Eur Heart J 2009;30(3):362–71.

47. Hadamitzky M, Achenbach S, Al-Mallah M, et al. Optimized prognostic score for coronary computed tomographic angiography. J Am Coll Cardiol 2013;62(5): 468–76.

48. Nørgaard BL, Gaur S, Fairbairn TA, et al. Prognostic value of coronary computed tomography angiographic derived fractional flow reserve: a systematic review and meta-analysis. Heart 2022;108(3):194–202.

49. Götberg M, Christiansen EH, Gudmundsdottir IJ, et al. Instantaneous wave-free ratio versus fractional flow reserve to guide PCI. N Engl J Med 2017;376(19): 1813–23.

50. Davies JE, Sen S, Dehbi HM, et al. Use of the instantaneous wave-free ratio or fractional flow reserve in PCI. N Engl J Med 2017;376(19):1824–34.

51. Min JK, Koduru S, Dunning AM, et al. Coronary CT angiography versus myocardial perfusion imaging for near-term quality of life, cost and radiation exposure: a pro-spective multicenter randomized pilot trial. Journal of cardiovascular computed tomography 2012;6(4):274–83.

52. McKavanagh P, Lusk L, Ball PA, et al. A comparison of cardiac computerized to-mography and exercise stress electrocardiogram test for the investigation of sta-ble chest pain: the clinical results of the CAPP randomized prospective trial. European Heart Journal-Cardiovascular Imaging 2015;16(4):441–8.

53. Douglas PS, Hoffmann U, Patel MR, et al. Outcomes of anatomical versus func-tional testing for coronary artery disease. N Engl J Med 2015;372(14):1291–300.

54. Newby DE, Newby DE, Adamson PD, et al. Coronary CT angiography and 5-year risk of myocardial infarction. N Engl J Med 2018;379(10):924–33.

55. Williams MC, Hunter A, Shah ASV, et al. Use of coronary computed tomographic angiography to guide management of patients with coronary disease. J Am Coll Cardiol 2016;67(15):1759–68.
56. Gueret P, Deux JF, Bonello L, et al. Diagnostic performance of computed tomography coronary angiography (from the prospective national multicenter multivendor EVASCAN Study). Am J Cardiol 2013;111(4):471–8.
57. Lowenstern A, Alexander KP, Hill CL, et al. Age-related differences in the noninvasive evaluation for possible coronary artery disease: insights from the prospective multicenter imaging study for evaluation of chest pain (PROMISE) trial. JAMA Cardiol 2020;5(2):193–201.
58. Pagidipati NJ, Coles A, Hemal K, et al. Sex differences in management and outcomes of patients with stable symptoms suggestive of coronary artery disease: insights from the PROMISE trial. Am Heart J 2019;208:28–36.
59. Foldyna B, Udelson JE, Karády J, et al. Pretest probability for patients with suspected obstructive coronary artery disease: re-evaluating Diamond–Forrester for the contemporary era and clinical implications: insights from the PROMISE trial. European Heart Journal-Cardiovascular Imaging 2019;20(5):574–81.
60. Reeh J, Therming CB, Heitmann M, et al. Prediction of obstructive coronary artery disease and prognosis in patients with suspected stable angina. Eur Heart J 2019;40(18):1426–35.
61. Douglas PS, Nanna MG, Kelsey MD, et al. Comparison of an initial risk-based testing strategy vs usual testing in stable symptomatic patients with suspected coronary artery disease: the precise randomized clinical trial. JAMA Cardiology 2023;8(10):904–14.
62. Udelson JE, Kelsey MD, Nanna MG, et al. Deferred testing in stable outpatients with suspected coronary artery disease: a prespecified secondary analysis of the precise randomized clinical trial. JAMA Cardiology 2023;8(10):915–24.

Optimal Medical Therapy for Stable Ischemic Heart Disease in 2024

Focus on Blood Pressure and Lipids

Timothy Abrahams, MBBS[a], Stephen J. Nicholls, MBBS, PhD[a], Adam J. Nelson, MBBS, MBA, MPH, PhD[a,b,*]

KEYWORDS

- Stable ischemic heart disease • Hypertension • Targets • Lipids • LDL-C
- Triglycerides

KEY POINTS

- Hypertension and hypercholesterolemia are 2 prevalent modifiable risk factors, and their management is central to optimal medical therapy in patients with ischemic heart disease.
- The benefits of blood pressure lowering are achieved regardless of agent. Although guidelines endorse an incremental benefit for beta-blockers in post-myocardial infarction patients, these data are not from a contemporary era and may not be as relevant today.
- A blood pressure target of between 120 to 130/80 mm Hg should be pursued in most patients.
- Low-density lipoprotein cholesterol (LDL-C) levels should be as low as feasible, but treatment should aim for a 50% reduction from baseline, with maximally tolerated statin therapy, and be intensified with ezetimibe and PSCK9 inhibitors if levels remain at or above 70 mg/dL.
- Modest triglyceride lowering with agents such as niacin and fibrates does not impart cardiovascular benefit; however, use of icosapent ethyl among patients with hypertriglyceridemia (≥135 mg/dL) may reduce cardiovascular events by up to 25%.

HYPERTENSION AND CORONARY ARTERY DISEASE

Hypertension affects one-third of the global population, making it the most common modifiable cardiovascular (CV) risk factor and a leading cause of death.[1] Between 25%

[a] Victorian Heart Institute, Monash University, Melbourne, Victoria, Australia; [b] Adelaide Medical School, University of Adelaide, Adelaide, South Australia
* Corresponding author. Victorian Heart Institute, Blackburn Road, Clayton, Melbourne, Victoria, Australia.
E-mail address: adam.nelson@monash.edu

Med Clin N Am 108 (2024) 441–453
https://doi.org/10.1016/j.mcna.2023.12.005
0025-7125/24/© 2023 Elsevier Inc. All rights reserved.

medical.theclinics.com

and 50% of the risk of coronary artery disease (CAD) may be attributed to the presence of hypertension alone.[2,3] Consequently almost three-quarters of patients with CAD have concomitant hypertension,[4] and the prevalence of both appears to be increasing.[5]

Pathophysiology

Multiple pathophysiologic processes suggest a causal relationship between hypertension and CAD,[6] likely mediated by endothelial dysfunction, oxidative stress, and inflammation, among other processes. The hemodynamic impact of established hypertension may compound stable CAD by affecting elements of the coronary supply and demand equation. First, elevated systolic blood pressure (SBP) increases impedance to left ventricular (LV) outflow, increasing LV wall tension, leading to hypertrophy and ultimately greater myocardial oxygen demand. Secondly, hypertension induces vascular remodeling marked by a loss of vascular elasticity, increased collagen deposition, and ultimately increased stiffness. Stiffening appears to preferentially impact the aorta,[7] causing an increase in pulse wave velocity, a loss of diastolic pressure augmentation, and a purported reduction in coronary blood flow.[8] Notably, arterial stiffness, a parameter that is readily measured noninvasively, is an important marker for adverse CV outcomes and among patients with stable CAD and is an independent determinant of ischemic threshold on treadmill testing.[9]

EFFECT OF HYPERTENSION ON ADVERSE CARDIOVASCULAR OUTCOMES

A plethora of data links prior diagnosis of hypertension with adverse outcomes after myocardial infarction (MI)[10] and among patients with CAD. In formulating the TIMI (thrombolysis in myocardial infarction) risk score for secondary prevention (TRS 2°P), hypertension among patients with CAD was independently associated with a 61% increased risk for CV death, MI, and ischemic stroke (aHR 1.61 95% confidence interval [CI] 1.34–1.93).[11]

Yet despite decades of data, a point of ongoing contention remains as to what normal blood pressure is, and where treatment thresholds and targets should land among patients with and without CAD. A meta-regression analysis using burden of proof risk function techniques suggested elevated levels of SBP pressure may impact CV outcomes in a dose-dependent manner from as low as 120 mm Hg when compared with a baseline value of 100 mm Hg[12]; Specifically in patients with CAD, post hoc analyses of trial data show higher levels of SBP (with and without a prior diagnosis of hypertension) clearly impart risk for adverse CV outcomes. In the ACTION trial comparing nifedipine with placebo on angina relief among 7665 patients with CAD, an SBP of 155 mm Hg or more compared with less than 155 mm Hg was associated with a 22% increased risk for all-cause death, MI, and stroke at 5 years follow-up hazard ratio [HR] 1.23 (95% CI 1.07–1.42).[13] The INVEST trial involving over 20,000 participants with hypertension and CAD found that on-treatment SBP of 140 mm Hg or more compared with SBP 110 to 139 mm Hg was associated with an adjusted 11% increased risk for all-cause death, MI, or stroke (aHR 1.11, 95% CI 1.00–1.22).[14] Underpinning these observations are mechanistic data from the CAMELOT trial comparing amlodipine versus enalapril versus placebo among participants with angiographic CAD.[15] There was a monotonic relationship between achieved SBP and atherosclerosis progression during follow-up; patients with on-treatment SBP of 120 to 140 mm Hg experienced neither net progression nor regression; values greater than 140 mm Hg were associated with progression, while values less than 120 mm Hg achieved regression.

Impact of Treating Hypertension on Adverse Cardiovascular Outcomes

Lowering blood pressure significantly reduces adverse CV outcomes across the spectrum of CV risk, consistent with the observed relationship between hypertension and adverse CV outcomes,. In a meta-analysis of over 120,000 participants across 74 trials of various classes of antihypertensives compared with control among patients with and without established stable ischemic heart disease (SIHD), an approximate 15% reduction in recurrent CAD events was observed (relative risk [RR] 0.85 (0.79–0.91)).[16] A similar magnitude of RR reduction was observed among primary and secondary prevention patients, which suggests that for a similar degree of blood pressure lowering, a greater absolute benefit is likely to be derived among those with CAD given their higher baseline risk for adverse outcomes. The same pooled analysis suggested a similar benefit from blood pressure lowering irrespective of agent used, implying the presence of only minimal (if any) class-specific pleotropic effects. However, a caveat exists and relates to patients shortly after an MI, in whom the use of a beta blocker compared with control was associated with a 31% RR reduction (RR 0.69 [0.62–0.76]) for adverse CV events. Notably, when restricting the analysis of beta blocker effects to only those participants enrolled remote from their MI (ie, >2 years), the proportionate risk reduction was of similar magnitude to other agents (RR 0.87 [0.78–1.02]). However, given these post-MI studies were performed before prompt (and more complete) revascularization where infarcts were larger with a greater risk for arrhythmia and ventricular rupture, it is unclear whether beta blockers retain their specific benefits in this population; nevertheless, they continue to attract a Class I recommendation in the European guidelines (**Table 1**).

Blood Pressure Goals

Most randomized controlled trials (RCTs) have compared an anti-hypertensive regimen with placebo or control (**Table 2**), while few have compared specific goals or targets with varying proportions of patients with established CAD included. In the Hypertension Optimal Treatment (HOT) trial, participants were randomized to 1 of 3 diastolic blood pressure (DBP) goals using a felodipine-based antihypertensive regimen: less than or equal to 90 mm Hg, less than or equal to 85 mm Hg, or less than or equal to 80 mm Hg.[17] Despite achieving meaningful differences in DBP between the groups, there was no overall difference in the rate of the primary outcome. However, among the 15% with established CAD, there was a monotonic (but nonsignificant) trend of fewer CV events with lower DBP, hinting at benefit with more intensive DBP targets, albeit to a level of 80 mm Hg (77 versus 68 versus 62 events). The ACCORD trial compared an intensive (SBP <120 mm Hg) versus standard BP goal (<140 mm Hg) and an intensive (HbA1c <6%) versus standard glycemic goal (HbA1c 7%–7.9%) using a factorial design among patients with Type II diabetes, of whom approximately 25% had concomitant CVD. The trial's premature termination obscured potential benefits of intensive BP control in diabetic patients, possibly because of the adverse effects of intensive glycemic control.[18] Consistent with this hypothesis, a later subanalysis of those receiving the intensive BP control (achieved SBP 119 mm Hg) in the permissive glycemic control arm experienced fewer CV events in follow-up compared with those allocated to a standard BP target (achieved SBP 133 mm Hg), HR 0.71, 95% CI 0.56 to 0.90.[19]

In line with the later interpretation of the ACCORD data is the more contemporary SPRINT trial, which randomized 9361 participants without diabetes and elevated CV risk (of whom 20% had established CV disease [CVD]) to the same targets of <120 mm Hg versus <140 mm Hg.[20] The overall trial showed a 25% reduction in the rate of the primary composite CV outcome (HR 0.75, 95% CI 0.64 to 0.89) among

Table 1
Recommendations from the American College of Cardiology/American Heart Association chronic coronary disease guidelines relevant to hypertension and lipids

Condition	Class of Recommendation	Level of Evidence	Recommendations
Hypertension	1	A	Nonpharmacologic strategies recommended as first-line therapy to lower BP in those with elevated BP (target 120–129/<80 mm Hg)
	1	B-R	In those with hypertension, BP target of <130/<80 mm Hg is recommended to reduce CVD events and all-cause death
	1	B-R	In those with hypertension (≥130/≥80 mm Hg) ARB or BB are first line for compelling indications (recent MI/angina) with additional anti-hypertensive medications (calcium channel blocker thiazides, mineralocorticoid receptor antagonist) as needed
Lipids	1	A	High-intensity statin therapy is recommended with the aim of achieving a ≥50% reduction in LDL-C to reduce major adverse CV events (MACE)
	2a	B-R	Very high risk and on maximally tolerated statin with LDL-C ≥70 mg/dL, ezetimibe can be beneficial to reduce MACE
	2a	A	Very high risk and on maximally tolerated statin and ezetimibe with LDL-C ≥70 mg/dL, a PCSK9 monoclonal antibody (mAb) can be beneficial to reduce MACE
	2b	B-R	Maximally tolerated statin therapy with LDL-C <100 mg/dL and TG 150–499 mg/dL after addressing secondary causes, icosapent ethyl may be considered to further reduce MACE and CV death
	2b	B-R	Not at very high risk on maximally tolerated statin with LDL-C ≥70 mg/dL, reasonable to add ezetimibe to reduce MACE
	2b	B-R	Maximally tolerated statin therapy with LDL-C ≥70 mg/dL, and in whom ezetimibe and PCSK9 mAb are deemed insufficient or not tolerated, it may be reasonable to add bempedoic acid or inclisiran (in place of PCSK9 mAb) to reduce LDL-C

ACC/AHA Chronic Coronary Disease 2023 Guidelines

participants receiving intensive treatment (achieved SBP 121 mm Hg) versus permissive treatment (achieved SBP 136 mm Hg), albeit with an excess of acute kidney injury and hypotension. There was no evidence of treatment heterogeneity among patients with established CVD (P=0.39) suggesting their higher event rates in follow-up compared with the overall population is likely to confer a greater absolute benefit from a lower treatment target. Given older patients are likely to be more vulnerable to the adverse event profile observed in the SPRINT trial, the STEP study tested a similar intervention among participants aged 60 to 80 years, of whom only 6% had established CVD.[21] At a median follow-up of just over 3 years there were fewer cardiovascular events in the intensive compared with standard arm (achieved SBP 128 mm Hg versus 136 mm Hg, HR 0.74, 95% CI 0.60–0.92) supporting a more intensive

Table 2 **Definition of very high risk for the purposes of intensive low-density lipoprotein cholesterol-lowering**	
Multiple major ASCVD events **OR** **One major ASCVD event and ≥ 2 high-risk conditions**	
Major ASCVD events	**High risk conditions**
Recent acute coronary syndrome (ACS) (within 12 months) History of MI (other than a recent ACS) History of ischemic stroke Symptomatic peripheral artery disease	Age >65 years old Familial hypercholesterolemia History of revascularisation Diabetes Hypertension Chronic kidney disease (eGFR 15–59) Current tobacco smoking LDL >100 mg/dL despite statin/ezetimibe History of congestive heart failure

approach to BP lowering even among older adults, albeit with only a minority reporting established CVD.

Although the totality of data supports incremental CV benefit for lower treatment targets to at least 120 mm Hg among high-risk patients, higher rates of hypotension, syncope, and acute kidney injury are observed, even if transient. Caution must be exercised when extrapolating these findings to patients with CAD, as they represented only a minority of the population enrolled; hence there exists an important gap in our understanding of how to best treat these patients. Nonetheless the European guidelines for patients with chronic coronary syndromes released in 2019 recommend an office BP target of 120 to 130 mm Hg, with a more permissive target of 130 to 140 mm Hg for those older than 65 years of age.[22] In contrast, the US guidelines for chronic coronary disease released in 2023,[23] which mainly reference the 2017 US hypertension guidelines, recommend a target of less than 130/80 mm Hg for all.

J-Curve of Blood Pressure and Cardiovascular Events

The pursuit of lower BP is associated with more treatment-related adverse events as described above (ie, hypotension, acute kidney injury, falls) but also a fear that CV outcomes may be negatively impacted through the presence of a J-shaped curve at very low BPs. Proponents of a mechanistic basis for this relationship point to modelling data whereby reduced diastolic pressure exceeds the capacity for autoregulation, thereby negatively impacting coronary perfusion, a phenomenon that may be conceptually more important among patients with obstructive CAD. An alternate explanation is reverse causality, whereby lower levels of DBP (and overall) BP likely reflect competing comorbidities such as age, cancer, and heart failure. Although no prospective trials have been done to explore the impact of very low DBP (ie, target < 60 mm Hg), the most robust analysis comes from the SPRINT data, in which a J shaped curve between baseline DBP and CV outcomes in both intensive and standard groups was observed.[24] However, there was no increase in absolute risk based on achieved DBP during hypertension treatment, suggesting that lower DBP were a marker for poor prognosis rather than a causal element.

Optimal Drug Choices and Key Subgroups

Optimal drug choices and key subgroups in hypertension management should consider individual patient profiles. Hypertension guidelines ubiquitously recommend a multidrug regimen at lower individual drug doses as opposed to a single drug at maximal tolerated dose. This approach leverages the complementary modes of action, which may be required to overcome the multiple pathways involved in the development of hypertension, and avoids side effects that are more common at higher doses. Multiple trials have established the safety and efficacy of calcium channel blockers, thiazides, angiotensin-converting enzymes (ACEs), angiotensin receptor blockers (ARBs), and beta blockers (BBs) for the management of hypertension, although the populations in these trials included varying proportions of patients with CAD.

The treatment aim is to balance target BP achievement with minimal side effects, considering existing conditions and comorbidities. Several key considerations and patient subgroups exist.

Recent myocardial infarction
As per the current guidelines, patients within 6 months of an MI should be commenced on a BB-containing regimen. Whether more contemporary data will change this recommendation remains to be seen. In patients with exertional symptoms, calcium channel blockers and/or BBs are preferred given their dual anti-anginal and antihypertensive actions and will assist in reducing pill burden.

Diabetes and/or chronic kidney disease
The presence of diabetes and/or chronic kidney disease (CKD) in the context of both CAD and hypertension should direct the clinician toward an ACE- or ARB-based regimen that is nephroprotective, particularly in the context of albuminuria.[25] Furthermore patients with CKD (and probably diabetes) may benefit from a more intensive target such as 120/80 mm Hg, which may slow the progression of nephrosclerosis.[26]

Older adults
Despite a prevalence of over 90% in older adults, management of hypertension among this group remains challenging in clinical practice; these individuals are frequently subject to the risk-treatment paradox, whereby their higher risk for adverse events results in less-intensive treatment than patients at lower risk. The STEP program demonstrated the benefits of lower treatment targets among older patients aged greater than 60 years, but only a minority had established atherosclerotic CVD (ASCVD). Similarly, a subanalysis of the SPRINT trial, which included approximately 3000 individuals aged at least 80 years of whom almost 25% had established CVD, also showed a significant reduction in CV events (HR 0.66, 95% CI 0.49–0.90) and mortality (HR 0.67, 95% CI 0.48–0.93) among those treated to a lower SBP target.[27] Acute kidney injury events were higher among more intensively treated patients; however, the rates of injurious falls (a feared sequel of iatrogenic hypotension in this age group) were similar in both arms. Subgroup analyses suggested those with lower cognitive function and lower physical function were less likely to benefit. Thus, although the guidelines allow a more permissive target of 140/80 mm Hg among patients older than 65 years, older adults with preserved cognitive and physical function appear to derive benefit from more intensive treatment.

LOW-DENSITY LIPOPROTEIN CHOLESTEROL AND CORONARY ARTERY DISEASE
Background

Substantial evidence has established the causal role of low-density lipoprotein cholesterol (LDL-C) in the development and progression of CAD. The statin experience elegantly demonstrates that a 40 mg/dL (1 mmol/L) reduction in LDL-C is associated with an approximate 23% reduction in the risk for a CV event. Recent advancements in nonstatin lipid-lowering treatments further underscore the importance of LDL-C lowering. These newer therapies reinforce the notion that substantial CV benefits can be attained by lowering LDL-C levels to even lower levels, regardless of the method employed.[28]

Guidelines and Risk Assessment

Successive guideline updates from the United States and Europe have focused on 2 pivotal areas for patients with CAD: lower treatment targets consistent with "lower is better," and identification of higher-risk patients. As the reduction in relative risk is constant, the highest absolute-risk patients will derive the greatest absolute benefit from intensive LDL-C lowering. Those with established CAD are considered at high risk and should be prescribed a high-intensity statin with the goal of 50% reduction in LDL-C from baseline, and if LDL-C is greater than or equal to 70 mg/dL, the addition of ezetimibe can be considered (class 2b). In patients with stable CAD considered at very high risk (see **Table 2**), the recommendation for ezetimibe is stronger (class 2A), and if still greater than or equal to 70 mg/dL following ezetimibe, a proprotein convertase subtilisin/kexin type 9 (PCSK9) inhibitor can subsequently be considered (class 2A). Inclisiran, a small interfering RNA (siRNA) to PCSK9 that lowers LDL-C levels by approximately 50% on top of statins, has received US Food and Drug Administration (FDA) approval and is in the later stages of its pivotal trials in the United States and Europe.[29] With its 6-monthly maintenance administration, inclisiran dosing could benefit patients struggling with daily medication adherence and has a class 2b recommendation for use if monoclonal PCSK9 inhibitors are not tolerated. Although US and European guidelines differ semantically, their core aim is consistent: intensifying therapy around the 70 mg/dL threshold to achieve an LDL-C level of less than 55 mg/dL, the latter being the specific target in European guidelines. One point of difference is that subsequent European consensus documents advocate for a target of 40 mg/dL among those experiencing a recurrent event within 2 years. Given the fiscal challenges of accessing more potent lipid lowering, CV clinicians must be proactive at identifying very high-risk features in their CAD patients and advocating on their patient's behalf for coverage of these more expensive (but indicated) agents.

Novel Approaches and Targets

Recent research underscores the "lower is better" principle for LDL-C levels, emphasizing prompt initiation of potent therapies. In the HUYGENS trial, participants with a vulnerable nonculprit plaque on intravascular imaging were randomized to receive evolocumab or placebo on top of high-intensity statin for 12 months.[30] At follow-up, participants receiving evolocumab experienced more fibrous cap thickening and a greater reduction in lipid arc, consistent with plaque stabilization. This finding supports the importance of maintaining very low LDL-C levels throughout the early post-MI period and highlights the value of early combination therapy in achieving targets. The historic approach of titration and stepwise addition of therapies promotes clinical inertia and missed opportunities. A paradigm shift toward early combination therapy, also shown to be of benefit with ezetimibe upfront in the RACING trial,[31] will be further explored in the EVOLVE MI trial, which will test the effect of an upfront multidrug regimen including a PCSK9 inhibitor in very high-risk patients compared with standard of care on CV outcomes (NCT05284747).

Emerging Therapies

Adherence to long-term medication in patients with established CAD remains challenging,[32] with as many as 50% of patients discontinuing statins within 18 months.[33] Statin intolerance is undoubtedly a contributor, and although n-of-1 studies have shown that most patients can tolerate some dose of statin,[34] large unmet treatment needs remain. In relation to statin intolerance, the recently completed CLEAR outcomes study comparing bempedoic acid with placebo demonstrated a 13% reduction in rate of the primary MACE composite (HR 0.87, 95% CI 0.79–0.96) among patients at high CV risk unable to take guideline-recommended doses of statins.[35] Although the LDL-C lowering is only modest as monotherapy, combined with ezetimibe, bempedoic acid can lower LDL-C by more than 40%, providing an oral alternative to PCSK9 inhibitors.[36] The fourth-generation oral CETP inhibitor obicetrapib, which is currently in later phase clinical development, has also been shown to reduce LDL-C levels by up to 50%, in combination with high-intensity statins.[37]

Challenges

Despite a wealth of evidence and guideline recommendations supporting more intensive lipid lowering regimens, data from the United States suggest almost 3 in 4 patients do not achieve target LDL-C levels,[38] and fewer than 10% are treated with nonstatin agents.[39] Furthermore, despite a level 1A guideline recommendation, contemporary US data from Medicare beneficiaries suggest less than one-third of patients have their LDL-C levels checked within 3 months of an MI.[40] Compelling arguments have been made to promote LDL-C level measurement to a performance and quality metric[41] and to include it as part of a routine precardiac catheterization blood draw as is done for estimated glomerular filtration rate (eGFR), for example.[42] Regardless of the approach, patients with CAD should have their LDL-C levels checked within 6 to 12 weeks of treatment change and every 6 to 12 months if otherwise stable.

TRIGLYCERIDES AND STABLE CORONARY ARTERY DISEASE
Background

Interest in the relationship between triglycerides and CV risk has oscillated for several decades, at times elevated to independent risk factor status worthy of pursuing treatment, and at others merely an epiphenomenon of low levels of high-density lipoprotein cholesterol (HDL-C). Current understanding points to apolipoprotein-B containing triglyceride-rich lipoproteins as key risk contributors, rivaling LDL-C in atherogenic potential.[43] Hence triglycerides must remain of interest to the cardiologist.

Guidelines and Triglyceride Lowering

Therapies that have been trialed to date (eg, niacin, fenofibrate, mixed omega 3 fatty acids) lower triglycerides only modestly, without clear CV benefits. Accordingly, pharmacologic lowering of modestly elevated levels of triglycerides (200–499 mg/dL) is not currently recommended for CV risk reduction. This position has recently been supported by the results of the PROMINENT trial of pemafibrate, which did not reduce CV events among participants at high CV risk compared with placebo and despite reducing triglycerides by 25%, it did not reduce apolipoprotein-B overall.[44] Thus, unless prescribed to reduce the risk of pancreatitis (ie, among patients with triglyceride levels > 500 mg/dL), fibrates have no role in reducing CV risk and can be ceased to avoid polypharmacy. Several therapies are entering later-phase clinical development and, based on genomic studies identifying targets implicated in metabolism of triglyceride-rich lipoproteins, may lower triglyceride levels by up to 80%. Whether lowering of this magnitude will meaningfully impact CV outcomes remains to be determined.

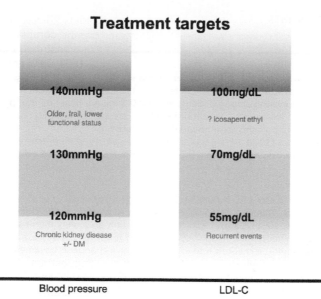

Fig. 1. Treatment targets for blood pressure and LDL-C.

Risk Marker

Although definitive evidence for triglyceride lowering remains elusive, elevated triglyceride levels remain key indicators of residual CV risk in patients on statin therapy. Several societies now recommend the use of icosapent ethyl (a highly purified ester of eicosapentanoic acid, EPA) after the REDUCE-IT trial demonstrated a 25% reduction in the primary composite endpoint compared with placebo among patients with triglycerides greater than 150 mg/dL (HR 0.75, 95% CI 1.68–0.93).[45] Interaction testing revealed no evidence of treatment heterogeneity, suggesting the 5789 patients (71%) who had established CVD (over half of whom had prior MI) benefitted equally from icosapent ethyl. Icosapent ethyl reduces triglycerides by a similarly modest amount (approximately 20%), suggesting its benefit is not well explained by triglyceride lowering alone and instead may be attributed to multiple pleiotropic mechanisms including EPA's anti-inflammatory, antithrombotic and antioxidant effects.[46] The REDUCE-IT trial was published after the US and European cholesterol guidelines; thus icosapent ethyl does not appear in either document. However, consensus statements from the American College of Cardiology and other professional societies in addition to the Chronic Coronary Syndromes guidelines recommend icosapent ethyl to REDUCE-IT like patients such as those with triglyceride levels greater than 150 mg/dL and LDL less than 100 mg/dL on statin.

SUMMARY

Control of modifiable risk factors remains central to a definition of optimal medical therapy in stable CAD; undertaking revascularization without addressing hypertension and hypercholesterolemia is akin to emptying the bath without turning the tap off. As successive guidelines have recommended lower treatment targets, many patients will be on multidrug regimens for hypertension and hypercholesterolemia. With a plethora of evidence demonstrating few people achieve BP and LDL-C treatment targets individually let alone together, models of care will be needed to overcome this large implementation gap (**Fig. 1**).

CLINICS CARE POINTS

Hypertension
- Higher SBP increases myocardial oxygen demand, drives atherosclerosis, and is strongly linked to arterial stiffness, which is a determinant of ischemic threshold
- Benefits of BP lowering among patients with CAD appear independent of agent. Historical data point to an incremental benefit of beta blockers with a recent MI (<2 years), although recent data to support this recommendation are lacking.
- A goal of less than 130/80 mm Hg should be targeted among most patients; however, tighter control (SBP approximately 120 mm Hg) may be of incremental benefit if tolerated without adverse effects.

Dyslipidemia
- All patients with stable CAD should be on a maximally tolerated dose of statin targeting an LDL-C of less than 70 mg/dL and a 50% reduction from baseline. Clinicians must diligently identify the presence of features that fulfill the definition of very high-risk status, which permits the commencement of a PCSK9 inhibitor if levels remain at least 70 mg/dL.
- LDL-C levels should be checked 6 to 12 weeks after a change in treatment and every 6 to 12 months when clinically stable.
- Triglycerides remain an important marker of residual risk, and although there is no evidence to support fibrates to lower triglyceride levels for CV benefit, icosapent ethyl should be considered in those with triglyceride levels greater than 150 mg/dL and LDL-C less than 100 mg/dL on statin therapy.

DISCLOSURE

T. Abrahams has no disclosures. S.J. Nicholls has received research support from AstraZeneca, United Kingdom, Amgen, United States, Anthera, CSL Behring, United States, Cerenis, Eli Lilly, Esperion, United States, Resverlogix, Novartis, Switzerland, InfraRedx, United States, and Sanofi-Regeneron; and is a consultant for Amgen, Akcea, AstraZeneca, Boehringer Ingelheim, CSL Behring, Eli Lilly, Esperion, Kowa, Merck, Takeda, Pfizer, Sanofi-Regeneron, Novo Nordisk, CSL Sequiris, and Vaxxinity. A.J. Nelson has received research support from Amgen, Eli Lilly, Novartis and Boehringer Ingelheim; and is a consultant for Amgen, AstraZeneca, Boehringer Ingelheim, Eli Lilly, Merck, Sanofi, Novo Nordisk, CSL Sequiris, and Vaxxinity.

REFERENCES

1. Collaborators GBDRF. Global burden of 87 risk factors in 204 countries and territories, 1990-2019: a systematic analysis for the Global Burden of Disease Study 2019. Lancet 2020;396(10258):1223–49.
2. Kannel WB. Some lessons in cardiovascular epidemiology from Framingham. Am J Cardiol 1976;37(2):269–82.
3. Lewington S, Clarke R, Qizilbash N, et al. Age-specific relevance of usual blood pressure to vascular mortality: a meta-analysis of individual data for one million adults in 61 prospective studies. Lancet 2002;360(9349):1903–13.
4. Khot UN, Khot MB, Bajzer CT, et al. Prevalence of conventional risk factors in patients with coronary heart disease. JAMA 2003;290(7):898–904.
5. Chen Y, Zhou ZF, Han JM, et al. Patients with comorbid coronary artery disease and hypertension: a cross-sectional study with data from the NHANES. Ann Transl Med 2022;10(13):745.
6. Fuchs FD, Whelton PK. High Blood Pressure and Cardiovascular Disease. Hypertension 2020;75(2):285–92.

7. Nelson AJ, Worthley SG, Cameron JD, et al. Cardiovascular magnetic resonance-derived aortic distensibility: validation and observed regional differences in the elderly. J Hypertens 2009;27(3):535–42.
8. Nelson AJ, Puri R, Nicholls SJ, et al. Aortic distensibility is associated with both resting and hyperemic coronary blood flow. Am J Physiol Heart Circ Physiol 2019;317(4):H811–9.
9. Kingwell BA, Waddell TK, Medley TL, et al. Large artery stiffness predicts ischemic threshold in patients with coronary artery disease. J Am Coll Cardiol 2002;40(4):773–9.
10. Chen G, Hemmelgarn B, Alhaider S, et al. Meta-analysis of adverse cardiovascular outcomes associated with antecedent hypertension after myocardial infarction. Am J Cardiol 2009;104(1):141–7.
11. Bohula EA, Bonaca MP, Braunwald E, et al. Atherothrombotic risk stratification and the efficacy and safety of vorapaxar in patients with stable ischemic heart disease and previous myocardial infarction. Circulation 2016;134(4):304–13.
12. Razo C, Welgan CA, Johnson CO, et al. Effects of elevated systolic blood pressure on ischemic heart disease: a burden of proof study. Nat Med 2022;28(10):2056–65.
13. Clayton TC, Lubsen J, Pocock SJ, et al. Risk score for predicting death, myocardial infarction, and stroke in patients with stable angina, based on a large randomised trial cohort of patients. BMJ 2005;331(7521):869.
14. Bavry AA, Kumbhani DJ, Gong Y, et al. Simple integer risk score to determine prognosis of patients with hypertension and chronic stable coronary artery disease. J Am Heart Assoc 2013;2(4):e000205.
15. Nissen SE, Tuzcu EM, Libby P, et al. Effect of antihypertensive agents on cardiovascular events in patients with coronary disease and normal blood pressure: the CAMELOT study: a randomized controlled trial. JAMA 2004;292(18):2217–25.
16. Law MR, Morris JK, Wald NJ. Use of blood pressure lowering drugs in the prevention of cardiovascular disease: meta-analysis of 147 randomised trials in the context of expectations from prospective epidemiological studies. BMJ 2009;338:b1665.
17. Hansson L, Zanchetti A, Carruthers SG, et al. Effects of intensive blood-pressure lowering and low-dose aspirin in patients with hypertension: principal results of the Hypertension Optimal Treatment (HOT) randomised trial. HOT Study Group. Lancet 1998;351(9118):1755–62.
18. Group AS, Cushman WC, Evans GW, et al. Effects of intensive blood-pressure control in type 2 diabetes mellitus. N Engl J Med 2010;362(17):1575–85.
19. Margolis KL, O'Connor PJ, Morgan TM, et al. Outcomes of combined cardiovascular risk factor management strategies in type 2 diabetes: the ACCORD randomized trial. Diabetes Care 2014;37(6):1721–8.
20. Group SR, Wright JT Jr, Williamson JD, et al. A Randomized Trial of Intensive versus Standard Blood-Pressure Control. N Engl J Med 2015;373(22):2103–16.
21. Zhang W, Zhang S, Deng Y, et al. Trial of intensive blood-pressure control in older patients with hypertension. N Engl J Med 2021;385(14):1268–79.
22. Knuuti J, Wijns W, Saraste A, et al. 2019 ESC guidelines for the diagnosis and management of chronic coronary syndromes. Eur Heart J 2020;41(3):407–77.
23. Writing Committee M, Virani SS, Newby LK, et al. 2023 AHA/ACC/ACCP/ASPC/NLA/PCNA guideline for the management of patients with chronic coronary disease: a report of the American Heart Association/American College of Cardiology Joint Committee on Clinical Practice Guidelines. J Am Coll Cardiol 2023;82(9):833–955.

24. Beddhu S, Chertow GM, Cheung AK, et al. Influence of baseline diastolic blood pressure on effects of intensive compared with standard blood pressure control. Circulation 2018;137(2):134–43.

25. ElSayed NA, Aleppo G, Aroda VR, et al. 10. Cardiovascular disease and risk management: standards of care in diabetes-2023. Diabetes Care 2023; 46(Suppl 1):S158–90.

26. Kidney Disease: Improving Global Outcomes Blood Pressure Work Group. KDIGO 2021 clinical practice guideline for the management of blood pressure in chronic kidney disease. Kidney Int 2021;99(3S):S1–87.

27. Pajewski NM, Berlowitz DR, Bress AP, et al. Intensive vs standard blood pressure control in adults 80 years or older: a secondary analysis of the systolic blood pressure intervention trial. J Am Geriatr Soc 2020;68(3):496–504.

28. Silverman MG, Ference BA, Im K, et al. Association between lowering LDL-C and cardiovascular risk reduction among different therapeutic interventions: a systematic review and meta-analysis. JAMA 2016;316(12):1289–97.

29. Ray KK, Wright RS, Kallend D, et al. Two phase 3 trials of inclisiran in patients with elevated LDL cholesterol. N Engl J Med 2020;382(16):1507–19.

30. Nicholls SJ, Kataoka Y, Nissen SE, et al. Effect of evolocumab on coronary plaque phenotype and burden in statin-treated patients following myocardial infarction. JACC Cardiovasc Imaging 2022;15(7):1308–21.

31. Kim BK, Hong SJ, Lee YJ, et al. Long-term efficacy and safety of moderate-intensity statin with ezetimibe combination therapy versus high-intensity statin monotherapy in patients with atherosclerotic cardiovascular disease (RACING): a randomised, open-label, non-inferiority trial. Lancet 2022;400(10349):380–90.

32. Nelson AJ, Pagidipati NJ, Bosworth HB. Improving medication adherence in cardiovascular disease. Nat Rev Cardiol 2024. https://doi.org/10.1038/s41569-023-00972-1.

33. Lin I, Sung J, Sanchez RJ, et al. Patterns of statin use in a real-world population of patients at high cardiovascular risk. J Manag Care Spec Pharm 2016;22(6):685–98.

34. Wood FA, Howard JP, Finegold JA, et al. N-of-1 trial of a statin, placebo, or no treatment to assess side effects. N Engl J Med 2020;383(22):2182–4.

35. Nissen SE, Lincoff AM, Brennan D, et al. Bempedoic Acid and cardiovascular outcomes in statin-intolerant patients. N Engl J Med 2023;388(15):1353–64.

36. Ballantyne CM, Laufs U, Ray KK, et al. Bempedoic acid plus ezetimibe fixed-dose combination in patients with hypercholesterolemia and high CVD risk treated with maximally tolerated statin therapy. Eur J Prev Cardiol 2020;27(6):593–603.

37. Nelson AJ, Sniderman AD, Ditmarsch M, et al. Cholesteryl ester transfer protein inhibition reduces major adverse cardiovascular events by lowering apolipoprotein B levels. Int J Mol Sci 2022;23(16).

38. Aggarwal R, Chiu N, Libby P, et al. Low-density lipoprotein cholesterol levels in adults with coronary artery disease in the US, January 2015 to March 2020. JAMA 2023;330(1):80–2.

39. Nelson AJ, Haynes K, Shambhu S, et al. High-intensity statin use among patients with atherosclerosis in the U.S. J Am Coll Cardiol 2022;79(18):1802–13.

40. Colantonio LD, Wang Z, Jones J, et al. Low-density lipoprotein cholesterol testing following myocardial infarction hospitalization among Medicare beneficiaries. JACC (J Am Coll Cardiol): Advances 2023;3(1):100753.

41. Virani SS, Aspry K, Dixon DL, et al. The importance of low-density lipoprotein cholesterol measurement and control as performance measures: a joint clinical

perspective from the National Lipid Association and the American Society for Preventive Cardiology. Am J Prev Cardiol 2023;13:100472.

42. Ranard LS, Duffy EY, Kirtane AJ. The case for inclusion of a lipid panel in the standard precatheterization laboratory blood draw-stating what should be obvious. JAMA Cardiol 2023;8(7):629–30.

43. Ference BA, Kastelein JJP, Ray KK, et al. Association of triglyceride-lowering LPL variants and LDL-C-lowering LDLR variants with risk of coronary heart disease. JAMA 2019;321(4):364–73.

44. Das Pradhan A, Glynn RJ, Fruchart JC, et al. Triglyceride lowering with pemafibrate to reduce cardiovascular risk. N Engl J Med 2022;387(21):1923–34.

45. Bhatt DL, Steg PG, Miller M, et al. Cardiovascular risk reduction with icosapent ethyl for hypertriglyceridemia. N Engl J Med 2019;380(1):11–22.

46. Mason RP, Eckel RH. Mechanistic insights from REDUCE-IT strengthen the case against triglyceride lowering as a strategy for cardiovascular disease risk reduction. Am J Med 2021;134(9):1085–90.

Optimal Medical Therapy for Stable Ischemic Heart Disease: Focus on Anti-anginal Therapy

Brett M. Montelaro, MD[a], Rand Ibrahim, MD[a], Marc Thames, MD[b], Puja K. Mehta, MD[b,c],*

KEYWORDS

- Angina • Coronary flow reserve • Myocardial ischemia • Coronary artery disease

KEY POINTS

- Angina is the most common symptom of ischemic heart disease and occurs when the coronary arteries are unable to supply sufficient blood flow to meet the metabolic needs of the myocardium.
- Anti-anginal therapies work through various mechanisms such as reducing myocardial oxygen demand by limiting increases in heart rate, reducing myocardial oxygen demand through direct effects on the myocardium, and altering myocardial work and oxygen consumption through effects on the peripheral circulation.
- Common agents for management of angina include β-blockers, calcium channel blockers, nitrates, and ranolazine.
- To achieve adequate symptom control, therapy should be individualized, combined, and titrated as maximally tolerated, based on patient hemodynamics, left ventricular function, comorbidities, and intolerances/adverse effects.

Funding: This work was supported in part by a developmental grant on Specialized Center of Research Excellence in Sex Differences (SCORE) from the NIH (1U54AG062334–01), 1R01HL157311, and Mrs. Marcia Taylor. Acknowledgments: We thank Esha Dave, MS for her help with figures and tables in this manuscript.

[a] Division of Cardiology, Department of Medicine, J. Willis Hurst Internal Medicine Residency Training Program, Emory University School of Medicine, Atlanta, GA, USA; [b] Division of Cardiology, Department of Medicine, Emory University Division of Cardiology, Atlanta, GA, USA; [c] Women's Translational Cardiovascular Research, Emory Women's Heart Center, Emory Clinical Cardiovascular Research Institute, 1750 Haygood Drive, 2nd Floor, Office #243, Atlanta, GA 30322, USA

* Corresponding author. Women's Translational Cardiovascular Research, Emory Women's Heart Center, Emory Clinical Cardiovascular Research Institute, 1750 Haygood Drive, 2nd Floor, Office #243, Atlanta, GA 30322.
E-mail address: pkmehta@emory.edu

Med Clin N Am 108 (2024) 455–468
https://doi.org/10.1016/j.mcna.2023.12.006
0025-7125/24/© 2023 Elsevier Inc. All rights reserved.

medical.theclinics.com

INTRODUCTION

The management of chronic coronary disease (CCD) is well established as one of the medical community's largest global health care challenges. An estimated 244 million people worldwide live with CCD, and it remains the leading cause of death in the United States.[1] Lifestyle changes and aggressive risk factor modification play a critical role in the management of CCD, but have a limited impact on symptoms in those with established disease. An estimated 10.8 million Americans live with angina pectoris, the principal manifestation of atherosclerotic coronary artery disease (CAD), and 9 to 15 billion dollars are spent on the management of angina.[1-3] The occurrence of angina pectoris has an enormous psychological impact on patients with CCD and the goal of the physician is to minimize the frequency and duration of anginal episodes. This review will focus on the pathophysiologic basis for symptoms of angina and how current guideline-directed therapies contribute to prevention or reduction of anginal episodes.

PATHOPHYSIOLOGY

Stable angina pectoris should be defined as symptoms of myocardial ischemia that occur with exertion or emotional upset. Angina results when, for a variety of reasons, coronary flow rate is inadequate to meet the metabolic needs of the left ventricular myocardium.[4] When this mismatch occurs, it results in ischemia and the release of substances from the myocardium which activate nerve endings that are responsible for the sensation of angina. Normally, coronary blood flow is auto regulated to match myocardial demand, by dilation or constriction of the vessels of the microcirculation, vessels too small to be seen on coronary angiography. These vessels dilate as myocardial metabolic rate increases, increasing blood flow up to 4-times or 5-times resting levels.

The ratio of maximal myocardial blood flow to resting myocardial blood flow is termed the "coronary flow reserve (CFR)." Seminal studies conducted in the 1970s established an association between reduction in cross-sectional area due to epicardial coronary stenosis and CFR (**Fig. 1**); more recent evidence has illustrated the

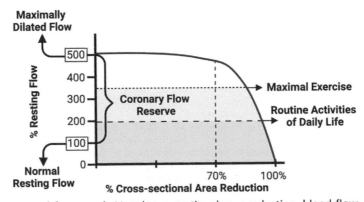

Fig. 1. Conceptual framework: Vessel cross-sectional area reduction, blood flow, and coronary flow reserve. When there is a reduction in coronary artery diameter, it leads to a reduction in cross-sectional area, and compromises flow. For example, a 50% stenosis of the coronary artery leads to a 75% reduction in the cross-sectional area. Coronary flow reserve (CFR) is defined as the ratio of maximal myocardial blood flow to resting myocardial blood flow. CFR is an integrated measure of flow through the epicardial vessels and the microcirculation. (Created with BioRender.com.)

importance of microcirculatory dysfunction as a contributor to reduced CFR and stable angina. However, epicardial and microcirculatory impairment of coronary blood flow are not the only contributors to impaired CFR and symptoms of stable angina. Broadly, pathologic factors that reduce myocardial oxygen supply and/or increase myocardial oxygen demand interfere with the normal physiologic process by which increased myocardial metabolic rate is balanced by increased coronary blood flow. These pathophysiologic processes lead to supply-demand mismatch and symptoms of myocardial ischemia at lower myocardial metabolic rates (**Fig. 2**). For example, pathologic states that increase coronary venous pressure, such as heart failure and left ventricular hypertrophy, lower the driving pressure for coronary blood flow, and may contribute to angina. Other pathologic processes—including anemia, arrythmias, thyrotoxicosis, and aortic stenosis—increase myocardial metabolic demand (**Box 1**).

COMMON OPTIONS FOR MEDICAL THERAPY

Because angina results from an imbalance between myocardial metabolic rate and coronary blood flow, all pharmacologic antianginal therapies work by attenuating the myocardial metabolic rate increase in response to increasing physical exercise or emotional upset. Myocardial metabolic rate can be estimated by the product of the heart rate and the systolic blood pressure (termed "the rate pressure product," or the "double product"); increasing left ventricular preload also contributes to myocardial metabolic rate, though less substantially than heart rate and systolic blood

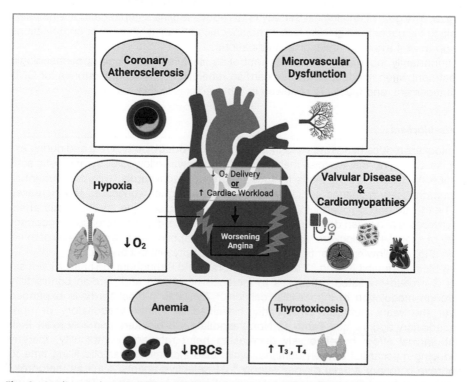

Fig. 2. Cardiac and noncardiac contributors to myocardial ischemia and angina pectoris. Factors that increase cardiac metabolic demand and/or reduce oxygen delivery can precipitate angina. (Created with BioRender.com.)

> **Box 1**
> **Factors of coronary flow reserve**
>
> Length of stenosis
>
> Alteration in flow-mediated coronary vasomotion
>
> Effects of the sympathetic nerves and circulating substances on the caliber of both diseased and non-diseased vessels
>
> Oxygen carrying capacity of the blood
>
> Myocardial oxygen demand (preload, afterload, sympathetic nervous system, thyroid status, etc.)
>
> Platelets, which can transiently worsen stenoses due to localized adherence and aggregation at sites of pre-existing stenosis

pressure. Of the available medical therapies for angina, beta blockers work by limiting heart rate and systolic blood pressure increase in response to exercise and/or emotional upset, calcium channel blockers (CCBs) work by attenuating systolic blood pressure increase, and nitrates work by attenuating systolic blood pressure and left ventricular preload increases. Ranolazine works by reprogramming the regulation of myocardial metabolic rate. An overview of antianginal agents available in the United States is presented in **Table 1** with their predominant mechanisms highlighted in **Fig. 3**. The goal of antianginal therapy is to reduce angina symptoms to a level tolerable to the patient, which may require no specific antianginal therapy or combinations of up to all 4 available antianginal medications.

Importantly, optimizing risk factor control by lifestyle changes and pharmacologic treatment when needed, as well as cardiac rehabilitation, are cornerstones for CCD management, and these are reviewed in other articles in this volume.

Beta-Blockers

β-blockers reduce heart rates and thus the double product, both at rest and during exercise. During normal exercise there is vagal withdrawal followed by sympathetic activation. Vagal withdrawal leads to some degree of tachycardia, with recruitment of sympathetically mediated additional tachycardia at higher workloads. The increases in heart rate and myocardial contractility during exercise have an enormous effect on myocardial oxygen demand. By limiting the tachycardia and increases in contractility of exercise, β-blockers reduce myocardial metabolic rate at a given level of exertion (**Fig. 4**), allowing patients to tolerate more activity without angina.

β-blockers inhibit β1 and β2 adrenoreceptors found throughout the heart, which act via G-protein–mediated processes to increase heart rate and cardiac contractility through modulation of intracellular calcium.[5] Available β-blockers have expanded over the years but can be broadly classified as either vasodilatory or non-vasodilatory agents (see **Table 1**). Non-vasodilatory ß-blockers primarily exert their anti-anginal effect by effectively decreasing heart rate and contractility, thereby reducing myocardial oxygen demand, while also increasing diastolic filling time to improve coronary arterial oxygen supply.[6] ß1 selective agents, such as metoprolol and atenolol, are the most commonly utilized agents in this class. The vasodilatory ß-blockers, such as carvedilol and nebivolol, also have concomitant alpha-blocking properties, which leads to a reduction in blood pressure and thus afterload.[6–9]

Table 1
Common anti-anginal medications and hemodynamic effects

Class	Dosage	Mechanism of Action				ESC COR/LOE	ACC/AHA COR/LOE	Important Considerations
		HR	BP	CC	SVR			
Beta Blockers[a]								• Indicated post-MI and systolic dysfunction
Non-vasodilatory		↓↓	→	→	—			• Avoid concurrent use with non-DHB CCB
• Atenolol	50–200 mg							• Caution in those with ADHF
• Metoprolol	25–400 mcg					I-A	IB-R	• Common AE: bradycardia, bronchoconstriction, postural hypotension, fatigue, sexual dysfunction, heart block
• Nadolol	40–80 mg							• Contraindicated in cardiogenic shock, AV blockade, severe peripheral disease
• Propranolol	80–320 mg							
• Bisoprolol	5–20 mg							
Vasodilatory		↓	↓↓	→	→			
• Carvedilol	25–50 mg							
• Nebivolol	5–40 mg							
Calcium Channel Blockers[a]								• Indicated for vasospastic angina
Non-dihydropyridine		↓↓	→	→	→			• DHB are suitable those with angina and hypertension
• Diltiazem	120–360 mg					I-A	IB-R	• Caution in those with hypotension, sick sinus rhythm, heart block, and aortic stenosis
• Verapamil	180–480 mg							• Common AE: bradycardia (non-DHB), dizziness, reflex tachycardia, edema, headache, flushing
Dihydropyridine		→	↓↓	—/↓	→			• Contraindicated in cardiogenic shock, sick sinus syndrome, severe AS, obstructive cardiomyopathy
• Amlodipine	2.5–10 mg					I-A		
• ER Nifedipine	30–120 mg							
Nitrates								• Short-acting indicated for acute or unstable angina, whereas long-acting useful for vasospastic angina
Short-Acting		—	→	→	→			• Contraindicated in those with severe hypotension, anemia, right ventricular infarction
• Sublingual Nitroglycerin	0.3–0.6mcg					I-B	IB-NR	• Caution for development of tolerance
• Isosorbide dinitrate	10–60 mg							• Common AE: nausea, low blood pressure, dizziness, headaches
Long-Acting[a]		—	→	→	→			
• Isosorbide mononitrate	30–240 mg					IIa-B	IB-R	

(continued on next page)

Table 1
(continued)

Class	Dosage	Mechanism of Action				ESC COR/ LOE	ACC/ AHA COR/ LOE	Important Considerations
		HR	BP	CC	SVR			
Ranolazine[b]	500–1000 mg	—	—	—	—	IIa-B	IB-R	• Useful for chronic stable angina when other medications are not sufficient or well tolerated • Caution in those with liver damage and with prolonged QT intervals • Common AE: dizziness, headache, nausea • Drug interactions with PDE5 inhibitors (eg, sildenafil) and cytochrome P450 3A4 (digoxin, simvastatin)
Ivabradine[b]	5–15 mg	↓	—/↓	—	—	IIa-B	N/A	• Useful for chronic stable angina when other medications are not sufficient or well tolerated • Useful to control heart rate when other agents are not sufficient • Caution in those with severe bradycardia, second or third AV block, ADHF • Common AE: dizziness, arrythmias, irregular rhythms, and heart rate • Drug interactions with antiretroviral therapies and QTc prolonging agents (macrolides, antifungals, antipsychotics)

Abbreviations: ADHF, acute decompensated heart failure; AE, adverse event; AS, aortic stenois; AV, atrioventricular; BP, blood pressure; CC, cardiac contractility; COR, Class (strength) of Recommendation; HR, heart rate; LOE, level (quality) of evidence; SVR, Systemic vascular resistance.

[a] First Choice Agent.

[b] Second Choice Agent.

Taken from Virani SS, Newby LK, Arnold SV, et al. 2023 AHA/ACC/ACCP/ASPC/NLA/PCNA Guideline for the Management of Patients With Chronic Coronary Disease: A Report of the American Heart Association/American College of Cardiology Joint Committee on Clinical Practice Guidelines. Circulation. 2023;148(9):e9-e119; and Modified from Fihn SD, Gardin JM, Abrams J, et al. 2012 ACCF/AHA/ACP/AATS/PCNA/SCAI/STS Guideline for the diagnosis and management of patients with stable ischemic heart disease: a report of the American College of Cardiology Foundation/American Heart Association Task Force on Practice Guidelines, and the American College of Physicians, American Association for Thoracic Surgery, Preventive Cardiovascular Nurses Association, Society for Cardiovascular Angiography and Interventions, and Society of Thoracic Surgeons. J Am Coll Cardiol. 2012;60(24):e44-e164, and ESC 2019 Guidelines on Chronic Coronary Syndromes.[14]

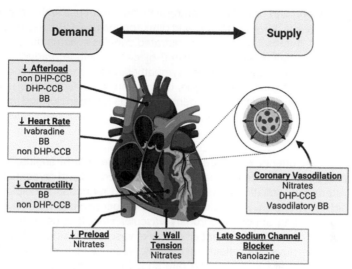

Fig. 3. Physiologic targets of common anti-anginal therapies. Anti-anginal therapies target various factors, such as heart rate, preload, afterload, contractility, and wall tension, to improve blood supply and myocardial demand mismatch. BB, beta blocker; DHP-CCB, dihydropyridine-calcium channel blocker. (Created with BioRender.com.)

Nebivolol also stimulates the release of nitric oxide and has anti-oxidant properties,[10] leading to vasodilation and decreased peripheral vascular resistance.[11]

β-blockers are first-line therapy in patients with history of myocardial infarction (MI) or left ventricular systolic dysfunction (LVSD).[12–14] Even with the lack of mortality benefit in those with CAD without prior myocardial infarction or LVSD, these agents remain a first-line option as their efficacy in the management of angina has been well-established.[13–15] They are also useful to manage conditions that contribute to sinus tachycardia and angina pectoris (eg, thyrotoxicosis). When considering combination therapy, the concurrent use of β-blockers and non-dihydropyridine CCBs should be avoided and if needed, used with caution, given additive effects on atrioventricular

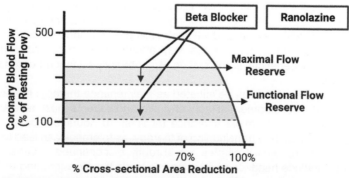

Fig. 4. Coronary blood flow: Beta-blockers and ranolazine. Antianginals such as beta-blockers reduce myocardial oxygen demand that is needed for routine activities and during exercise. By inhibiting late sodium channels in the heart and improving calcium handling, ranolazine also improves supply-demand mismatch. (Created with BioRender.com.)

(AV) nodal depression and reduction of inotropy.[6] Concurrent use with more vasodilatory anti-anginal agents, such as nitrates and dihydropyridine CCBs, has documented benefit, and recent studies have also demonstrated benefits in combination with ivabradine.[16,17] Adverse effects associated with ß-blockade include bradycardia, hypotension, bronchospasm, and impaired sympathetic response to hypoglycemia. Neuropsychiatric effects, including fatigue, depression, and sleep disturbances, are more commonly seen with lipophilic agents, such as propranolol and metoprolol, due to their ability to cross the blood–brain barrier.[6,18]

Calcium Channel Blockers

CCBs have multiple effects which are useful for management of angina, but mostly work by dilating peripheral arteries, thereby reducing afterload and myocardial oxygen demand. Systemic vasodilation and resulting afterload reduction is helpful in those with comorbid hypertension. By blocking coronary vasoconstriction, CCBs are particularly helpful in treating abnormal coronary vascular smooth muscle hyperactivity, which can result in clinically significant episodes of vasospastic angina.[19] While dihydropyridine CCBs have an effect on mainly vascular smooth muscle, non-dihydropyridine CCBs also reduce heart rate and, as in the case of verapamil, even contractility. The negative chronotropic and inotropic effects of this class of CCBs make concurrent use with ß-blockers relatively contraindicated, and they should additionally be avoided in those with LVSD or sensitivity to excess AV-nodal blockade.

Common side effects of CCBs include light-headedness, headaches, flushing, hypotension, and peripheral edema.[6] Both classes of CCBs seem to have similar efficacy in the treatment of symptomatic CCD, and current guidelines designate CCBs as first-line agents for stable angina.[13,14,20,21] Additionally, the concurrent use of dihydropyridine CCB and ß-blockers has been found to have superior efficacy as compared to either agent alone in treatment of angina that does not respond to single agent alone.[16] Given more limited data on other anti-anginal combination therapies, this pairing is frequently recommended as initial combination therapy for these patients.[14]

Nitrates

Nitrates are utilized in both immediate-release form and in long-acting form. Immediate-release tablets placed under the tongue are utilized to treat episodes of angina or to prevent exercise-induced angina if used shortly before exercise.[22] Long-acting nitrates are utilized to minimize angina during the period of time of greatest activity. Nitrates primarily act by inducing marked peripheral vasodilation, thereby reducing systolic blood pressure and left ventricular preload, and reducing myocardial metabolic rate. As with CCBs, nitrates may attenuate coronary vasoconstriction, which is particularly beneficial in the setting of abnormally enhanced coronary vasoreactivity (**Fig. 5**).[6]

Long-acting preparations can be initiated as maintenance therapy; however, titration is limited by the development of tachyphylaxis, and patients must have a substantial "nitrate-free" period to avoid tolerance (at least 10 hours per day).[6] This has implications for cessation or transitioning of therapy, as tolerance can lead to rebound or worsening of symptoms if nitrates are abruptly discontinued.[23] Other common adverse effects include headaches, flushing, systemic hypotension, and orthostasis. They should be avoided or used with caution in patients who are preload dependent, for example, those with severe aortic stenosis or hypertrophic obstructive cardiomyopathy. Additionally, nitrates are contraindicated in those taking phosphodiesterase inhibitors, as concurrent therapy can lead to hypotension.[6] Given their similar efficacy

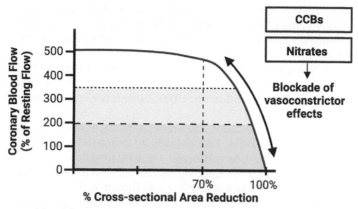

Fig. 5. Coronary blood flow: calcium channels blockers and nitrates. CCBs and nitrates block or attenuate coronary vasoconstriction, and thereby improving flow, and are first-line therapies for coronary vasospastic angina. They also lead to peripheral vasodilation and thus reduce afterload. (Created with BioRender.com.)

as compared to CCBs and β-blockers, guidelines include long-acting nitrates as a first-line agent in angina management.[13] In patients with angina refractory to a single agent, combination therapy with either β-blockers or non-dihydropyridine calcium channel blockers is recommended, as they help combat potential reflex tachycardia and increased contractility as a result of high-dose nitrate therapy.[6,16]

Ranolazine

Ranolazine is an anti-anginal agent which acts to reduce myocardial oxygen demand. However, it has a unique mechanism of action of blocking late inward sodium current, thereby reducing sodium-calcium exchange, which increases intracellular calcium, and thus improves supply-demand mismatch.[6,24] This agent also improves relaxation which facilitates coronary blood flow by reducing left ventricular end diastolic pressure. In ischemic cells, there is rapid activation of these late sodium channels, leading to calcium overload and mechanical dysfunction displayed as diastolic tension.[24] By reducing this intracellular exchange, ranolazine reduces diastolic wall tension and subsequent myocardial oxygen consumption, notably without reduction in chronotropy or inotropy.[6]

Several trials have demonstrated the efficacy of ranolazine in improving angina when added as an adjunct agent to typical first-line therapy.[13,14,24] It has also been shown to demonstrate significant anginal relief as monotherapy, with one study demonstrating similar efficacy as atenolol.[24] Ranolazine does not have significant effects on blood pressure or heart rates, and therefore is an important consideration in those whose hemodynamics may not tolerate previously mentioned agents. Adverse effects associated with ranolazine include QTc interval prolongation, dizziness, and constipation.[6,24] Use is also contraindicated in those with cirrhosis or who are on concurrent therapies that inhibit CYP3A4-dependent metabolism in the liver as this can lead to potential drug accumulation.[6,24]

Ivabradine

Ivabradine selectively inhibits the I_f channel in the sinoatrial node, effectively reducing heart rate in a rate-dependent manner.[6] This means that its effects become more pronounced as heart rates increase. This agent specifically targets heart rate without affecting inotropy (force of myocardial contractions). Ivabradine is beneficial in those with symptomatic left ventricular systolic dysfunction with resting heart rates $\geq$ 70 beats per minute.[25]

In addition, it has a potential role in angina management, given that it reduces myocardial oxygen demand by lowering heart rates. Notably, ivabradine was found to be non-inferior to atenolol and amlodipine, 2 commonly prescribed medications for angina management.[26]

Some common adverse effects include bradycardia (slow heart rate), visual disturbances, headache, and dizziness. Furthermore, an increased risk of atrial fibrillation and atrioventricular block has been observed, necessitating caution when using ivabradine in patients with these conditions. It is contraindicated to use ivabradine in combination with medications that inhibit CYP3A4 metabolism in the liver, as it can lead to increased levels of circulating ivabradine.[27] Based on the currently available data, European guidelines classify ivabradine as a second-line treatment option, while it is not FDA-approved for anti-anginal use in the United States. In clinical practice, ivabradine can be considered as part of combination therapy for patients with concurrent CCD and LVSD, who have high resting heart rates despite maximum tolerated β-blocker therapy. However, further studies are necessary to fully understand the role of ivabradine as a standalone therapy for chronic angina.

Selection of Anti-anginal Therapy

Among the first-line anti-anginal agents, such as β-blockers, CCBs, and nitrates, no single agent has demonstrated significant superiority in terms of major adverse cardiovascular events (MACE) or disease progression in CCD.[6,12,15,20,21,28,29] The mortality benefit of β-blockers following an acute coronary syndrome is well-established, while for patients with CCD who have not had a prior MI or left ventricular systolic dysfunction, no specific agent has shown statistically significant benefits.[30] This lack of superiority allows for greater flexibility in the initial selection of first-line therapies, and some experts even recommend avoiding a hierarchical approach altogether.[13,14,28] In cases where patients experience recurrent angina symptoms or have limited tolerance for the initial therapy, a second agent from a different class can be added to improve symptom control. It is important to closely follow patients during the titration process to assess efficacy, tolerability, and the occurrence of adverse effects.

Coronary Revascularization

The role of coronary revascularization in managing CCD symptoms has been extensively studied. Research has shown that for stable CAD without associated left ventricular systolic dysfunction or severe left main stenosis, there is no significant difference in MACE outcomes between medical therapy and more invasive strategies.[31–33] While a recent meta-analysis reiterated the absence of a mortality difference, it did indicate a reduction in spontaneous MI among those who underwent coronary revascularization.[34] Both groups experienced improvements in angina symptoms, with a larger effect observed in the invasive intervention group.[32,33] However, it should be noted that a considerable proportion of patients (20%–40%) may experience recurrent or persistent symptoms even after revascularization. A risk-benefit discussion with the patient is crucial in evaluating the appropriate course of action, weighing the potential benefits of invasive intervention against the risks, and the possibility of managing symptoms effectively with medical therapy alone.[13,14,34,35]

ISCHEMIA WITH NO OBSTRUCTIVE CORONARY ARTERIES

While obstructive CAD is a major cause of angina in CCD, there is a subgroup of patients, particularly women, who have chest pain from abnormal regulation of coronary blood flow as reflected by impaired CFR, despite having no obstructive epicardial stenosis. Their symptoms are attributed to coronary microvascular dysfunction (CMD), resulting in limited coronary vasodilation.[36–38] These patients are complex, with multiple factors that could impact the regulation of coronary blood flow at the level of the large and medium-sized vessels (where there is often atheroma), as well as the microcirculation. Endothelium-dependent and non-endothelium-dependent factors contribute to CMD. In the Women's Ischemia Syndrome Evaluation study of symptomatic women with chest pain and no obstructive CAD who underwent invasive coronary function testing, more than 50% had epicardial coronary endothelial dysfunction.[39] Previously these patients were referred to having a benign condition termed "cardiac syndrome X ," but it is now clear that having CMD is associated with adverse cardiovascular outcomes.[39–43] Diagnosis and management of CMD patients are beyond the scope of this review, but have been recently reviewed.[36,44–46] Since may patients with CMD have endothelial dysfunction in addition to low CFR, therapies that target the endothelium such as angiotensin-converting enzyme inhibitors (ACE-i) and statins are used in management. A large, multicenter, randomized controlled trial testing the impact of optimal medical therapy versus usual care in women with no obstructive CAD is underway: Women's Ischemia Trial to Reduce Events in Non-Obstructive CAD (WARRIOR) trial (NCT03417388) is testing optimal therapy with ACE-inhibition (or angiotensin receptor blockade) and high-intensity statin compared to usual care in women.[47] One interesting new strategy for angina management in patients with recurrent angina despite maximally tolerated anti-anginal therapy (either with CAD or CMD) that is currently being tested is the use of a device that is placed in the coronary sinus, called coronary sinus reducer (Neovasc Reducer), to alleviate symptoms.[48–50] Prior investigation has also demonstrated that compared to those with obstructive CAD, patients with CMD have heightened nociception (ie, more pain with adenosine infusion, with right ventricular pacing, and with contrast injection in the catheterization laboratory).[51,52] In those with persistent chest pain where a heightened nociceptive abnormality is suspected, low-dose tri-cyclic medications (such as imipramine or amitriptyline) or neuromodulatory strategies (such as spinal cord stimulator) can be considered with referral to anesthesia/pain specialist.[53–55]

SUMMARY

Our discussion has centered around the agents used to prevent or reduce angina pectoris, which is the most common symptom of CCD. To address this condition, medications are employed that largely act by reducing myocardial oxygen demand by reducing heart rate and systolic blood pressure. This framework not only provides a mechanistic rationale for the use of anti-anginal agents, but it can also assist in selecting the most appropriate agents based on their mechanisms of action. By understanding the pathophysiology of angina symptoms and available anti-anginal therapies, health care professionals can effectively prevent or minimize symptoms in patients with CCD.

DISCLOSURES

All authors have no conflicts of interest.

REFERENCES

1. Tsao CW, Aday AW, Almarzooq ZI, et al. Heart Disease and Stroke Statistics-2023 Update: A Report From the American Heart Association. Circulation 2023; 147(8):e93–621.
2. Javitz HS, Ward MM, Watson JB, et al. Cost of illness of chronic angina. Am J Manag Care 2004;10(11 Suppl):S358–69.
3. IHME) IfHMaE. GBD compare 2020. Available at: https://vizhub.healthdata.org/gbd-results./. Accessed August 7, 2023.
4. Ganz PGW. Coronary Blood Flow and Myocardial Ischemia. In: Braunwald EZ, Douglas, Libby Peter, editors. Braunwald: heart disease: a textbook of cardiovascular medicine. 6 edition. Philadelphia: W.B. Saunders Company; 2001. p. 1087–108.
5. do Vale GT, Ceron CS, Gonzaga NA, et al. Three Generations of beta-blockers: History, Class Differences and Clinical Applicability. Curr Hypertens Rev 2019; 15(1):22–31.
6. Husted SE, Ohman EM. Pharmacological and emerging therapies in the treatment of chronic angina. Lancet 2015;386(9994):691–701.
7. Sugioka K, Hozumi T, Takemoto Y, et al. Early recovery of impaired coronary flow reserve by carvedilol therapy in patients with idiopathic dilated cardiomyopathy: a serial transthoracic Doppler echocardiographic study. J Am Coll Cardiol 2005; 45(2):318–9.
8. Xiaozhen H, Yun Z, Mei Z, et al. Effect of carvedilol on coronary flow reserve in patients with hypertensive left-ventricular hypertrophy. Blood Press 2010; 19(1):40–7.
9. Togni M, Vigorito F, Windecker S, et al. Does the beta-blocker nebivolol increase coronary flow reserve? Cardiovasc Drugs Ther 2007;21(2):99–108.
10. Kalinowski L, Dobrucki LW, Szczepanska-Konkel M, et al. Third-generation beta-blockers stimulate nitric oxide release from endothelial cells through ATP efflux: a novel mechanism for antihypertensive action. Circulation 2003;107(21):2747–52.
11. Erdamar H, Sen N, Tavil Y, et al. The effect of nebivolol treatment on oxidative stress and antioxidant status in patients with cardiac syndrome-X. Coron Artery Dis 2009;20(3):238–44.
12. Sorbets E, Steg PG, Young R, et al. beta-blockers, calcium antagonists, and mortality in stable coronary artery disease: an international cohort study. Eur Heart J 2019;40(18):1399–407.
13. Virani SS, Newby LK, Arnold SV, et al. 2023 AHA/ACC/ACCP/ASPC/NLA/PCNA Guideline for the Management of Patients With Chronic Coronary Disease: A Report of the American Heart Association/American College of Cardiology Joint Committee on Clinical Practice Guidelines. Circulation 2023;148(9):e9–119.
14. Knuuti J, Wijns W, Saraste A, et al. 2019 ESC Guidelines for the diagnosis and management of chronic coronary syndromes. Eur Heart J 2020;41(3):407–77.
15. Andersson C, Shilane D, Go AS, et al. beta-blocker therapy and cardiac events among patients with newly diagnosed coronary heart disease. J Am Coll Cardiol 2014;64(3):247–52.
16. Belsey J, Savelieva I, Mugelli A, et al. Relative efficacy of antianginal drugs used as add-on therapy in patients with stable angina: A systematic review and meta-analysis. Eur J Prev Cardiol 2015;22(7):837–48.
17. Amosova E, Andrejev E, Zaderey I, et al. Efficacy of ivabradine in combination with Beta-blocker versus uptitration of Beta-blocker in patients with stable angina. Cardiovasc Drugs Ther 2011;25(6):531–7.

18. Cojocariu SA, Maştaleru A, Sascău RA, et al. Neuropsychiatric Consequences of Lipophilic Beta-Blockers. Medicina (Kaunas, Lithuania) 2021;57(2).
19. Lanza GA, Careri G, Crea F. Mechanisms of coronary artery spasm. Circulation 2011;124(16):1774–82.
20. Heidenreich PA, McDonald KM, Hastie T, et al. Meta-analysis of trials comparing beta-blockers, calcium antagonists, and nitrates for stable angina. JAMA 1999; 281(20):1927–36.
21. Ferrari R, Pavasini R, Camici PG, et al. Anti-anginal drugs-beliefs and evidence: systematic review covering 50 years of medical treatment. Eur Heart J 2019; 40(2):190–4.
22. Ohman EM. Chronic Stable Angina. N Engl J Med 2016;375(3):293.
23. Munzel T, Daiber A, Mulsch A. Explaining the phenomenon of nitrate tolerance. Circ Res 2005;97(7):618–28.
24. Rayner-Hartley E, Sedlak T. Ranolazine: A Contemporary Review. J Am Heart Assoc 2016;5(3):e003196.
25. Swedberg K, Komajda M, Bohm M, et al. Ivabradine and outcomes in chronic heart failure (SHIFT): a randomised placebo-controlled study. Lancet 2010; 376(9744):875–85.
26. Chen C, Kaur G, Mehta PK, et al. Ivabradine in Cardiovascular Disease Management Revisited: a Review. Cardiovasc Drugs Ther 2021;35(5):1045–56.
27. Tse S, Mazzola N. Ivabradine (Corlanor) for Heart Failure: The First Selective and Specific I f Inhibitor. P T 2015;40(12):810–4.
28. Ferrari R, Camici PG, Crea F, et al. Expert consensus document: A 'diamond' approach to personalized treatment of angina. Nat Rev Cardiol 2018;15(2): 120–32.
29. Balla C, Pavasini R, Ferrari R. Treatment of Angina: Where Are We? Cardiology 2018;140(1):52–67.
30. Byrne RA, Rossello X, Coughlan JJ, et al. 2023 ESC Guidelines for the management of acute coronary syndromes. Eur Heart J 2023;44(38):3720–826.
31. Group BDS, Frye RL, August P, et al. A randomized trial of therapies for type 2 diabetes and coronary artery disease. N Engl J Med 2009;360(24):2503–15.
32. Maron DJ, Hochman JS, Reynolds HR, et al. Initial Invasive or Conservative Strategy for Stable Coronary Disease. N Engl J Med 2020;382(15):1395–407.
33. Boden WE, O'Rourke RA, Teo KK, et al. Optimal medical therapy with or without PCI for stable coronary disease. N Engl J Med 2007;356(15):1503–16.
34. Vij A, Kassab K, Chawla H, et al. Invasive therapy versus conservative therapy for patients with stable coronary artery disease: An updated meta-analysis. Clin Cardiol 2021;44(5):675–82.
35. Crea F, Bairey Merz CN, Beltrame JF, et al. Mechanisms and diagnostic evaluation of persistent or recurrent angina following percutaneous coronary revascularization. Eur Heart J 2019;40(29):2455–62.
36. Mehta PK, Huang J, Levit RD, et al. Ischemia and no obstructive coronary arteries (INOCA): A narrative review. Atherosclerosis 2022;363:8–21.
37. Pargaonkar VS, Kimura T, Kameda R, et al. Invasive assessment of myocardial bridging in patients with angina and no obstructive coronary artery disease. EuroIntervention 2021;16(13):1070–8.
38. Hashikata T, Honda Y, Wang H, et al. Impact of Diastolic Vessel Restriction on Quality of Life in Symptomatic Myocardial Bridging Patients Treated With Surgical Unroofing: Preoperative Assessments With Intravascular Ultrasound and Coronary Computed Tomography Angiography. Circ Cardiovasc Interv 2021;14(10): e011062.

39. Wei J, Mehta PK, Johnson BD, et al. Safety of coronary reactivity testing in women with no obstructive coronary artery disease: results from the NHLBI-sponsored WISE (Women's Ischemia Syndrome Evaluation) study. JACC Cardiovasc Interv 2012;5(6):646–53.
40. Geltman EM, Henes CG, Senneff MJ, et al. Increased myocardial perfusion at rest and diminished perfusion reserve in patients with angina and angiographically normal coronary arteries. J Am Coll Cardiol 1990;16(3):586–95.
41. Hasdai D, Holmes DR Jr, Higano ST, et al. Prevalence of coronary blood flow reserve abnormalities among patients with nonobstructive coronary artery disease and chest pain. Mayo Clin Proc 1998;73(12):1133–40.
42. Rutledge T, Reis SE, Olson M, et al. History of anxiety disorders is associated with a decreased likelihood of angiographic coronary artery disease in women with chest pain: the WISE study. J Am Coll Cardiol 2001;37(3):780–5.
43. von Mering GO, Arant CB, Wessel TR, et al. Abnormal coronary vasomotion as a prognostic indicator of cardiovascular events in women: results from the National Heart, Lung, and Blood Institute-Sponsored Women's Ischemia Syndrome Evaluation (WISE). Circulation 2004;109(6):722–5.
44. Bairey Merz CN, Pepine CJ, Shimokawa H, et al. Treatment of coronary microvascular dysfunction. Cardiovasc Res 2020;116(4):856–70.
45. Mehta PK, Quesada O, Al-Badri A, et al. Ischemia and no obstructive coronary arteries in patients with stable ischemic heart disease. Int J Cardiol 2022;348:1–8.
46. Mathew RC, Bourque JM, Salerno M, et al. Cardiovascular Imaging Techniques to. Assess Microvascular Dysfunction 2020;13(7):1577–90.
47. Handberg EM, Merz CNB, Cooper-Dehoff RM, et al. Rationale and design of the Women's Ischemia Trial to Reduce Events in Nonobstructive CAD (WARRIOR) trial. Am Heart J 2021;237:90–103.
48. Stoller M, Traupe T, Khattab AA, et al. Effects of coronary sinus occlusion on myocardial ischaemia in humans: role of coronary collateral function. Heart 2013;99(8):548–55.
49. Verheye S, Jolicœur EM, Behan MW, et al. Efficacy of a device to narrow the coronary sinus in refractory angina. N Engl J Med 2015;372(6):519–27.
50. Ullrich H, Hammer P, Olschewski M, et al. Coronary Venous Pressure and Microvascular Hemodynamics in Patients With Microvascular Angina: A Randomized Clinical Trial. JAMA Cardiology 2023;8(10):979–83.
51. Lagerqvist B, Sylven C, Waldenstrom A. Lower threshold for adenosine-induced chest pain in patients with angina and normal coronary angiograms. Br Heart J 1992;68(3):282–5.
52. Frobert O, Arendt-Nielsen L, Bak P, et al. Pain perception and brain evoked potentials in patients with angina despite normal coronary angiograms. Heart 1996;75(5):436–41.
53. Cannon RO 3rd, Quyyumi AA, Mincemoyer R, et al. Imipramine in patients with chest pain despite normal coronary angiograms. N Engl J Med 1994;330(20):1411–7.
54. Gallone G, Baldetti L, Tzanis G, et al. Refractory Angina: From Pathophysiology to New Therapeutic Nonpharmacological Technologies. JACC Cardiovasc Interv 2020;13(1):1–19.
55. Cannon RO 3rd, Quyyumi AA, Schenke WH, et al. Abnormal cardiac sensitivity in patients with chest pain and normal coronary arteries. J Am Coll Cardiol 1990;16(6):1359–66.

A New Age for Secondary Prevention: Optimal Medical Therapy for Stable Ischemic Heart Disease Among Patients with Diabetes and/or Obesity

Nkiru Osude, MD, MS[a],*, Neha J. Pagidipati, MD, MPH[b]

KEYWORDS

- Prevention • ASCVD risk • T2D • GLP-1RA • SGLT-2 inhibitor

KEY POINTS

- Glucagon-like peptide-1 receptor agonists and sodium–glucose cotransporter-2 inhibitors have demonstrated efficacy in decreasing cardiovascular events (myocardial infarctions, strokes, and cardiovascular-related death) in patients with established cardiovascular disease and type 2 diabetes mellitus.
- Emerging data suggest cardiovascular benefit of semaglutide in patients with obesity and established cardiovascular disease without diabetes.
- The use of these agents by internists, primary care physicians, and cardiologists is critical to reducing the risk of recurrent events in this high-risk population.
- Vast under-use of these agents as well as disparities in use contribute to large gaps in care especially for minority populations; implementation efforts can help to close these gaps.

BACKGROUND

Ischemic heart disease is the leading cause of death in the United States, accounting for approximately one in four deaths.[1,2] Although many factors contribute to the risk for ischemic heart disease, diabetes and obesity are among the most potent.[3,4] Patients with diabetes experience up to 50% increased risk of all-cause mortality and cardiovascular (CV) death compared with those without diabetes.[5] Obesity has been associated with an increase in all-cause mortality for those with a body mass index (BMI) above 30 kg/m^2.[6] Indeed, ischemic heart disease is the leading cause of

[a] Cardiovascular Division, Duke University, 2301 Erwin Road, Durham, NC 27710, USA;
[b] Cardiovascular Division, 2301 Erwin Road, Durham, NC 27701, USA
* Corresponding author. 2301 Erwin Road, Durham NC 27710.
E-mail address: Nkiru.osude@duke.edu
Twitter: @NkiruOsude (N.O.)

Med Clin N Am 108 (2024) 469–487
https://doi.org/10.1016/j.mcna.2023.11.003
0025-7125/24/© 2023 Elsevier Inc. All rights reserved.

death in patients with diabetes mellitus and obesity.[7,8] With the incidence and prevalence of diabetes and obesity on the rise in the United States, secondary prevention therapies to decrease atherosclerotic CV disease (ASCVD) events have the potential to reach a large and at-risk population.[9]

In recent years, newer agents, including glucagon-like peptide-1 receptor agonists (GLP-1RAs) and sodium–glucose cotransporter-2 inhibitors (SGLT-2 inhibitors), have demonstrated a reduction in recurrent atherosclerotic CV risk in patients with type 2 diabetes mellitus (T2D) and established ischemic heart disease independent of their effects on glycemic control. However, there has been slow clinical uptake of GLP1-RAs and SGLT2 inhibitors in patients with type 2 diabetes and obesity with ischemic heart disease, even more so in certain underrepresented populations.[10,11] Lower utilization rates of these agents in patients with established ASCVD have been identified in non-Caucasian races and ethnicities and in those with less resources, contributing to disparities in outcomes in these populations.[12–18] Here, the authors review the use of SGLT2 inhibitors and GLP1-RA as optimal medical therapy for ASCVD secondary prevention in patients with obesity and/or diabetes. Other secondary prevention measures, diet, exercise, blood pressure control, and lipid management, are essential in conjunction with these agents but are outside the scope of this review. In this review, the authors highlight data for using these agents, practical aspects of use, and current inequities that, when improved, can decrease disparities in recurrent ASCVD outcomes.

Secondary Prevention Therapies Among Patients with Type 2 Diabetes

There has been a recent paradigm shift in diabetes management, such that if CV disease or elevated ASCVD risk is present, the American Diabetes Association recommends GLP-1RA or SGLT-2 inhibitor should be chosen as first-line therapy for the management of T2D for added CV disease benefit.[19] For the remainder of this review, the authors specifically highlight the medications in these classes that improve CV outcomes in patients with type 2 diabetes.

Glucagon-like Peptide-1 Receptor Agonists

GLP-1 is a peptide hormone released from gastrointestinal cells after food is ingested that increases insulin production and decreases glucagon release.[20,21] GLP-1RAs reduce the risk of ASCVD events among patients with T2D, such as myocardial infarctions (MIs) and strokes.[22] The CV effects of GLP-1RAs are thought to be mediated by the direct and indirect effects of their activation of the GLP-1 receptor on cardiomyocytes, blood vessels, and fat cells; however, the exact mechanism for which GLP-1RAs reduce CV outcomes remains unclear and is under investigation.[23,24]

In this review, the authors discuss GLP1-RAs that have demonstrated superiority in CV outcome trials (CVOTs), are currently on the market in the United States, and are recommended by the 2023 AHA/ACC/ACP/ASPC/PCNA Guideline for the Management of Patients with Chronic Coronary Disease. The GLP-1RAs that meet these criteria include liraglutide, semaglutide (subcutaneous), and dulaglutide. The guidelines provide a Class IA indication for the use of GLP-1RA with proven cardiovascular benefit to reduce major adverse cardiovascular events (MACE) in patients with established coronary disease and concurrent T2D.[22]

Liraglutide is a once-daily subcutaneous injectable GLP-1RA and was the first GLP-1RA to demonstrate CV outcomes superiority in the LEADER (Liraglutide Effect and Action in Diabetes: Evaluation of Cardiovascular Outcome Results) trial (**Table 1**). Among patients with established CVD and T2D, liraglutide decreased the risk of a composite outcome of 3-point MACE (3P-MACE), which included CV death, MI,

Table 1
Glucagon-like peptide-1 receptor agonist cardiovascular outcome trial results

Drug	CVOT	Inclusion Criteria	% Patients with Established CVD	MACE HR (95% CI)	CV Death HR (95% CI)	Nonfatal MI HR(95% CI)	Nonfatal Stroke HR(95% CI)
Liraglutide	LEADER[25]	Age ≥50 y with T2D, and with ≥1 CV coexisting condition OR ≥ 60 y with ≥ 1 CV risk factor	82%	0.87 (0.78–0.97) $P = .01$	(0.66–0.93) $P = .007$	0.88 (0.75–1.03) $P = .11$	0.89 (0.72–1.11) $P = .30$
Semaglutide (subcutaneous)	SUSTAIN 6[26]	Age ≥50 y with T2D and established CVD, chronic HF, or chronic kidney disease OR ≥ 60 y with ≥ 1 CV risk factor	85%	0.74 (0.58–0.95) $P < .001$ non-inferiority; $P = .02$ superiority	0.98 (0.65–1.48); $P = .92$	0.74 (0.51–1.08); $P = .12$	0.61 (0.38–0.99); $P = .04$
Dulaglutide	REWIND[45]	Age ≥50 y with T2D and vascular disease OR ≥ 55 y with ≥ 1 cardiorenal condition OR ≥ 60 y with ≥ 2 CV risk factors	31%	0.88 (0.79–0.99) $P = .026$	0.91 (0.78–1.06) $P = .21$	0.96 (0.79–1.16) $P = .65$	0.76 (0.61–0.95) $P = .017$

Abbreviations: CKD, chronic kidney disease; HF, heart failure.

and stroke; however, no significant difference was observed for heart failure (HF) hospitalizations.[25] Semaglutide is commercially available in several forms, including both subcutaneous and oral routes of administration. Semaglutide 1 mg weekly SC was evaluated in SUSTAIN 6 (Trial to Evaluate Cardiovascular and Other Long Term Outcomes with Semaglutide in Subjects with Type 2 Diabetes) and demonstrated a reduction in MACE that was primarily driven by a 39% decrease in nonfatal stroke.[26] Similar to liraglutide, a decrease in HF hospitalizations was not seen in SUSTAIN-6.[26] Oral semaglutide was found to be non-inferior to placebo concerning MACE, but the trial was not powered to show superiority.[27] Dulaglutide, a weekly subcutaneous injectable GLP-1RA, was evaluated in the REWIND (Researching Cardiovascular Events with a Weekly Incretin in Diabetes) trial, which showed a 12% reduction in 3P-MACE in both secondary and primary prevention populations.[28]

In 2021, an updated meta-analysis that included eight completed GLP-1RA CVOTs showed a 14% risk reduction in MACE which was consistent across the class and across subgroups.[29] To prevent one MACE event, the overall number needed to treat with a mean follow of 3 years is 65 patients. In addition, GLP1-RAs demonstrated an 18% reduction in worsening kidney function.[29] Based on this meta-analysis, it is reasonable to postulate that the MACE benefit with GLP-1RA is a class benefit.[30] That being said, we generally prioritize the commercially available GLP-1RA agents discussed above (liraglutide, semaglutide, dulaglutide) because they have clear CV benefit.

Practical issues with prescribing glucagon-like peptide-1 receptor agonist

Information on target dosing, titrations, and impact on hemoglobin A1c and weight are outlined in **Table 2**. As GLP-1RAs facilitate endogenous insulin secretion, the risk of hypoglycemia when taken in isolation is low. However, the risk of hypoglycemia increases when used in combination with insulin and/or sulfonylureas.[31] In patients with relatively well-controlled glycemic status, adjustments to these concomitant medications may need to be made when initiating GLP-1RAs.[32]

Gastrointestinal side effects (nausea, vomiting, and diarrhea) are the most common side effects associated with GLP-1RAs, occurring in 10% to 50% of patients in clinical trials.[32,33] These gastrointestinal symptoms are caused by the action of the GLP-1 hormone on slowing gastrointestinal motility, which is part of the physiologic effect of the hormone.[34] Of note, these effects are most substantial at drug initiation and

Table 2
Glucagon-like peptide-1 receptor agonist dosing and metabolic impact

Medication	HbA1c Reduction (%)	Weight Reduction (kg)	Initial Dose	Up-Titration	Target Dose (for CVD Protection)
Liraglutide	−0.40% (1.8 mg)	−2.5 kg (1.8 mg)	0.6 mg	Increase by 0.6 mg monthly	1.8 mg
Semaglutide Subcutaneous injection	−1.1% (0.5 mg) −1.4% (1.0 mg)	−3.6 kg (0.5 mg) −4.9 kg (1.0 mg)	0.25 mg weekly	Increase by 0.25 mg monthly	1.0 mg
Dulaglutide	−0.51%	−1.46 kg	0.75 mg weekly	Increase to 1.5 mg after 1 mo	1.5 mg

Data obtained from CVOT results of LEADER, SUSTAIN 6, and REWIND data Refs.[25,45,46]

typically subside with continued use. With all GLP-1RAs, we recommend "start low and titrate slow" to improve gastrointestinal tolerability. GLP-1RAs should be used with caution in patients with gastroparesis.[31] In September 2023, The Food and Drug Administration (FDA) added ileus as an adverse reaction to the safety label; ileus was not seen in the clinical trials, and because the reactions are reported voluntarily from an unknown population size, it is difficult to estimate the frequency of this reaction.[35] Pancreatitis has been associated with GLP-1RAs, yet causality has not been established. If a clinical concern of pancreatitis is suspected, GLP-1RAs should be discontinued. Injection site reactions (cellulitis, necrosis, abscess) have been described and occur at a slightly higher rate than local reactions seen with insulin injections.[33,36]

Emerging therapies

There are several phase II, phase III, and CVOTs trials underway evaluating both combination therapy with and oral variations of GLP-1RAs.[37–42] Tirzepatide, a once-weekly subcutaneous injectable that combines agonism of GLP-1 and GIP (glucose-dependent insulinotropic polypeptide), leads to larger hemoglobin A1c and weight reduction when compared head-to-head to semaglutide 1 mg. The CV benefits of tirzepatide are unknown and are currently being examined with SURPASS-CVOT, comparing non-inferiority and superiority of the CV outcomes of tirzepatide against dulaglutide (**Table 3**).[37] CVOTs that are planned for additional agents are outlined in **Table 3**.

Sodium–Glucose Cotransporter Type 2 Inhibitors

The sodium–glucose cotransporter type 2 is expressed in the proximal tubule and controls the reabsorption of most of the filtered glucose load. SGLT2 inhibitors have been shown to reduce the risk of ASCVD among secondary prevention patients with type 2 diabetes, in addition to HF and kidney disease benefits.[43] The exact mechanism of how SGLT-2 inhibitors are cardioprotective is poorly understood; however, it is postulated to be cardioprotective via three main mechanisms: natriuresis/osmotic diuresis, reduction in oxidative stress, and increase in ketone production. SGLT-2 inhibitors do not decrease the intravascular volume, but rather by natriuresis decrease the interstitial fluid that reduces the likelihood of volume expansion that precedes HF hospitalizations.[44] SGLT-2 inhibitors also work directly on the heart, independent of reductions in plasma glucose, to promote autophagy, which reduces oxidative stress and enhances cardiac cellular function.[44] Finally, by reducing plasma glucose levels, SGLT-2 inhibitors increase ketone production, an additional energy source to the myocardium.[45]

The 2023 *Guideline for the Management of Patients with Chronic Coronary Disease* provides a Class IA recommendation for the use of SGLT-2 inhibitors in patients with T2D and chronic coronary disease.[22] In addition, the same guidelines also recommend SGLT-2 inhibitor use in patients with HF, irrespective of diabetes status, to decrease the risk of CV death, HF hospitalizations, and improve quality of life: A Class IA indication for SGLT-2 inhibitors in patients chronic coronary disease and HF with left ventricular ejection fraction (LVEF) ≤40% in the Chronic Coronary Disease Guidelines[22], *and a* Class IIa indication is given for patients with HF with preserved ejection fraction (LVEF >40%) irrespective of diabetes status.[22] In contrast, the *2023 Focused Update of the 2021 European Society of Cardiology Guidelines for Diagnosis and Treatment of Acute and Chronic Heart Failure* recommend empagliflozin and dapagliflozin in patients with HF with mildly preserved or reduced ejection fraction as a Class I LOE:A recommendation based on the results seen in two CVOTs in these populations.[46–48]

Table 3
Ongoing or planned cardiovascular outcome trials in patients with diabetes and/or obesity

Ongoing Trial	Drug Class	Inclusion Criteria	Intervention	Primary Outcome	Estimated Completion Date
SUMMIT[38] (A Study of Tirzepatide in Participants With Heart Failure With Preserved Ejection Fraction and Obesity) NCT 04847557	Subcutaneous GIP/GLP-1RA	Stable HFpEF (NYHA II-IV), elevated NT-pro-BNP, • BMI ≥30 (kg/m²), KCCQ CSS ≤80, eGFR <70 mL/min/1.73 m² or HF decompensation within 12 mo, 6MWD 100–425 m	Tirzepatide vs placebo	Hierarchical composite of all-cause mortality, heart failure events, 6MWD, and KCCQ clinical summary score Change from baseline in exercise capacity as measured by 6MWD	July 2024
SURPASS-CVOT[35] (A Study of Tirzepatide Compared With Dulaglutide on Major Cardiovascular Events in Participants With Type 2 Diabetes) NCT04255433	Subcutaneous GIP/GLP-1RA	T2D diagnosis, confirmed ASCVD, HbA1c ≥ 7.0% to ≤10.5%, BMI ≥25 kg/m²	Tirzepatide vs Dulaglutide	Time to first event composite (CV death, nonfatal MI, nonfatal stroke)	October 2024
ACHIEVE-4[37] (A Study of Daily Orforglipron Compared with Insulin Glargine in Participants with Type 2 Diabetes and Obesity or Overweight at Increased Cardiovascular Risk) NCT05803421	Oral GLP-1RA	T2D diagnosis, HbA1c ≥ 7.0% to ≤10.5%, increased risk for CV events, stable weight before screening, BMI ≥25 kg/m²	Orforglipron vs Insulin Glargine	Time to first event (myocardial infarction, stroke, hospitalization for unstable angina, CV death)	September 2025

Trial	Intervention	Population	Comparison	Primary Outcome	Completion
SURMOUNT- MMO[39] (A Study of Tirzepatide on the Reduction on Morbidity and Mortality in Adults With Obesity) NCT05556512	Subcutaneous GIP/GLP-1RA	BMI ≥27 kg/m², ≥40 y of age Established CVD or PAD or presence of CV risk factors	Tirzepatide vs placebo	Time to first event composite (all-cause death, nonfatal myocardial, nonfatal stroke, coronary revascularization, or HF events)	October 2027
REDEFINE 3[40] (A Research Study to See Effects of CagriSema on Heart Disease in People Living with Obesity and Diseases in Heart and Blood Vessels) NCT05669755	Subcutaneous GLP-1RA/Amylin Analogue	BMI ≥30 kg/m², established CVD OR patients with T2D, HbA1c ≥ 7.0% to ≤10%, with treatment with life style intervention or oral antidiabetic drugs or basal insulin	Cagrilintide-semaglutide vs placebo	Time to first occurrence of MACE (CV death, nonfatal MI, nonfatal stroke)	October 2027

Abbreviations: 6MWD, 6-min walk test distance; BMI, body mass index; CV, cardiovascular; CVD, cardiovascular disease; eGFR, estimated glomerular filtration rate; HbA1c, hemoglobin A1c; HF, heart failure; HFpEF, heart failure with prereved ejection fraction; GIP, glucose-dependent insulinotropic polypeptide; KCCQ, Kansas City Cardiomyopathy Questionnaire clinical summary score category.

Here, the authors focus on SGLT-2 inhibitors that have demonstrated superiority in CVOTs, are currently on the market in the United States, and are recommended by 2023 AHA/ACC/ACP/ASPC/PCNA Guideline for the Management of Patients with Chronic Coronary Disease. The agents that meet these criteria include empagliflozin, canagliflozin, dapagliflozin, and sotagliflozin (which is a dual SGLT-1/SGLT-2 inhibitor).

Empagliflozin was initially evaluated in the EMPA-REG OUTCOME (Empagliflozin Cardiovascular Outcome Event Trial in Type 2 Diabetes Mellitus Patients) trial, a randomized, double-blind, placebo-controlled trial in which patients with T2D and established CVD were treated with once-daily empagliflozin 10 mg or 25 mg versus placebo (**Table 4**).[49] At the trial end, empagliflozin led to a 14% reduction in 3P-MACE, 38% relative risk reduction in CV death, 32% risk reduction in all-cause mortality, 35% risk reduction in HF hospitalization, and 44% reduction in eGFR decline in further analyses.[49,50] Canagliflozin was evaluated in the CANVAS program (The Canagliflozin Cardiovascular Assessment Study), which integrated data from two companion double-blind, randomized, placebo-controlled trials (CANVAS and CANVAS–Renal) aimed to understand CV safety, CV, and renal protection. The primary outcome, 3P-MACE, demonstrated a 14% risk reduction; a 27% risk reduction in the progression of albuminuria and regression of albuminuria occurred in the canagliflozin group. There was also a lower rate of HF hospitalizations and renal composite (40% reduction in eGFR, need for dialysis, and death from renal causes) seen in the canagliflozin group, without statistical significance.[51] Dapagliflozin was evaluated in DECLARE-TIMI CVOT which evaluated two primary outcomes: 3-P MACE and a CV death and HF hospitalization composite. Dapagliflozin was non-inferior with regard to 3P-MACE but was superior with respect to the composite of CV death and HF hospitalization.

Sotagliflozin is a once-daily SGLT-1 and SGLT-2 inhibitor which provides dual antagonism of glucose co-transporters in the kidney (SGLT-2) and the small intestine (SGLT-1).[52] Despite terminating early due to loss of funding, the SCORED (Sotagliflozin in Patients with Diabetes and Chronic Kidney Disease) trial showed superiority in the outcome of total number of CV deaths, HF hospitalizations, and urgent visits for HF (0.74[0.63–0.88] $P < .001$).[53] Dosing and metabolic targets are found in **Table 5**.

A 2019 SGLT-2 inhibitor meta-analysis, which included EMPA-REG OUTCOME, CANVAS Program, and DECLARE-TIMI, found that there was a class reduction of HF hospitalizations and progression of renal disease; a reduction in MACE was only seen in patients with ASCVD and not in patients without ASCVD.[54] A 2020 SGLT-2 inhibitor meta-analysis (SCORED was not included) showed an overall class benefit for reducing HF hospitalizations and tendency for kidney disease progression.[43] There was, however, heterogeneity in the impact on other CV outcomes. These meta-analyses suggest a class benefit for HF and kidney outcomes, but not for MACE or CV death. However, ertugliflozin is the only SGLT2 inhibitor without demonstrated kidney benefit, and therefore, we choose empagliflozin, canagliflozin, dapagliflozin, or sotagliflozin over this agent.[55]

Prescribing considerations

The most common adverse effect associated with SGLT-2 inhibitors are genitourinary infections; these infections are predominantly mild to moderate and can be treated in the ambulatory setting.[56–59] Excess glucose in the urine can facilitate predominantly genital mycotic infections (balanitis and vulvovaginitis) and, in some cases, bacterial urinary tract infections. Patients should be advised on maintaining genital hygiene.[60,61]

Table 4
Sodium–glucose cotransporter-2 inhibitor cardiovascular outcome trial results

Drug	CVOT	Key Inclusion Criteria (Not including T2D)	% Patients with Established CVD	MACE HR (95% CI)	CV Death HR (95% CI)	Nonfatal MI HR (95% CI)	Nonfatal Stroke HR (95% CI)	HF Hospitalization HR (95% CI)
Empagliflozin	EMPA-REG OUTCOME[53]	Age ≥18 y with BMI <45 and ≥ eGFR 30 mL/min1.73 m² with established CVD	99%	0.86 (0.74–0.99) $P < .001$; $P = .04$ superiority	0.62 (0.49–0.77); $P < .001$	0.87 (0.70–1.09)	1.24 (0.92–1.67)	0.65 (0.509–0.85) $P = .002$
Canagliflozin	CANVAS[55]	Age ≥50 y with ≥2 CVD risk factors OR Age ≥30 with symptomatic ASCVD	65.6%	0.86 (0.75–0.97) $P < .001$; $P = .02$ for superiority	0.87 (0.72–1.06)	0.85 (0.69–1.05)	0.87 (0.69–1.09)	0.67 (0.52–0.87)
Dapagliflozin	DECLARE-TIMI[56]	Age ≥40 y with T2D and established CVD OR Age men ≥55 y or age ≥60 y in women with CVD risk factors	40.6%	0.93 (0.84–1.03) $P = .17$	0.98 (0.82–1.17)	0.89 (0.77)-1.01)[a]	1.01 (0.84–1.21)	0.73 (0.61–0.88)
Sotagliflozin	SCORED[58]	Age ≥18 with CKD with CVD risk factors	48.9%	Not reported	0.9 (0.73–112)	Not provided	Not provided	0.67 (0.55–0.82) $P<.001$

Abbreviations: BMI, body mass index; HF, heart failure; eGFR, estimated glomerular filtration rate, CV, cardiovascular; CVD, cardiovascular disease.
[a] DECLARE-TIMI reported as myocardial infarction and stroke did not distinguish between fatal and nonfatal event rates

Table 5
Sodium–glucose cotransporter-2 inhibitors dosing and metabolic impact

Medication	HbA1c Reduction (%)	Weight Reduction (kg)	Initial Dose	Up-Titration	Target Dose (for CVD Protection)
Empagliflozin	−0.24% (10 mg) −0.36% (25 mg) at 206 wk	Not provided	10 mg or 25 mg (no difference)	Can increase to 25 mg for metabolic considerations	10 mg
Canagliflozin	−0.58% (mean difference)	−1.6 kg (mean difference)	100 mg or 300 mg	Can increase to 300 mg after 13 wk	100 mg or 300 mg
Dapagliflozin	Not provided	Not provided	10 mg	N/A	10 mg
Sotagliflozin	−0.60% (patients with egFR >30) −0.56% (patients with egFr < 30)	−1.4 kg	200 mg	Increase by 200 mg after 2 wk based on tolerability	400 mg

Reviewed in this table are results from EMPA-REG OUTCOME, DECLARE-TIMI, CANVAS, SCORED CVOT data Refs.[53,55,56,58]

Volume depletion can also occur due to osmotic diuresis, and it is characteristically seen as lightheadedness, increased thirst, and orthostatic hypotension.[44] Euglycemic diabetic ketoacidosis (DKA) is a rare complication of SGLT2 inhibitor use and is estimated to occur in 0.003% to 0.1% of patients.[62] Caution should be taken in patients with prior episodes of DKA, during times of fasting or decreased oral intake (before surgery), or in individuals on ketogenic diets.

In 2017, the FDA issued a Boxed Warning for canagliflozin because of increased risk of lower extremity infection and atraumatic amputation seen in the CANVAS program.[63] A subsequent trial of canagliflozin, CREDENCE (Canagliflozin and Renal Outcomes in Type 2 Diabetes and Nephropathy), demonstrated no increased risk of amputation. Subsequent SGLT-2 inhibitor trials have not shown this increased amputation risk, despite diligent and rigorous collection and adjudication of peripheral artery disease potential events. Thus, the FDA boxed warning was removed in 2020.[64]

Canagliflozin has been associated with an increased incidence of bone fractures, potentially related to a drug-related decrease in bone mineral density.[65,66] Fractures can occur as early as 12 weeks after drug initiation and can occur with minor trauma.[67] This adverse effect was not seen with other SGLT-2 inhibitors.

Secondary Prevention Therapies Among Patients with Obesity

Although obesity is a significant contributor to CV risk factors, including hypertension, T2D, hyperlipidemia, and sleep disorders, it also independently increases the risk of coronary artery disease, MIs, stroke, HF, and mortality.[68,69] Obesity is pro-inflammatory and accelerates atherosclerosis by lipid deposition and atherothrombosis formation through insulin resistance and inflammation. Obesity-induced systemic inflammation increases low-density lipoprotein oxidation, which promotes plaque formation.[3]

Despite these links, lifestyle interventions have not demonstrated a reduction in CV outcomes in patients with obesity and T2D.[70] Look AHEAD (Action for Health in Diabetes) was a randomized clinical trial that addressed whether an intensive lifestyle intervention decreased CV outcomes (CV death, nonfatal MI, and nonfatal stroke) among individuals with overweight or obesity and T2D. In the initial year, the intervention group had substantially reduced weight, waist circumference, hemoglobin A1c, and increased physical fitness compared with the control group; however, the differences between the groups decreased over time. The study was terminated at a median follow-up of 9.6 years due to futility as the primary composite CV outcome showed no significant difference.[70] Because weight loss was not maintained in this trial, the futility of the intervention does not necessarily imply a lack of CV benefit with maintained weight loss. Bariatric surgery, on the other hand, was associated with decreases all-cause mortality, CV deaths, MIs, and strokes in the non-randomized SOS (Swedish Obese Subjects) Study.[71] SOS was a surgical, matched, prospective study that compared bariatric surgery (gastric bypass, gastric banding, vertical banded gastroplasty) to usual care in adults with a BMI above 34 in men and 38 in women.[71] In addition to substantial weight reduction, bariatric surgery was associated with a reduced number of CV deaths (HR [95% CI]: 0.47 [0.29–0.76]; $P = .002$) and reduced number of total (both fatal and nonfatal) strokes and MIs (unadjusted HR [95% CI]: 0.56 [0.35–0.88]; $P = .01$).[71]

Although bariatric surgery is associated with improved CV outcomes, socioeconomic and racial disparities exist in surgery referrals and after referrals are placed, similar disparities remain in those who obtain the surgery.[72] Barriers to bariatric surgery after referral include the time and number of appointments required for preoperative testing, perceived fear of surgical complications, and insurance approval. Fewer than 1% of eligible patients receive bariatric surgery.[72] There is a real and present need for nonoperative ways to lose and sustain weight loss with the additive benefit of reduction of MACE.

Anti-obesity medications are aiming to fill this need as CVOTs are ongoing. SGLT-2 inhibitors promote weight loss by inhibiting renal glucose absorption and can produce modest weight loss of 1.5 to 3 kg, as seen in the SGLT-2 CVOTs. However, SGLT-2 inhibitors have not been tested in the secondary ASCVD prevention population with obesity but without diabetes.[73] GLP-1RAs and related classes have demonstrated substantial weight loss in patients with obesity, with or without diabetes. Whether this weight loss itself leads to CV benefit, however, is unknown.

The SELECT (Semaglutide Effects on Cardiovascular Outcomes in People) trial is shedding light on this critical issue. Published in 2023, SELECT was the first CVOT to address whether a GLP-1RA (semaglutide 2.4 mg weekly) improves CV outcomes among patients with overweight or obesity and known ASCVD, but without diabetes.[74] It showed a 20% relative risk reduction (1.5% absolute risk reduction) in MACE over a median follow-up of 34 months. Interestingly, mean change in body weight was only −8.51% with semaglutide versus placebo over 104 weeks, much lower than the average −12.4% weight loss seen in the STEP1 (Semaglutide Treatment Effect in People with Obesity) trial over 68 weeks.[75] Further, the separation of curves for the MACE outcome in SELECT occurred almost immediately, presumably before patients had an opportunity to lose substantial weight. Further details on the possible impact of weight loss versus other potential mechanisms for CV benefit with semaglutide are eagerly awaited. In addition, several CVOTs with emerging anti-obesity medications such as tirzepatide, orforglipron, retatrutide, and cagrisema are planned and are summarized in **Table 3**.

Disparate Use and Disparities in Care

Despite their significant evidence base, the use of GLP-1RAs and SGLT-2 inhibitors in appropriate populations is alarmingly poor. In 2021, an inquiry of medical claims data for more than 155,000 patients with T2D and ASCVD demonstrated that 9.9% of eligible patients were on GLP-1RAs or SGLT-2 inhibitors.[76] Cost-related barriers have been associated with the poor adoption of these two classes of medications, specifically high out-of-pocket (OOP) costs. In a Medicare Advantage and commercial insurance population, OOP costs for GLP-1RAs range from $25 to $118 each month, with SGLT-2 inhibitors from $23 to $91 each month.[77] Although annual prescriptions for GLP-1RAs and SGLT-2 inhibitors have continued to rise with the expansion of approved indications, current prescription rates remain very low.[78,79]

In addition, persistent, pervasive disparities remain across the spectrum of CV disease preventive care by race, ethnicity, and socioeconomic status.[80] Recurrent ASCVD events are seen in higher rates in racial and ethnic monitories, women, and those in disadvantaged neighborhoods.[14,15] Black race, Asian race, and female gender have been associated with lower rates of SGLT-2 inhibitor use, whereas higher median income is associated with higher rates of SGLT-2 inhibitor use.[81] Black race, Asian race, and Hispanic ethnicity are associated with lower GLP-1RA use, whereas female sex and higher zip-code linked median household incomes are associated with higher GLP-1RA use.[17] When accounting for system-level factors, all racial/ethnic minorities have lower odds of being prescribed these medications than their Caucasian counterparts.[18,82]

Systematic implementation programs may help to increase prescribing rates in all populations. COORDINATE-Diabetes was a randomized cardiology clinic-level trial of a multifaceted intervention (including assessment of gaps, development of care pathways, and audit and feedback) versus usual care to improve prescription of three evidence-based therapies for patients with ASCVD and T2D. The intervention was associated with a 23.4% increase in prescription of all three groups of therapies (high-intensity statins, angiotensin-converting enzyme inhibitors (ACEi) or antiotensin receptor blockers (ARBs), and SGLT2 inhibitors and/or GLP-1RA).[83]

SUMMARY

Patients with type 2 diabetes and obesity are at increased risk for recurrent ASCVD events. In the last decade, several CV outcomes trials have shown that options for secondary prevention are no longer isolated to risk factor modification and bariatric surgery. GLP-1RAs and SGLT-2 inhibitors are effective medications to reduce ASCVD events, promote weight reduction, decrease HF hospitalizations, and slow progression of kidney disease.

In deciding whether to initiate an SGLT2 inhibitor versus a GLP-1RA in a patient with known ASCVD and obesity and/or diabetes, the following factors should be kept in mind. The mechanisms of action of these two classes of agents are very different, and therefore, their CV benefit is expected to be additive rather than duplicative.[84] Thus, high-risk secondary prevention patients who are eligible for both therapies, particularly those with diabetes, should be considered for both. However, known barriers to using multiple medications, including cost and polypharmacy, may preclude usage of both classes in the same patient. When this is case, we favor starting SGLT2 inhibitors in patients with chronic kidney disease and/or HF and starting GLP1-RA in patients with ASCVD and/or obesity.[85] In reality, these therapies are so under-used in clinical practice, particularly in vulnerable populations that initiating either of these classes is preferable to initiating neither. As additional agents come down the pipeline, we need to ensure appropriate and equitable use of these evidence-based therapies across all populations.

CLINICS CARE POINTS

- Glucagon-like peptide-1 receptor agonists (GLP-1RAs) and sodium–glucose cotransporter-2 inhibitors (SGLT-2 inhibitors) reduce cardiovascular events among patients with T2D and atherosclerotic cardiovascular disease (ASCVD), and the benefits are independent of their A1c reductions.

- GLP1RA should be used in patients with T2D and a history of ASCVD as these have been shown to decrease cardiovascular death, myocardial infarctions, and stroke.

- SGLT2 inhibitors should be used in patients with T2D and a history of ASCVD as they have been shown to decrease HF hospitalizations and progression of kidney disease and decrease MACE in a secondary prevention population

- Emerging data suggest that semaglutide 2.4 mg can decrease MACE among patients with obesity and ASCVD.

- Data-driven implementation programs can help to improve equitable use of GLP-1RAs and SGLT-2 inhibitors.

DISCLOSURE

N. Osude: NIH, United States funded grant T32HL069749. N.J. Pagidipati: Research support from Alnylam, Amgen, United States, Boehringer Ingelheim, Germany, Eggland's Best, Eli Lilly, Novartis, Switzerland, Novo Nordisk, Denmark, Verily Life Sciences, United States. Consultation/Advisory Panels for Bayer, Boehringer Ingelheim, CRISPR Therapeutics, Eli Lilly, Esperion, AstraZeneca, Merck, Novartis, and Novo Nordisk.

Executive Committee member for trials sponsored by Novo Nordisk and by Amgen. DSMB for trials sponsored by J+J and Novartis. Medical advisory board for Miga Health.

REFERENCES

1. Benjamin EJ, Muntner P, Alonso A, et al. Heart disease and stroke Statistics—2019 update: A report from the American heart association | circulation. Circulation 2019. Available at: https://www.ahajournals.org/doi/10.1161/CIR.0000000000000659#d1e3747. Accessed July 26, 2023.
2. Tsao CW, Aday AW, Almarzooq ZI, et al. Heart disease and stroke Statistics—2023 update: A report from the American heart association | circulation. Circulation 2023. Available at: https://www.ahajournals.org/doi/10.1161/CIR.0000000000001123?utm_campaign=sciencenews22-23&utm_source=science-news&utm_medium=phd-link&utm_content=phd-01-25-23. Accessed July 25, 2023.
3. Powell-Wiley TM, Poirier P, Burke LE, et al. Obesity and cardiovascular disease: A scientific statement from the american heart association. Circulation 2021; 143(21):e984–1010.
4. Mohammadi H, Ohm J, Discacciati A, et al. Abdominal obesity and the risk of recurrent atherosclerotic cardiovascular disease after myocardial infarction. Eur J Prev Cardiol 2020;27(18):1944–52.
5. Barnett KN, Ogston SA, McMurdo MET, et al. A 12-year follow-up study of all-cause and cardiovascular mortality among 10,532 people newly diagnosed with type 2 diabetes in Tayside, Scotland. Diabet Med 2010;27(10):1124–9.
6. Berrington de Gonzalez A, Hartge P, Cerhan JR, et al. Body-mass index and mortality among 1.46 million white adults. N Engl J Med 2010;363(23):2211–9.
7. Das SR, Everrett BM, Birtcher KK, et al. 2018 ACC expert consensus decision pathway on novel therapies for cardiovascular risk reduction in patients with type 2 diabetes and atherosclerotic cardiovascular disease: A report of the american college of cardiology task force on expert consensus decision pathways - ScienceDirect. J Am Coll Cardiol 2018;72(24):3200–23. Available at: https://www.sciencedirect.com/science/article/pii/S0735109718384985. Accessed July 25, 2023.
8. The GBD 2015 Obesity Investigators. Health effects of overweight and obesity in 195 countries over 25 years. N Engl J Med 2017;377(1):13–27.
9. Cameron NA, Petito LC, McCabe M, et al. Quantifying the sex-race/ethnicity-specific burden of obesity on incident diabetes mellitus in the united states, 2001 to 2016: MESA and NHANES. J Am Heart Assoc 2021;10(4):e018799.
10. Arnold SV, de Lemos JA, Rosenson RS, et al. Use of guideline-recommended risk reduction strategies among patients with diabetes and atherosclerotic cardiovascular disease. Circulation 2019;140(7):618–20.
11. Arnold SV, Inzucchi SE, Tang F, et al. Real-world use and modeled impact of glucose-lowering therapies evaluated in recent cardiovascular outcomes trials: An NCDR® research to practice project. Eur J Prev Cardiol 2017;24(15):1637–45.
12. Peters SAE, Colantonio LD, Dai Y, et al. Trends in recurrent coronary heart disease after myocardial infarction among US women and men between 2008 and 2017. Circulation 2021;143(7):650–60.
13. Sardu C, Paolisso G, Marfella R. Impact of sex differences in incident and recurrent coronary events and all-cause mortality. J Am Coll Cardiol 2021;77(6):829–30.
14. An J, Zhang Y, Muntner P, et al. Recurrent atherosclerotic cardiovascular event rates differ among patients meeting the very high risk definition according to

age, sex, race/ethnicity, and socioeconomic status. J Am Heart Assoc 2020;9(23): e017310. Available at: https://www.ncbi.nlm.nih.gov/pmc/articles/PMC7763778/. Accessed September 11, 2023.

15. Brown AF, Liang L, Vassar SD, et al. Neighborhood disadvantage and ischemic stroke: The cardiovascular health study (CHS). Stroke 2011;42(12):3363–8.

16. Batchelor W, Kandzari DE, Davis S, et al. Outcomes in women and minorities compared with white men 1 year after everolimus-eluting stent implantation: Insights and results from the PLATINUM diversity and PROMUS element plus post-approval study pooled analysis. JAMA Cardiol 2017;2(12):1303–13.

17. Eberly LA, Yang L, Essien UR, et al. Racial, ethnic, and socioeconomic inequities in glucagon-like peptide-1 receptor agonist use among patients with diabetes in the US. JAMA Health Forum 2021;2(12):e214182. Available at: https://www.ncbi. nlm.nih.gov/pmc/articles/PMC8796881/. Accessed September 25, 2023.

18. Mahtta D, Ramsey DJ, Lee MT, et al. Utilization rates of SGLT2 inhibitors and GLP-1 receptor agonists and their facility-level variation among patients with atherosclerotic cardiovascular disease and type 2 diabetes: Insights from the department of veterans affairs. Diabetes Care 2022;45(2):372–80.

19. ElSayed NA, Aleppo G, Aroda VR, et al. 2. classification and diagnosis of diabetes: Standards of care in diabetes-2023. Diabetes Care 2023;46(Suppl 1): S19–40.

20. Rameshrad M, Razavi BM, Lalau J, et al. An overview of glucagon-like peptide-1 receptor agonists for the treatment of metabolic syndrome: A drug repositioning. Iran J Basic Med Sci 2020;23(5):556–68. Available at: https://www.ncbi.nlm.nih. gov/pmc/articles/PMC7374997/. Accessed July 27, 2023.

21. Marx N, Husain M, Lehrke M, et al. GLP-1 receptor agonists for the reduction of atherosclerotic cardiovascular risk in patients with type 2 diabetes. Circulation 2022;146(24):1882–94.

22. Virani SS, Newby LK, Arnold SV, et al. 2023 AHA/ACC/ACCP/ASPC/NLA/PCNA guideline for the management of patients with Chronic Coronary disease: A report of the american heart association/american college of cardiology joint committee on clinical practice guidelines. J Am Coll Cardiol 2023;S0735–6.

23. Khan MS, Fonarow GC, McGuire DK, et al. Glucagon-like peptide 1 receptor agonists and heart failure: The need for further evidence generation and practice guidelines optimization. Circulation 2020;142(12):1205–18.

24. Ussher JR, Drucker DJ. Cardiovascular biology of the incretin system. Endocr Rev 2012;33(2):187–215. Available at: https://www.ncbi.nlm.nih.gov/pmc/ articles/PMC3528785/. Accessed July 27, 2023.

25. Marso SP, Daniels GH, Brown-Frandsen K, et al. Liraglutide and cardiovascular outcomes in type 2 diabetes. N Engl J Med 2016;375(4):311–22.

26. Marso SP, Bain SC, Consoli A, et al. Semaglutide and cardiovascular outcomes in patients with type 2 diabetes. N Engl J Med 2016;375(19):1834–44.

27. Husain M, Birkenfeld AL, Donsmark M, et al. Oral semaglutide and cardiovascular outcomes in patients with type 2 diabetes. N Engl J Med 2019;381(9):841–51.

28. Gerstein HC, Colhoun HM, Dagenais GR, et al. Dulaglutide and cardiovascular outcomes in type 2 diabetes (REWIND): A double-blind, randomised placebo-controlled trial. Lancet 2019;394(10193):121–30.

29. Sattar N, Lee MMY, Kristensen SL, et al. Cardiovascular, mortality, and kidney outcomes with GLP-1 receptor agonists in patients with type 2 diabetes: A systematic review and meta-analysis of randomised trials. Lancet Diabetes Endocrinol 2021;9(10):653–62.

30. McGuire DK, Pagidipati NJ. GLP1 receptor agonists: From antihyperglycaemic to cardiovascular drugs. Lancet Diabetes Endocrinol 2021;9(10):640–1.
31. Filippatos TD, Panagiotopoulou TV, Elisaf MS. Adverse effects of GLP-1 receptor agonists. Rev Diabet Stud 2014;11(3):202–30. Available at: https://www.ncbi.nlm.nih.gov/pmc/articles/PMC5397288/. Accessed September 28, 2023.
32. 9. pharmacologic approaches to glycemic treatment: Standards of medical care in diabetes-2022. Diabetes Care 2022;45(Suppl 1):S125–43.
33. Shyangdan DS, Royle P, Clar C, et al. Glucagon-like peptide analogues for type 2 diabetes mellitus. Cochrane Database Syst Rev 2011;2011(10):CD006423.
34. Halim MA, Degerblad M, Sundbom M, et al. Glucagon-like peptide-1 inhibits prandial gastrointestinal motility through myenteric neuronal mechanisms in humans. J Clin Endocrinol Metab 2018;103(2):575–85.
35. U.S food & drug administration: Drug safety-related labeling changes (SrLC). Available at: https://www.accessdata.fda.gov/Available at: https://www.accessdata.fda.gov/scripts/cder/safetylabelingchanges/index.cfm?event=searchdetail.page&DrugNameID=2183. Updated 2023. Accessed October 9, 2023.
36. Joshi GP, Abdelmalak BB, Weigel WA, et al. American society of anesthesiologists consensus-based guidance on preoperative management of patients (adults and children) on glucagon-like peptide-1 (GLP-1) receptor agonists. American Society of Anesthesiologists Web site. 2023. https://www.asahq.org/about-asa/newsroom/news-releases/2023/06/american-society-of-anesthesiologists-consensus-based-guidance-on-preoperative. Accessed August 3, 2023.
37. A study of tirzepatide (LY3298176) compared with dulaglutide on major cardiovascular events in participants with type 2 diabetes - full text view - ClinicalTrials.gov. . . https://classic.clinicaltrials.gov/ct2/show/NCT04255433. Accessed August 11, 2023.
38. A study of retatrutide (LY3437943) in participants with obesity and cardiovascular disease - full text view - ClinicalTrials.gov. . . https://classic.clinicaltrials.gov/ct2/show/NCT05882045?term=retatrutide&draw=2&rank=1. Accessed September 28, 2023.
39. A study of daily oral orforglipron (LY3502970) compared with insulin glargine in participants with type 2 diabetes and obesity or overweight at increased cardiovascular risk - tabular view - ClinicalTrials.gov. . . https://classic.clinicaltrials.gov/ct2/show/record/NCT05803421. Accessed September 28, 2023.
40. A study of tirzepatide (LY3298176) in participants with heart failure with preserved ejection fraction and obesity - full text view - ClinicalTrials.gov. . . https://classic.clinicaltrials.gov/ct2/show/NCT04847557. Accessed September 28, 2023.
41. A study of tirzepatide (LY3298176) on the reduction on morbidity and mortality in adults with obesity - full text view - ClinicalTrials.gov. . . https://classic.clinicaltrials.gov/ct2/show/NCT05556512. Accessed September 28, 2023.
42. Table view | REDEFINE 3: A research study to see the effects of CagriSema on heart disease in people living with obesity and diseases in the heart and blood vessels | ClinicalTrials.gov. . . https://clinicaltrials.gov/study/NCT05669755?intr=Cagrilintide%20and%20semaglutide&rank=6&tab=table. Accessed September 28, 2023.
43. McGuire DK, Shih WJ, Cosentino F, et al. Association of SGLT2 inhibitors with cardiovascular and kidney outcomes in patients with type 2 diabetes: A meta-analysis. JAMA Cardiol 2021;6(2):148–58.
44. Packer M, Wilcox CS, Testani JM. Critical analysis of the effects of SGLT2 inhibitors on renal tubular sodium, water and chloride homeostasis and their role in influencing heart failure outcomes | circulation. Circulation 2023;. https://www.

ahajournals.org/doi/full/10.1161/CIRCULATIONAHA.123.064346?af=R. Accessed August 16, 2023.

45. Saucedo-Orozco H, Voorrips SN, Yurista SR, et al. SGLT2 inhibitors and ketone metabolism in heart failure. J Lipid Atheroscler 2022;11(1):1–19. https://www.ncbi.nlm.nih.gov/pmc/articles/PMC8792821/. Accessed October 9, 2023.

46. Marx N, Federici M, Schütt K, et al. 2023 ESC Guidelines for the management of cardiovascular disease in patients with diabetes. Eur Heart J. 2023;44(39):4043-4140.

47. Solomon SD, McMurray JJV, Claggett B, et al. Dapagliflozin in heart failure with mildly reduced or preserved ejection fraction. N Engl J Med 2022;387(12):1089–98.

48. Anker SD, Butler J, Filippatos G, et al. Empagliflozin in heart failure with a preserved ejection fraction. N Engl J Med 2021;385(16):1451–61.

49. Zinman B, Wanner C, Lachin JM, et al. Empagliflozin, cardiovascular outcomes, and mortality in type 2 diabetes. N Engl J Med 2015;373(22):2117–28.

50. Wanner C, Inzucchi SE, Lachin JM, et al. Empagliflozin and progression of kidney disease in type 2 diabetes. N Engl J Med 2016;375(4):323–34.

51. Neal B, Perkovic V, Mahaffey KW, et al. Canagliflozin and cardiovascular and renal events in type 2 diabetes. N Engl J Med 2017;377(7):644–57.

52. Vallianou NG, Christodoulatos GS, Kounatidis D, et al. Sotagliflozin, a dual SGLT1 and SGLT2 inhibitor: In the heart of the problem. Metabol Open 2021;10:100089. https://www.ncbi.nlm.nih.gov/pmc/articles/PMC7989208/. Accessed Oct 9, 2023.

53. Bhatt DL, Szarek M, Pitt B, et al. Sotagliflozin in patients with diabetes and chronic kidney disease. N Engl J Med 2021;384(2):129–39.

54. Zelniker TA, Wiviott SD, Raz I, et al. SGLT2 inhibitors for primary and secondary prevention of cardiovascular and renal outcomes in type 2 diabetes: A systematic review and meta-analysis of cardiovascular outcome trials. Lancet 2019;393(10166):31–9.

55. Cannon CP, Pratley R, Dagogo-Jack S, et al. Cardiovascular outcomes with ertugliflozin in type 2 diabetes. N Engl J Med 2020;383(15):1425–35.

56. Hollander P, Liu J, Hill J, et al. Ertugliflozin compared with glimepiride in patients with type 2 diabetes mellitus inadequately controlled on metformin: The VERTIS SU randomized study. Diabetes Ther 2018;9(1):193–207.

57. Bailey CJ, Gross JL, Hennicken D, et al. Dapagliflozin add-on to metformin in type 2 diabetes inadequately controlled with metformin: A randomized, double-blind, placebo-controlled 102-week trial. BMC Med 2013;11:43.

58. Nyirjesy P, Zhao Y, Ways K, et al. Evaluation of vulvovaginal symptoms and candida colonization in women with type 2 diabetes mellitus treated with canagliflozin, a sodium glucose co-transporter 2 inhibitor. Curr Med Res Opin 2012;28(7):1173–8.

59. Unnikrishnan AG, Kalra S, Purandare V, et al. Genital infections with sodium glucose cotransporter-2 inhibitors: Occurrence and management in patients with type 2 diabetes mellitus. Indian Journal of Endocrinology and Metabolism 2018;22(6):837. Available at: https://journals.lww.com/indjem/fulltext/2018/22060/genital_infections_with_sodium_glucose.22.aspx. Accessed Oct 9, 2023.

60. Prevention and management of genital mycotic infections in the setting of sodium-glucose cotransporter 2 inhibitors - kristin engelhardt, McKenzie ferguson, jennifer L. rosselli, 2021, Available at: https://journals.sagepub.com/doi/full/10.1177/1060028020951928. Accessed Aug 16, 2023.

61. McGovern AP, Hogg M, Shields BM, et al. Risk factors for genital infections in people initiating SGLT2 inhibitors and their impact on discontinuation. BMJ

Open Diabetes Research and Care 2020;8(1):e001238. Available at: https://drc. bmj.com/content/8/1/e001238. Accessed Aug 16, 2023.

62. Dizon S, Keely EJ, Malcolm J, et al. Insights into the recognition and management of SGLT2-inhibitor-associated ketoacidosis: It's not just euglycemic diabetic ketoacidosis. Can J Diabetes 2017;41(5):499–503.

63. FDA drug safety communication: FDA confirms increased risk of leg and foot amputations with the diabetes medicine canagliflozin (invokana, invokamet, invokamet XR). 2017. https://www.fda.gov/media/104870/download#:~:text=%5B5%2D16%2D2017%5D,of%20leg%20and%20foot%20amputations.

64. FDA removes boxed warning about risk of leg and foot amputations for the diabetes medicine canagliflozin (invokana, invokamet, invokamet XR). 2020. https://www.fda.gov/media/104870/download#:~:text=%5B5%2D16%2D2017%5D,of%20leg%20and%20foot%20amputations.

65. Watts NB, Bilezikian JP, Usiskin K, et al. Effects of canagliflozin on fracture risk in patients with type 2 diabetes mellitus. J Clin Endocrinol Metab 2016;101(1): 157–66.

66. Research, Center for Drug Evaluation. FDA drug safety communication: FDA revises label of diabetes drug canagliflozin (invokana, invokamet) to include updates on bone fracture risk and new information on decreased bone mineral density. FDA; 2019. Available at: https://www.fda.gov/drugs/drug-safety-and-availability/fda-drug-safety-communication-fda-revises-label-diabetes-drug-canagliflozin-invokana-invokamet. Accessed August 16, 2023.

67. Research, Center for Drug Evaluation. FDA drug safety communication: FDA revises label of diabetes drug canagliflozin (invokana, invokamet) to include updates on bone fracture risk and new information on decreased bone mineral density. FDA; 2019. Available at: https://www.fda.gov/drugs/drug-safety-and-availability/fda-drug-safety-communication-fda-revises-label-diabetes-drug-canagliflozin-invokana-invokamet. Accessed October 9, 2023.

68. Xu H, Cupples LA, Stokes A, et al. Association of obesity with mortality over 24 years of weight history: Findings from the framingham heart study. JAMA Netw Open 2018;1(7):e184587.

69. Adams KF, Schatzkin A, Harris TB, et al. Overweight, obesity, and mortality in a large prospective cohort of persons 50 to 71 years old. N Engl J Med 2006; 355(8):763–78.

70. Cardiovascular effects of intensive lifestyle intervention in type 2 diabetes. N Engl J Med 2013;369(2):145–54.

71. Sjöström L, Peltonen M, Jacobson P, et al. Bariatric surgery and long-term cardiovascular events. JAMA 2012;307(1):56–65.

72. Hlavin C, Sebastiani RS, Scherer RJ, et al. Barriers to bariatric surgery: A mixed methods study investigating obstacles between clinic contact and surgery. Obes Surg 2023;33(9):2874–83.

73. Brown E, Wilding JPH, Barber TM, et al. Weight loss variability with SGLT2 inhibitors and GLP-1 receptor agonists in type 2 diabetes mellitus and obesity: Mechanistic possibilities. Obes Rev 2019;20(6):816–28.

74. Lincoff AM, Brown-Frandsen K, Colhoun HM, et al. Semaglutide and cardiovascular outcomes in obesity without diabetes. N Engl J Med 2023. https://doi.org/10.1056/NEJMoa2307563.

75. Wilding JPH, Batterham RL, Calanna S, et al. Once-weekly semaglutide in adults with overweight or obesity. N Engl J Med 2021;384(11):989–1002.

ᴐs in evidence-based therapy use in
ᴐ diabetes mellitus and atheroscle-
2021;10(2):e016835.

ᴐn of out-of-pocket costs and
ᴐLP-1 RA in patients with
Netw Open 2023;6(6):

ᴐ use of sodium-glucose co-
ᴐ receptor agonists by cardiol-
J Am Heart Assoc 2022;11(9):

ᴐt al. Use of lipid-, blood pressure-, and
ᴐ patients with type 2 diabetes and athero-
ᴐAMA Netw Open 2022;5(2):e2148030.

ᴐez F. Health disparities across the continuum of
ᴐp 2022;24(9):1129–37.

ᴐya ND, et al. Association of race/ethnicity, gender, and
ᴐwith sodium-glucose cotransporter 2 inhibitor use among
ᴐes in the US. JAMA Netw Open 2021;4(4):e216139.

ᴐlegre JA, Madden E, Tummalapalli SL, et al. Association of race
ᴐwith prescription of SGLT2 inhibitors and GLP1 receptor agonists
ᴐents with type 2 diabetes in the veterans health administration system.
2022;328(9):861–71.

ᴐdipati NJ, Nelson AJ, Kaltenbach LA, et al. Coordinated care to optimize cardiovascular preventive therapies in type 2 diabetes: A randomized clinical trial.
JAMA 2023;329(15):1261–70.

84. ElSayed NA, Aleppo G, Aroda VR, et al. 10. cardiovascular disease and risk management: Standards of care in diabetes-2023. Diabetes Care 2023;46(Suppl 1):
S158–90.

85. Das SR, Everett BM, Birtcher KK, et al. 2020 expert consensus decision pathway
on novel therapies for cardiovascular risk reduction in patients with type 2 diabetes: A report of the american college of cardiology solution set oversight committee. J Am Coll Cardiol 2020;76(9):1117–45.

...JAMA. 2022;328(9):...

...Risk factors for ... prevention ...
JAMA. 2022;328(9):...

... Edwards MA, Fields S, ...
... 158:90 ...

... Davis ..., ...
... level disparities ...
... Arch ... ...
Circulation. ...

Optimal Medical Therapy for Chronic Coronary Disease in 2024: Focus on Antithrombotic Therapy

Parth P. Patel, MD[a], Alexander C. Fanaroff, MD, MHS[b],*

KEYWORDS

- Antithrombotic therapy • Chronic coronary disease • Coronary artery disease

KEY POINTS

- Antiplatelet therapy is indicated for the secondary prevention of recurrent ischemic events in patients with chronic coronary disease.
- Aspirin is the most commonly used antiplatelet agent in this population.
- Clinical trials have evaluated more potent antithrombotic regimens and have generally shown that they reduce ischemic risk but increase bleeding risk compared with aspirin alone.
- Special populations without prior acute coronary syndrome or revascularization— including certain patients with diabetes, chronic kidney disease stage 3b, and/or coronary artery calcium score > 1000—may be at equivalent risk to patients with chronic coronary disease and could be considered candidates for antiplatelet therapy.

INTRODUCTION

Patients with previous myocardial infarction (MI) are at high risk of recurrent MI, stroke, and cardiovascular death, with a 5-year risk of nearly 40%. Although the highest risk period is immediately following an MI, among patients who survive a year after MI, the risk of cardiovascular events remains approximately 5% per year.[1,2] Antiplatelet therapy has been shown in rigorous clinical trials to improve long-term prognosis after MI and limit progression of coronary artery disease (CAD) in patients with chronic coronary disease (CCD), but more than 40% of patients with prior MI are not treated with an

a Department of Medicine, University of Pennsylvania, Philadelphia, PA, USA; b Division of Cardiovascular Medicine, Penn Cardiovascular Outcomes, Quality, and Evaluative Research Center, Leonard Davis Institute for Health Economics, University of Pennsylvania, Philadelphia, PA, USA
* Corresponding author. 3400 Civic Center Boulevard, Perelman Center for Advanced Medicine, South 11-103, Philadelphia, PA 19104.
E-mail address: alexander.fanaroff@pennmedicine.upenn.edu

Med Clin N Am 108 (2024) 489–507
https://doi.org/10.1016/j.mcna.2023.11.004
0025-7125/24/© 2023 Elsevier Inc. All rights reserved.

antiplatelet agent.[3] Because some patients may stop long-term follow-up with a cardiologist in the years after an MI, primary care providers are in a critical position to help improve outcomes for patients with CCD through continued aggressive secondary prevention using antithrombotic therapy.

This review briefly describes the pathophysiology of acute coronary syndromes (ACSs) and the mechanism of action of antiplatelet agents, before covering clinical trials of antithrombotic agents (including antiplatelets and anticoagulants) for the secondary prevention of MI. The authors specifically focus on patients with CCD, which they define (consistent with consensus guidelines) as patients who.

- Have been discharged after ACS or percutaneous coronary intervention (PCI) and stabilized from all acute cardiovascular issues. Consistent with populations enrolled in pivotal trials testing antiplatelet agents, patients with CCD include those who had an ACS greater than 1 year prior or PCI greater than 6 months prior
- Have left ventricular systolic dysfunction and known or suspected CAD
- Have stable angina medically managed with or without positive results on an imaging test
- Have angina symptoms and evidence of coronary vasospasm or microvascular angina
- Have CAD based on the results of an imaging study (ie, stress test or coronary computed tomographic angiography)

The authors conclude with recommendations for long-term management of antithrombotic therapy for secondary prevention, with a focus on counseling and shared decision-making.

Importantly, though recent trials have called into question the risk–benefit trade-off of using antiplatelet therapy for the primary prevention of cardiovascular disease and guidelines no longer recommend the routine use of aspirin for primary prevention, patients with CCD are at substantially higher risk of recurrent cardiovascular events than those without CCD and recommendations regarding the use of antiplatelet therapy for primary prevention do not apply to patients with CCD.

RATIONALE FOR ANTITHROMBOTIC THERAPY IN SECONDARY PREVENTION

CAD is characterized by the development of atherosclerotic plaque in coronary artery endothelium, a process defined by the formation of enlarging plaques driven by macrophage absorption of low-density lipoprotein cholesterol.[4] Ultimately, a mature atherosclerotic plaque is characterized by a lipid-rich core covered by a cap of smooth muscle cells and fibrous tissue. Over time, this plaque can stay stable, grow by continued absorption of LDL by intra-plaque macrophages, or rupture with exposure of the lipid-rich core and subendothelial layer. When plaques rupture, tissue factor is exposed, activating factor Xa, which activates thrombin, which activates platelets via protease-activated receptor 1. Simultaneously, von Willebrand factor and collagen are exposed on the surface of the subendothelial layer, activating platelets via glycoprotein Ia/IIa and Ib. Activated platelets secrete thromboxane A2 and adenosine diphosphate (ADP), which attract more activated platelets. Activated platelets adhere to each other, forming a platelet plug that is stabilized by fibrin to form a thrombus. Rapid thrombus formation leads to an abrupt reduction in coronary blood flow distal to the thrombotic lesion, leading to myocardial ischemia or infarction.[4] Given the centrality of platelet activation and thrombosis to this process, antiplatelet agents (and to a lesser extent, anticoagulants) have been natural targets for reducing recurrent MI.

ASPIRIN

For decades, aspirin has served as the foundation of secondary prevention of CAD.[5] Aspirin is a synthetic derivative of salicylic acid, a compound derived from willow plants and used for medicinal purposes for over thousands of years.[6] In the 1960s, aspirin was found to inhibit platelet aggregation via irreversible inhibition of cyclooxygenase 1 (COX 1). Inhibition of COX1 prevents generation of thromboxane A_2 **(Fig. 1)**, a potent platelet-activating molecule.[7–10]

The first trials showing aspirin's efficacy in secondary prevention were completed in the 1970s **(Table 1)**. In 1974, Cardiff I, a study of 1239 men, demonstrated aspirin 300 mg daily (vs placebo) started within 3 months of index MI led to a 25% relative reduction in 1-year post-MI mortality, though this difference was not statistically significant.[11] In 1979, Cardiff II randomized 1628 patients (15% women) with recent (<21 days) MI to aspirin 300 mg three times daily versus placebo. Compared with placebo, aspirin led to an absolute reduction of the composite of 1-year death and nonfatal MI by 6.5% (14.7 vs 21.2%).[12,13] Although both Cardiff studies enrolled patients shortly after index MI, subsequent studies showed that later initiation of aspirin after MI also reduced adverse post-MI outcomes. In 1980, The Coronary Drug Project Aspirin Study, enrolling 1529 men (of whom three-quarters were enrolled at least 5 years after index MI), demonstrated a decreased risk of mortality with aspirin versus placebo (5.8% vs 8.3%), although the difference was not statistically significant.[14] These trials, along with their contemporaries (AMIS, persantine-aspirin reinfarction study [PARIS], German-Austrian aspirin trial [GAMIS]), had weaknesses, namely inclusion of a demographic of largely young white men, variable time of aspirin initiation after index MI, a higher dose of aspirin (300–1500 mg daily) than used in contemporary practice, small sample size, and a lack of consistent statistically significant results demonstrating decreases in primary outcomes of cardiovascular death necessitating further studies.[15–17]

Ultimately, several meta-analyses solidified aspirin's role in the secondary prevention of CAD.[18–20] The most recent of these three, published in 2022, included 18,788 patients with previous MI enrolled in 12 trials. In these trials, antiplatelet therapy versus placebo reduced the composite of vascular death, nonfatal MI, and nonfatal stroke for patients treated with antiplatelet therapy versus placebo more than 27-month follow-up by 3.5% points. This absolute risk reduction translates to 18 fewer MIs, 14 fewer vascular deaths, and 5 fewer strokes per 1000 patients treated with antiplatelet agents

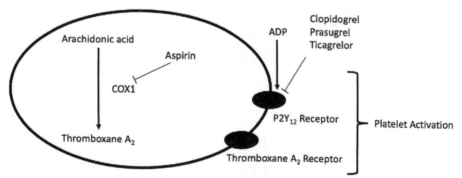

Fig. 1. Mechanism of action of aspirin and P2Y12 inhibitors. Aspirin inhibits cyclooxensase 1 (COX1) preventing the synthesis of thromboxane A2, a potent platelet activator. Clopidogrel, prasugrel, and ticagrelor inhibit the P2Y12 subtype of ADP receptor, preventing it from binding the platelet activator ADP.

Table 1
Major trials studying antithrombotic therapy in chronic coronary disease

Study Name (Year)	Primary Study Question, Comparators, and Outcomes	Patient Population, Study Size	Outcomes and Mean Follow-Up
Aspirin in Secondary Prevention			
Cardiff I (1974)	Does aspirin reduce mortality after MI? *Groups:* 300 mg aspirin daily or placebo *Primary outcome:* Overall mortality	Men physicians who had previous MI at least 3 mo prior (n = 1239)	*Primary outcome:* Aspirin vs placebo (8.3% vs 10.9%) *Median follow-up:* 12 mo
Cardiff II (1979)	Does aspirin reduce mortality after MI? *Groups:* 300 mg aspirin three times daily or placebo *Primary outcome:* Overall mortality *Secondary outcome:* Composite of 1-y death and nonfatal MI	Patients with previous MI (50% with MI ≤ 21 d before enrollment) (n = 1682)	*Primary outcome:* Aspirin vs placebo (12.3% vs 14.8%; *P* > .05) *Secondary outcome:* Aspirin vs placebo (14.7 vs 21.2%; *P* < .05) *Follow-up:* 12 mo
The Coronary Drug Aspirin Project Study (1976)	Does aspirin reduce mortality after MI? *Groups:* 324 mg three times daily or placebo *Primary outcome:* Overall mortality	Men with previous MI (75% had an MI > 5 y before enrollment) (n = 1529)	*Primary outcome:* aspirin vs placebo (5.8% vs 8.3%; *P* > .05) *Mean follow-up:* 22 mo
AMIS (1980)	Does aspirin reduce mortality after MI? *Groups:* 500 mg aspirin twice daily or placebo *Primary outcome:* Overall mortality *Secondary outcome:* Nonfatal MI	Patients with MI in the prior 8 wk to 60 mo (n = 4524)	*Primary outcome:* aspirin vs placebo (9.6% vs 8.8%; *P* > .05) *Secondary outcome:* Aspirin vs placebo (6.3% vs 8.1%; *P* < .05) *Follow-up:* 36 mo
PARIS (1980)	Does aspirin reduce coronary events and MI after previous MI? *Groups:* 324 mg aspirin daily with dipyridamole 75 mg three times daily, 324 mg aspirin three times daily, or placebo *Primary outcome:* all-cause mortality, coronary death, and total coronary events	Patients with MI in the prior 8 wk to 60 mo (n = 2026)	*Primary outcome:* dipyridamole plus aspirin vs aspirin alone vs placebo (10.7% vs 10.5% vs 12.8%; *P* > .05) *Mean follow-up:* 41 mo

GAMIS (1980)	Does aspirin reduce coronary death after MI? *Groups:* 1500 mg daily or placebo *Primary outcome:* coronary death	Patients with MI in the 30–42 d prior (n = 946)	*Primary outcome:* aspirin vs placebo (12% vs 22%; P > .05)
ADAPTABLE (2021)	Is 81 mg of aspirin non-inferior to 325 mg of aspirin in secondary prevention? *Groups:* 81 mg daily or 325 mg aspirin daily *Primary outcome:* Composite of all-cause death, MI, or stroke at 12 mo *Safety outcome:* Occurrence of major bleeding requiring blood transfusion at 12 mo	Patients with prior MI, prior coronary revascularization, prior coronary angiogram with ≥ 75% coronary stenosis, history of chronic ischemic heart disease, or CAD (n = 15,076)	*Primary outcome:* 7.3% vs 7.5%, 81 mg vs 325 mg (P=.75) *Safety outcome:* 0.6% vs 0.6%, 81 mg vs 325 mg (P=.41) *Median follow-up:* 26 mo
Long-term dual antiplatelet therapy			
CHARISMA (2006)	Is clopidogrel plus aspirin (DAPT) more effective than aspirin alone in long-term secondary prevention? *Groups:* clopidogrel 75 mg daily plus aspirin vs aspirin alone Aspirin dose: 75–162 mg daily *Primary outcome:* Composite of CV death, MI, stroke *Safety outcome:* Severe bleeding (GUSTO definition)	One of the following: • Previous documented CVD disease • Two major, three minor, or one major, and two minor risk factors Major: diabetes, ABI < 0.9, asymptomatic carotid stenosis ≥ 70%, ≥ 1 carotid plaque Minor: SBP ≥ 150 mm Hg despite 3 mo of therapy, primary hypercholesterolemia, current smoking > 15 cigarettes/day, male ≥ 65, female ≥ 70 (n = 15,603)	*Primary outcome:* Clopidogrel plus aspirin vs aspirin alone (6.8% vs 7.3%; P = .22) *Safety outcome:* Clopidogrel plus aspirin: (1.7% vs 1.3%; P=.09) *Median follow-up:* 27 mo

(continued on next page)

Table 1
(continued)

Study Name (Year)	Primary Study Question, Comparators, and Outcomes	Patient Population, Study Size	Outcomes and Mean Follow-Up
PRODIGY (2012)	Is short-term DAPT as effective as long-term DAPT after PCI? *Groups:* Short duration DAPT (6 mo) or longer DAPT (24 mo). Clopidogrel dose: 75 mg daily Aspirin dose: 80–160 mg daily *Primary outcome:* Composite of death, MI, CVA *Safety outcome:* BARC type II, III, V bleeding	Patients who received a PCI with a stent ≤ 30 d before enrollment (n = 1970)	*Primary outcome:* Short vs long-term DAPT (10.0% vs 10.1%; P=.91) *Safety outcome:* Short vs long-term DAPT (3.5% vs 7.4%; P < .001) *Follow-up:* 24 mo
DES-LATE (2014)	Is short-term DAPT as effective as long-term DAPT after PCI? *Groups:* clopidogrel 75 mg daily with aspirin vs aspirin alone Aspirin dose: 100–200 mg daily *Primary outcome:* composite of CV death, MI, stroke *Safety outcome:* TIMI major bleeding	Patients with a drug eluting stent placed ≥ 12 mo before enrollment (n = 5045)	*Primary outcome:* DAPT vs aspirin (4.4% vs 5.1%; P > .05) *Safety outcome:* DAPT vs aspirin (1.4% vs 1.1%; P=.20) *Mean follow-up:* 42 mo
DAPT (2014)	Is 30 mo of DAPT after PCI safer and more effective than 12 mo? *Groups:* DAPT for 30 mo after PCI (65% clopidogrel 70 mg daily, 35% prasugrel 10 mg daily) vs DAPT for 12 mo plus aspirin and placebo after the initial 12 mo Aspirin dose: 75–162 mg daily	Patients with PCI 12 mo prior, no contraindication to DAPT, who were free of death, MI, stroke, repeat coronary revascularization, major bleeding, stent thrombosis and were compliant with DAPT over the 12 mo following PCI (n = 9961)	*Primary outcome:* 30 mo of DAPT vs placebo arm (4.3 vs 5.9%; P < .001) *Safety outcome:* 30 mo of DAPT vs placebo arm (2.5% vs 1.6%; P=.001) *Follow-up:* 30 mo

	Primary outcome: Major adverse cardiovascular and cerebrovascular events at 30 mo from index procedure *Safety outcome:* Moderate or severe GUSTO bleeding at 30 mo from index procedure		
PEGASUS (2015)	Is ticagrelor-based DAPT safer and more effective than aspirin alone in patients with MI > 1 y prior? *Groups:* DAPT with ticagrelor 90 mg twice daily, DAPT with ticagrelor 60 mg daily, or aspirin alone Aspirin dose: 75–150 mg daily *Primary outcome:* composite of CV death, MI, or stroke *Safety outcome:* TIMI major bleeding	Patients with a previous MI (1–3 y prior) (n = 21,162)	*Primary outcome:* ticagrelor 90 mg vs ticagrelor 60 mg vs aspirin alone (7.8% vs 7.9% vs 9.0%) Ticagrelor 90 vs aspirin (P=.008) Ticagrelor 60 vs aspirin (P=.004) *Safety outcome:* Ticagrelor 90 mg vs ticagrelor 60 mg vs aspirin (2.6% vs 2.3% vs 1.1%) Both groups vs placebo (P < .001) *Median follow-up:* 33 mo
THEMIS (2019)	Is ticagrelor-based DAPT safer and more effective than aspirin alone in patients with CCD and diabetes without a history of MI? *Groups:* DAPT with ticagrelor twice daily (90 mg twice daily transitioned to 60 mg mid-trial) vs aspirin alone Aspirin dose: 75–150 mg *Primary outcome:* composite of CV	Patients with CCD and T2DM; patients with previous MI or stroke were excluded (n = 19,920)	*Primary outcome:* Ticagrelor vs placebo (7.7% vs 8.5%; P=.04) *Safety outcome:* Ticagrelor vs placebo (2.2% vs 1.0%; P < .001) *Median follow-up:* 40 mo

(continued on next page)

Table 1
(continued)

Study Name (Year)	Primary Study Question, Comparators, and Outcomes	Patient Population, Study Size	Outcomes and Mean Follow-Up
	death, MI, or stroke *Safety outcome:* TIMI major bleeding		
Long-term single antiplatelet therapy			
CAPRIE (1996)	Is clopidogrel safer and more effective than aspirin in secondary prevention? *Groups:* clopidogrel 75 mg daily vs aspirin 325 mg daily *Primary outcome:* Composite of ischemic stroke, MI, or vascular death	Patients with prior ischemic stroke, MI, or symptomatic PAD (*n* = 19,185)	*Primary outcome:* Clopidogrel vs aspirin (5.3% vs 5.8%; *P* = .043) *Median follow-up:* 23 mo
HOST-EXAM (2023)	Is clopidogrel safer and more effective than aspirin in secondary prevention? *Groups:* clopidogrel 75 mg daily vs aspirin 100 mg daily *Primary outcome:* Composite of cardiac death, MI, ischemic stroke, readmission due to	Patients who had previous PCI and completed DAPT for 12 ± 6 mo after PCI (*n* = 5438)	*Primary outcome:* Clopidogrel vs aspirin (7.9% vs 11.9%; *P* < .001) *Safety outcome:* Clopidogrel vs aspirin (4.5% vs 6.1%; *P*=.016) *Follow-up:* 69 mo

ACS, and stent thrombosis
Safety outcome:
BARC type 2 or greater bleeding

Dual pathway inhibition using anticoagulation and antiplatelet regimens

OAC ALONE (2018)	Is anticoagulation alone as effective as anticoagulation plus aspirin for in patients with AF and CCD? *Groups:* OAC with antiplatelet therapy vs OAC alone *OACs:* dabigatran (110 or 150 mg twice daily), rivaroxaban (10 or 15 mg once daily), apixaban (2.5 or 5 mg twice daily), and edoxaban (30 or 60 mg once daily) *Antiplatelets:* aspirin (81–324 mg/day) or clopidogrel (75 mg/day) *Primary Outcome:* Composite of all-cause mortality, MI, stroke, and systemic embolism *Safety outcome:* Major bleeding (ISTH criteria)	Patients with AF who underwent PCI > 12 mo before enrollment (*n* = 696; terminated due to slow enrollment)	*Primary outcome:* Combination therapy vs OAC alone (13.6% vs 15.7%; *P*=.20) *Safety outcome* Combination therapy vs OAC alone (10.4% vs 7.8%; *P*=.22) *Follow-up:* 30 mo
AFIRE (2019)	Is anticoagulation alone as effective as anticoagulation plus aspirin for in patients with AF and CCD? *Groups:* rivaroxaban monotherapy vs rivaroxaban and antiplatelet therapy Rivaroxaban dose: 15 mg daily (10 mg daily for Cr clearance < 50) once daily Antiplatelet: 70% aspirin, 27% P2Y12 inhibitor *Primary outcome:* Composite of stroke, systemic embolism, MI, unstable angina requiring revascularization, and	Patients with known atrial fibrillation and CCD (no PCI or CABG in last year before enrollment) (*n* = 2236)	*Primary outcome:* Rivaroxaban alone vs combination therapy (4.1%/patient-year vs 5.8%/patient-year; *P* < .0001) *Safety outcome:* Rivaroxaban alone vs combination therapy (1.6%/patient-year vs 2.8%/patient-year; *P*=.01) *Follow-up:* 24 mo

(continued on next page)

Table 1
(continued)

Study Name (Year)	Primary Study Question, Comparators, and Outcomes	Patient Population, Study Size	Outcomes and Mean Follow-Up
	death from any cause *Safety outcome:* Major bleeding (ISTH criteria)		
COMPASS (2020)	Does adding very-low dose rivaroxaban to aspirin or replacing aspirin with very-low dose rivaroxaban improve outcomes in patients with CCD? *Groups:* rivaroxaban 2.5 mg twice daily plus aspirin 100 mg daily vs rivaroxaban 2.5 mg twice daily vs aspirin 100 mg daily *Primary outcome:* Composite of CV death, stroke, MI, and fatal bleeding *Safety outcome:* Major Bleeding (ISTH criteria)	Patients with stable atherosclerosis who have a history of CAD or PAD (n = 27,395)	*Primary outcome:* Rivaroxaban plus aspirin vs rivaroxaban alone vs aspirin alone (4.1% vs 4.9% vs 5.4%; combination therapy vs aspirin alone: P < .001; rivaroxaban alone vs aspirin alone: P=.12) *Safety outcome:* Rivaroxaban plus aspirin vs rivaroxaban alone vs aspirin alone (3.1% vs 2.8% vs 1.9%; P < .001 for both rivaroxaban groups compared with aspirin Mean follow-up: 23 mo

Abbreviation: ABI, ankle-brachial index; BARC, bleeding academic research consortium; GUSTO, global use of streptokinase and t-PA for occluded coronary arteries; ISTH, International Society on Thrombosis and Haemostasis; OAC, oral anticoagulation; SBP, systolic blood pressure; TIMI, thromblysis in myocardial infarction.

versus placebo. Treatment with antiplatelet therapy was associated with an increase of three major bleeds per 1000 patients treated. In an indirect comparison, the meta-analysis compared the effect on vascular events of various doses of aspirin versus placebo, finding that the risk reduction versus placebo was similar when aspirin dose was 500 to 1500 mg daily, 160 to 325 mg daily, and 75 to 160 mg daily.[20]

Given the paucity of strong evidence favoring one dose of aspirin over another, the ADAPTABLE trial studied optimal aspirin dosing. ADAPTABLE randomized 15,076 patients with established atherosclerotic cardiovascular disease to 81 mg versus 325 mg aspirin daily and found that the rate of the composite of death, hospitalization for MI, and hospitalization for stroke was similar between groups (7.3% vs 7.5% for 81 vs 325 mg).[21] Although the bleeding risk was similar for patients randomized to high-dose versus low-dose aspirin in ADAPTABLE, previous trials and meta-analyses have noted significantly increased bleeding risk with a higher dose of aspirin.[22] Together, these results indicate that low-dose aspirin is just as effective as high-dose aspirin to prevent ischemic events while potentially being safer.

P2Y12 INHIBITORS

Although aspirin reduced the risk of recurrent ischemic events in the trials discussed above, residual risk among aspirin-treated patients was far from eliminated. ADP is another potent stimulant of platelet aggregation, and the P2Y12 inhibitors were developed to inhibit ADP-induced platelet activation.[23,24] P2Y12 inhibitors work by binding to and inhibiting the P2Y12 subtype of the ADP receptor, preventing ADP-induced platelet aggregation and fibrin cross-linking. The second-generation P2Y12 inhibitor, clopidogrel, is a prodrug that must be metabolized by the cytochrome P450 system before irreversibly binding and inhibiting the P2Y12 receptor. Metabolism is relatively slow, and onset of full antiplatelet effect takes greater than 2 hours. Moreover, up to 14% of patients are poor clopidogrel metabolizers, and clopidogrel is less effective in these individuals. For these reasons, the third-generation P2Y12 inhibitors prasugrel and ticagrelor were developed. Like clopidogrel, prasugrel is a prodrug that is metabolized into an active metabolite that irreversibly binds the P2Y12 receptor; unlike clopidogrel, metabolism of prasugrel into its active metabolite is rapid and there are no known poor metabolizers of prasugrel. Owing to the increased risk of bleeding, prasugrel is not recommended in patients greater than 75 year old or with a prior stroke. By contrast, ticagrelor reversibly binds to and allosterically inhibits the P2Y12 receptor. Unlike prasugrel and clopidogrel, ticagrelor must be taken twice daily and causes dyspnea in some patients. In addition, ticagrelor has a quicker offset of action. Given this and its reversible binding, any missed doses of ticagrelor have a higher risk of leaving patients unprotected compared with clopidogrel and prasugrel.

Dual Antiplatelet Therapy

In 2006, the first major trial testing the efficacy of long-term dual antiplatelet therapy (DAPT) for secondary prevention was CHARISMA. CHARISMA enrolled 15,603 patients with established atherosclerotic vascular disease (prior MI, prior stroke, or symptomatic peripheral artery disease) or multiple vascular risk factors; 78% of trial participants had established vascular disease.[25] Participants were randomized to DAPT (aspirin plus clopidogrel) versus aspirin alone and followed for a median of 28 months. There was no difference between groups in the primary composite endpoint of vascular death, nonfatal MI, and nonfatal stroke (6.8 vs 7.3%; relative risk [RR] 0.93, 95% CI 0.83–1.05), though DAPT reduced a secondary composite endpoint of death, MI, stroke, or hospitalization for ischemic events (16.7 vs 17.9%; RR 0.92, 95% CI 0.82–1.00). Moreover, in the subpopulation of patients with established atherosclerotic cardiovascular disease (ASCVD), DAPT reduced the primary composite outcome (6.9 vs 7.9%; RR 0.88, 95% CI 0.77–1.00). DAPT increased moderate and severe bleeding compared with aspirin alone.

In contrast to CHARISMA, PEGASUS enrolled a population of patients who all had prior MI. PEGASUS randomized 21,162 patients with MI 1 to 3 years before to ticagrelor 60 mg twice daily, ticagrelor 90 mg twice daily, or placebo; all were taking aspirin. Over 3-year follow-up, both ticagrelor doses reduced the rate of the composite of cardiovascular death, MI, or stroke (7.8% for 60 mg vs 7.9% for 90 mg vs 9.0% for placebo; hazard ratio [HR] 0.85, 95% CI 0.75 to 0.96 for 90 mg vs placebo; HR 0.84, 95% CI 0.74 to 0.95 for 60 mg vs placebo); however, both doses also increased the risk of major bleeding (2.3% for 60 mg vs 2.6% for 90 mg vs 1.1% for placebo, $P < .001$).[26] Later, the THEMIS trial tested ticagrelor-based DAPT in patients with diabetes and established CCD without a history of MI (60% with prior PCI, 29% with prior coronary artery bypass grafting surgery).[27] THEMIS randomized 19,220 patients who were taking aspirin to placebo versus ticagrelor 90 mg twice daily (subsequently switched to 60 mg twice daily once the results of PEGASUS were published) and followed them for a median of 39.9 months. Patients randomized to ticagrelor had a lower incidence of the composite of cardiovascular death, MI, and stroke (7.7 vs 8.5%; HR 0.90, 95% CI 0.81–0.99) but a higher incidence of major bleeding (2.2 vs 1.0%; HR 2.32, 95% CI 1.82–2.94).

Other trials have evaluated prolonged DAPT after PCI. The DAPT trial enrolled 9661 patients who had tolerated clopidogrel- or prasugrel-based DAPT for 12 months after PCI (65% clopidogrel, 35% prasugrel) and randomized them either to continue their P2Y12 inhibitor or to placebo (plus open-label aspirin) for an additional 18 months. Patients randomized to continue P2Y12 inhibitors had significantly lower rates of stent thrombosis (0.4% vs 1.4%; HR 0.29, 95% CI 0.17–0.48) and the composite of death, MI, or stroke (4.3% vs 5.9%; HR 0.71, 95% CI 0.59–0.85).[28] The incidence of moderate or severe bleeding was higher in the DAPT group (2.5 vs 1.6%; HR 1.61, 95% CI 1.21–2.16).

Other studies examining longer term DAPT have failed to find a clinical benefit. In the PRODIGY study, 1970 patients undergoing PCI were randomized to DAPT with aspirin and clopidogrel for 24 months or DAPT for 6 months followed by indefinite single antiplatelet therapy with aspirin. At 2-year follow-up, the incidence of the composite of death, MI, and stroke was similar between the arms and the 24-month DAPT arm had higher risk of clinically relevant bleeding (7.4 vs 3.5%, $P=.00018$).[29] Similarly, the DES-LATE trial, which enrolled 5045 Korean patients who had undergone PCI to clopidogrel-based DAPT versus aspirin alone at a median of 13.3 months after their procedure, found no difference in the incidence of the composite of cardiovascular death, MI, and stroke between arms at 2- and 4-year follow-up.[30] Other, more recent trials, have tested even shorter durations of DAPT following PCI and have generally shown that shorter durations do not significantly increase the risk of ischemic events while decreasing bleeding events.[31–33] However, these trials have been powered to detect a difference between groups in the incidence of clinically relevant bleeding events, which are more common than ischemic events, and cannot supersede larger trials intended to evaluate the effect of longer term DAPT on ischemic events.

P2Y12 Inhibitor Monotherapy

In addition to trials evaluating DAPT versus aspirin, two major trials have evaluated clopidogrel monotherapy versus aspirin. The first of these trials, CAPRIE, randomized 19,185 patients with significant vascular disease to clopidogrel versus aspirin, with mean follow-up of 1.9 years. Compared with aspirin, clopidogrel reduced the RR of ischemic stroke, MI, or vascular death by 8.7% (5.3 vs 5.8%, P=.04); the rates of any bleeding, severe bleeding, and intracranial hemorrhage were the same in patients randomized to aspirin and clopidogrel.[34] Although this trial tested the long-term use of clopidogrel monotherapy versus aspirin, modern patients who meet CAPRIE's CAD inclusion criteria (MI within 35 days of enrollment) would be treated with DAPT, which makes CAPRIE difficult to interpret in the modern context.

More recently, the HOST-EXAM trial again suggested the superiority of clopidogrel versus aspirin for secondary prevention. HOST-EXAM randomized 5438 Korean patients who had completed 6 to 18 months of DAPT after PCI to continue either aspirin or clopidogrel monotherapy. Over a median 5.8 year follow-up, patients randomized to clopidogrel had a lower incidence of the composite of cardiac death, MI, ischemic stroke, readmission due to ACS, and stent thrombosis (7.9 vs 11.9%, HR 0.66, 95% CI 0.55–0.79) and a lower incidence of clinically relevant bleeding (4.5 vs 6.1%, HR 0.74, 95% CI 0.57–0.94).[35] Although this study must be interpreted with caution as it enrolled an entirely east Asian population, the finding of clopidogrel's superiority versus aspirin for both ischemic and bleeding outcomes is consistent with the results of CAPRIE. Together, CAPRIE and HOST-EXAM provide compelling evidence for use of clopidogrel over aspirin for secondary prevention of recurrent ischemic events, though more evidence from diverse, contemporary populations is necessary. Additional studies are also need to demonstrate the benefit of clopidogrel in broader populations of patients with CCD, as CAPRIE primarily included a subgroup of patients with recent MI and HOST-EXAM specifically evaluated patients who tolerated DAPT after PCI.

ANTICOAGULANTS
Vascular-Dose Rivaroxaban

The involvement of both platelets and the coagulation cascade in coronary thrombosis, the role of thrombin as a potent platelet activator, and the advent of safe and effective Factor Xa inhibitors led to the idea of dual pathway inhibition or the use of antiplatelet and anticoagulant drugs together to reduce thrombosis.[36] In patients with CCD, dual pathway inhibition was tested in the COMPASS trial, which randomized 27,395 high-risk patients with CCD to either aspirin, very low-dose rivaroxaban (2.5 mg twice daily), or aspirin plus very low-dose rivaroxaban. Median follow-up was 23 months. COMPASS included patients with CCD plus either age $\geq$ 65 years, evidence of vascular disease affecting more than one territory, or $\geq$ 2 additional risk factors (current smoking, diabetes mellitus, chronic kidney disease [CKD], heart failure, or prior ischemic stroke). Dual pathway inhibition with aspirin plus rivaroxaban reduced the incidence of the composite of cardiovascular death, stroke, and MI compared with aspirin (4.1 vs 5.4%; HR 0.76, 95% CI 0.66–0.86); there was no significant difference in the rate of ischemic events between patients randomized to dual pathway inhibition and rivaroxaban alone (4.9 vs 5.4%, HR 0.90, 95% CI 0.79–1.03). Major bleeding occurred in 3.1% of patients randomized to rivaroxaban plus aspirin, 2.8% of patients randomized to rivaroxaban alone, and 1.9% of patients randomized to aspirin alone.[37]

Adding Aspirin to Anticoagulation in Patients with Atrial Fibrillation and Chronic Coronary Disease

Patients with atrial fibrillation (AF) and CCD represent a unique population with indications for both full-dose anticoagulation and antiplatelet therapy, as well as high risk for both ischemic and bleeding events.[38] Multiple trials have established that the combination of a direct oral anticoagulant (DOAC) plus a P2Y12 inhibitor offers the best balance of protection from coronary and cerebrovascular ischemic events among patients with recent ACS or PCI, but the risk–benefit trade-off is different in patients with CCD.[39,40]

The AFIRE trial enrolled 2236 Japanese patients with AF who had PCI or CABG greater than 1 year prior or angiographically documented CAD. Patients were randomized to either anticoagulation-dose rivaroxaban alone or anticoagulation-dose rivaroxaban plus a single antiplatelet agent (70% aspirin, 27% P2Y12 inhibitor) and median follow-up was 24 months. The trial was stopped early due to a higher rate of all-cause death in the rivaroxaban plus antiplatelet therapy arm. Ultimately, rivaroxaban alone was found to be non-inferior to combination therapy for the prevention of the composite of stroke, systemic embolism, MI, unstable angina requiring revascularization, and all-cause death (4.1 vs 5.8% per patient-year; HR 0.72, 95% CI 0.55–0.95), and superior for the incidence of major bleeding (1.6 vs 2.8% per patient-year; HR 0.59, 95% CI 0.39–0.89).[41]

Although the AFIRE study provides compelling evidence for the safety and efficacy of DOAC monotherapy for management of CCD in patients with concomitant AF and this clinical evidence is supported by in vitro evidence of the factor Xa inhibitors' antiplatelet effects, questions remain. AFIRE enrolled exclusively East Asian patients, and the anticoagulation dose used in the trial (15 mg daily) is lower than the approved dose in the United States (20 mg daily).

TRANSLATING EVIDENCE TO CLINICAL PRACTICE
Individualized Patient Decisions: Weighing Ischemic Versus Bleeding Risk

As a general rule, increasing potency or duration of antithrombotic therapy will increase the risk of bleeding while decreasing the risk of major ischemic events.[42] Individual bleeding and ischemic events may be of varying severity, but a major bleeding event has approximately the same effect on quality of life as a recurrent MI, and a clinically relevant non-major bleeding event has approximately half the effect on quality of life as a recurrent MI.[43,44] Some analyses have combined bleeding and ischemic events into one composite "net clinical benefit" endpoint, but this may not reflect the priorities of individual patients, nor does it reflect the idea that some patients may be at higher bleeding risk and lower ischemic risk, or vice versa. Optimal decision-making with respect to antithrombotic therapy for secondary prevention in CCD requires that clinicians weigh a patient's individualized risk of bleeding and ischemic events, and integrate this information with patients' preferences to arrive at a treatment plan through a shared decision-making process.

One option for quantitatively assessing a patient's risk of ischemic and bleeding events among patients with a prior stent is the DAPT score. The DAPT score includes age (0 points for < 65, −1 for 65–74, and −2 for ≥ 75), cigarette smoking in the year before PCI (+1), MI as the indication for recent PCI (+1), diabetes mellitus (+1), prior MI or PCI (+1), use of a second-generation paclitaxel-eluting stent (+1), stent diameter less than 3 mm (+1), heart failure or left ventricular ejection fraction (LVEF) less than 30% (+2), and vein graft PCI (+2). The points are summed to arrive at a DAPT score; a score of less than 2 is associated with greater harm than benefit of continued DAPT beyond 12 months, and a score of ≥ 2 is associated with more benefit than harm.[45] Clinicians can use scores like the DAPT score to individualize antithrombotic treatment plans, integrating the score with clinical judgment and patient preferences. Although there are not similar scores for replacing aspirin with a P2Y12 inhibitor or adding low-dose rivaroxaban to aspirin for dual pathway inhibition, similar principles apply: Older patients, those with a history of bleeding, and those with fewer risk factors for recurrent ischemic events may derive less benefit and more harm from more potent antithrombotic therapy, whereas younger patients and those with more vascular risk factors may derive more benefit and less harm.

In addition, given that patients with coronary stents have an added layer of complexity dependent on the types and locations of stents implanted, PCPs should not hesitate to consult interventional cardiologists for assistance with managing antithrombotic therapy in this population.

Expanding the Definition of Secondary Prevention

Although the trials discussed above largely focused on patients with either prior MI, prior PCI, or other established vascular disease, some patient populations may have risk of recurrent cardiovascular events similar to patients with CCD: those with extensive coronary calcium on noninvasive imaging, those with diabetes and multiple other risk factors, and those with CKD and multiple other risk factors.

Coronary calcification identified on cross-sectional imaging is a marker of coronary atherosclerosis. In a study of 6814 patients, those with no prior ASCVD events but coronary artery calcium (CAC) score greater than 1000 were found to have a risk of the composite of cardiovascular death, nonfatal MI, and nonfatal stroke that was similar to the risk of high-risk patients enrolled in contemporary secondary prevention trials.[46] Similarly, patients with diabetes plus ≥2 major vascular risk factors (age > 65 years in men or > 55 years in women, hypertension, smoking, low high-density lipoprotein cholesterol, family history of premature ASCVD events, ankle-brachial index < 0.9, elevated lipoprotein(a), high-sensitivity C-reactive protein greater than 2, CAC score greater than 100) have a risk of future ischemic events comparable to true secondary prevention patients.[47] Likewise, patients with at least CKD stage 3b and ≥2 major risk factors have a similarly high risk,[48,49] and patients with both diabetes and CKD are at extreme risk (>30% 10-year risk).[47]

Higher risk in patients with CAC greater than 1000, diabetes and CKD, or diabetes or CKD with major vascular risk factors indicates that the risk–benefit ratio for antithrombotic therapies in these patients favors antithrombotic treatment more than it does in traditional primary prevention patients. As such, after shared decision-making, antithrombotic therapy may be considered in these very high-risk primary prevention populations just as it would be in true secondary prevention populations.

GUIDELINE RECOMMENDATIONS

The 2023 American College of Cardiology (ACC)/American Heart Association (AHA) guidelines for the management of CCD make specific recommendations regarding antithrombotic therapy.[50] The guidelines strongly recommend (class I, level of evidence [LOE] A) low-dose aspirin (75–100 mg) to reduce atherosclerotic events in all patients with CCD and no indication for anticoagulation. Consistent with the DAPT and PEGASUS trials, they give a weaker recommendation (class 2b, LOE A) in favor of continuing DAPT beyond 12 months and up to 3 years in patients with previous MI and low bleeding risk, and recommend against (class 3, LOE A) DAPT in patients without recent ACS or a PCI-related indication for DAPT (consistent with CHARISMA). For patients with CCD and an indication for anticoagulation, the guidelines recommend (class 2b, LOE B-R) considering discontinuation of aspirin therapy and continuation of DOAC in patients who had PCI or ACS greater than 1 year before to reduce bleeding risk based on the AFIRE trial. Last, the guidelines indicate that it is reasonable (class 2a, LOE B-R) to add low-dose rivaroxaban 2.5 mg twice daily to aspirin in patients with high risk of recurrent ischemic events and low-to-moderate bleeding risk, as in the COMPASS trial.

The 2021 European Society of Cardiology guidelines for management of CCD similarly recommend (class I, LOE A) low-dose aspirin in patients with previous MI or PCI and indicate that low-dose aspirin may be considered (class IIb, LOE C) in patients without prior MI or PCI but definitive evidence of CAD on imaging.[51] They note that clopidogrel 75 mg daily is recommended in patients with aspirin intolerance (class I, LOE B) and, unlike the ACC/AHA guidelines, state that clopidogrel may be considered in preference to aspirin in patients with CCD and peripheral artery disease, prior stroke, or prior transient ischemic attack (class IIb, LOE B). They indicate that adding a second antithrombotic drug to aspirin (including clopidogrel 75 mg daily, prasugrel 10 mg daily, ticagrelor 60 mg twice daily, or rivaroxaban 2.5 mg twice daily) should be considered (class IIa, LOE A) for long-term secondary prevention in patients at high risk of ischemic events without high bleeding risk and may be considered (class IIb, LOE A) in patients at moderately increased risk of ischemic events without high bleeding risk. For patients with AF and CCD, the European Society of Cardiology (ESC) guidelines indicate that DOACs should be used for anticoagulation (class I, LOE A) and that aspirin may be considered in addition to a DOAC in patients with a history of MI and high risk of recurrent ischemic events without high bleeding risk.

SUMMARY

In this contemporary review, the authors highlight the importance of antithrombotic therapy in secondary prevention of CCD. Major trials established the benefit of antiplatelet therapy in patients with CCD, and consensus guidelines strongly recommend low-dose aspirin for all patients with CCD and no indication for anticoagulation. The evidence for more potent antiplatelet therapy (including prolonged DAPT or dual pathway inhibition with aspirin plus very low-dose rivaroxaban) is mixed, with some trials demonstrating a reduction in ischemic events with more potent antithrombotic therapy in patients at particularly high risk for vascular events but higher risk of bleeding events. Both bleeding and ischemic events are of importance to patients, and antithrombotic therapy must be individualized to each patient, taking into account that patient's bleeding risk, ischemic risk, and personal preferences. Other strategies, including the use of P2Y12 inhibitor monotherapy instead of aspirin, show promise, but more evidence is needed.

CLINICS CARE POINTS

- Aspirin is a first-line antithrombotic therapy for secondary prevention in chronic coronary disease (CCD), but clopidogrel monotherapy may reduce ischemic events with similar risk of bleeding.
- Low-dose aspirin (75–100 mg daily) should be used in preference to higher dose aspirin.
- Dual antiplatelet therapy (DAPT) and dual pathway inhibition with very low-dose rivaroxaban reduce ischemic risk in patients with CCD but increase bleeding risk.
- The DAPT score uncouples ischemic and bleeding risk, helping clinicians with shared decision-making with patients about secondary prevention using antithrombotic therapy
- Certain patient populations without a prior coronary event have exceptionally high risks of future coronary events, equivalent to those with CCD. These populations include patients with diabetes or chronic kidney disease stage 3b with major risk factors or patients with coronary artery calcium greater than 1000. Clinicians should consider treating these patients as if they have CCD.

DISCLOSURE

The authors report no disclosures relevant to the content of this manuscript.

REFERENCES

1. Li S, Peng Y, Wang X, et al. Cardiovascular events and death after myocardial infarction or ischemic stroke in an older Medicare population. Clin Cardiol 2019;42(3): 391–9.
2. Jernberg T, Hasvold P, Henriksson M, et al. Cardiovascular risk in post-myocardial infarction patients: nationwide real world data demonstrate the importance of a long-term perspective. Eur Heart J 2015;36(19):1163–70.
3. Aggarwal R, Chiu N, Pankayatselvan V, et al. Prevalence of angina and use of medical therapy among US adults: A nationally representative estimate. Am Heart J 2020;228:44–6.
4. Libby P, Theroux P. Pathophysiology of Coronary Artery Disease. Circulation 2005;111(25):3481–8.
5. Fihn SD, Gardin JM, Abrams J, et al. ACCF/AHA/ACP/AATS/PCNA/SCAI/STS Guideline for the Diagnosis and Management of Patients With Stable Ischemic Heart Disease: A Report of the American College of Cardiology Foundation/American Heart Association Task Force on Practice Guidelines, and the American College of Physicians, American Association for Thoracic Surgery, Preventive Cardiovascular Nurses Association, Society for Cardiovascular Angiography and Interventions, and Society of Thoracic Surgeons. Circulation 2012;126(25). https://doi.org/10.1161/CIR.0b013e318277d6a0.
6. Rezabakhsh A, Mahmoodpoor A, Soleimanpour H. Historical perspective of aspirin: A journey from discovery to clinical practice Ancient and modern history. J Cardiovasc Thorac Res 2021;13(2):179–80.
7. Hemler M, Lands WE. Purification of the cyclooxygenase that forms prostaglandins. Demonstration of two forms of iron in the holoenzyme. J Biol Chem 1976; 251(18):5575–9.
8. DeWitt DL, el-Harith EA, Kraemer SA, et al. The aspirin and heme-binding sites of ovine and murine prostaglandin endoperoxide synthases. J Biol Chem 1990; 265(9):5192–8.
9. Roth GJ, Majerus PW. The mechanism of the effect of aspirin on human platelets. I. Acetylation of a particulate fraction protein. J Clin Invest 1975;56(3):624–32.
10. Hamberg M, Svensson J, Samuelsson B. Thromboxanes: a new group of biologically active compounds derived from prostaglandin endoperoxides. Proc Natl Acad Sci 1975;72(8):2994–8.
11. Elwood PC, Cochrane AL, Burr ML, et al. A Randomized Controlled Trial of Acetyl Salicylic Acid in the Secondary Prevention of Mortality from Myocardial Infarction. BMJ 1974;1(5905):436–40.
12. Elwood PC, Sweetnam PM. Aspirin and secondary mortality after myocardial infarction. Lancet 1979;2(8156–8157):1313–5.
13. Elwood PC. British studies of aspirin and myocardial infarction. Am J Med 1983; 74(6):50–4.
14. Aspirin in coronary heart disease. The Coronary Drug Project Research Group. Circulation 1980;62(6 Pt 2):V59–62.
15. Persantine-aspirin reinfarction study. Design, methods and baseline results. By the persantine-aspirin reinfarction study research group. Circulation 1980;62(3 Pt 2):II1–42.

16. A Randomized, Controlled Trial of Aspirin in Persons Recovered From Myocardial Infarction. JAMA 1980;243(7):661.
17. Breddin K, Loew D, Lechner K, et al. The German-Austrian aspirin trial: a comparison of acetylsalicylic acid, placebo and phenprocoumon in secondary prevention of myocardial infarction. On behalf of the German-Austrian Study Group. Circulation 1980;62(6 Pt 2):V63–72.
18. Antiplatelet Trialists' Collaboration. Secondary prevention of vascular disease by prolonged antiplatelet treatment. Antiplatelet Trialists' Collaboration. Br Med J Clin Res Ed 1988;296(6618):320–31.
19. Collaborative overview of randomised trials of antiplatelet therapy–I: Prevention of death, myocardial infarction, and stroke by prolonged antiplatelet therapy in various categories of patients. Antiplatelet Trialists' Collaboration. BMJ 1994; 308(6921):81–106.
20. Antithrombotic Trialists' Collaboration. Collaborative meta-analysis of randomised trials of antiplatelet therapy for prevention of death, myocardial infarction, and stroke in high risk patients. BMJ 2002;324(7329):71–86.
21. Jones WS, Mulder H, Wruck LM, et al. Comparative Effectiveness of Aspirin Dosing in Cardiovascular Disease. N Engl J Med 2021;384(21):1981–90.
22. Campbell CL, Smyth S, Montalescot G, et al. Aspirin Dose for the Prevention of Cardiovascular Disease: A Systematic Review. JAMA 2007;297(18):2018.
23. Hollopeter G, Jantzen HM, Vincent D, et al. Identification of the platelet ADP receptor targeted by antithrombotic drugs. Nature 2001;409(6817):202–7.
24. Féliste R, Delebassée D, Simon MF, et al. Broad spectrum anti-platelet activity of ticlopidine and PCR 4099 involves the suppression of the effects of released ADP. Thromb Res 1987;48(4):403–15.
25. Bhatt DL, Fox KAA, Hacke W, et al. Clopidogrel and aspirin versus aspirin alone for the prevention of atherothrombotic events. N Engl J Med 2006;354(16):1706–17.
26. Bonaca MP, Bhatt DL, Cohen M, et al. Long-term use of ticagrelor in patients with prior myocardial infarction. N Engl J Med 2015;372(19):1791–800.
27. Bhatt DL, Steg PG, Mehta SR, et al. Lancet 2019;394(10204):1169–80.
28. Mauri L, Kereiakes DJ, Yeh RW, et al. Twelve or 30 months of dual antiplatelet therapy after drug-eluting stents. N Engl J Med 2014;371(23):2155–66.
29. Valgimigli M, Campo G, Monti M, et al. Short- Versus Long-Term Duration of Dual-Antiplatelet Therapy After Coronary Stenting: A Randomized Multicenter Trial. Circulation 2012;125(16):2015–26.
30. Park SJ, Park DW, Kim YH, et al. Duration of Dual Antiplatelet Therapy after Implantation of Drug-Eluting Stents. N Engl J Med 2010;362(15):1374–82.
31. Baber U, Dangas G, Angiolillo DJ, et al. Ticagrelor alone vs. ticagrelor plus aspirin following percutaneous coronary intervention in patients with non-ST-segment elevation acute coronary syndromes: TWILIGHT-ACS. Eur Heart J 2020;41(37):3533–45.
32. Hahn JY, Song YB, Oh JH, et al. Effect of P2Y12 Inhibitor Monotherapy vs Dual Antiplatelet Therapy on Cardiovascular Events in Patients Undergoing Percutaneous Coronary Intervention: The SMART-CHOICE Randomized Clinical Trial. JAMA 2019;321(24):2428.
33. Han Y, Xu B, Xu K, et al. Six Versus 12 Months of Dual Antiplatelet Therapy After Implantation of Biodegradable Polymer Sirolimus-Eluting Stent: Randomized Substudy of the I-LOVE-IT 2 Trial. Circ Cardiovasc Interv 2016;9(2).
34. CAPRIE Steering Committee. A randomised, blinded, trial of clopidogrel versus aspirin in patients at risk of ischaemic events (CAPRIE). CAPRIE Steering Committee. Lancet 1996;348(9038):1329–39.

35. Kang J, Park KW, Lee H, et al. Aspirin Versus Clopidogrel for Long-Term Maintenance Monotherapy After Percutaneous Coronary Intervention: The HOST-EXAM Extended Study. Circulation 2023;147(2):108–17.

36. Povsic TJ, Roe MT, Ohman EM, et al. A randomized trial to compare the safety of rivaroxaban vs aspirin in addition to either clopidogrel or ticagrelor in acute coronary syndrome: The design of the GEMINI-ACS-1 phase II study. Am Heart J 2016;174:120–8.

37. Eikelboom JW, Connolly SJ, Bosch J, et al. Rivaroxaban with or without Aspirin in Stable Cardiovascular Disease. N Engl J Med 2017;377(14):1319–30.

38. Fanaroff AC, Lopes RD. The role of triple antithrombotic therapy in patients with atrial fibrillation undergoing percutaneous coronary intervention. Prog Cardiovasc Dis 2021;69:11–7.

39. Capodanno D, Di Maio M, Greco A, et al. Safety and Efficacy of Double Antithrombotic Therapy With Non–Vitamin K Antagonist Oral Anticoagulants in Patients With Atrial Fibrillation Undergoing Percutaneous Coronary Intervention: A Systematic Review and Meta-Analysis. J Am Heart Assoc 2020;9(16):e017212.

40. Pilgrim T, Vranckx P, Valgimigli M, et al. Risk and timing of recurrent ischemic events among patients with stable ischemic heart disease, non–ST-segment elevation acute coronary syndrome, and ST-segment elevation myocardial infarction. Am Heart J 2016;175:56–65.

41. Yasuda S, Kaikita K, Akao M, et al. Antithrombotic Therapy for Atrial Fibrillation with Stable Coronary Disease. N Engl J Med 2019;381(12):1103–13.

42. Fanaroff AC, Hasselblad V, Roe MT, et al. Antithrombotic agents for secondary prevention after acute coronary syndromes: A systematic review and network meta-analysis. Int J Cardiol 2017;241:87–96.

43. Lewis EF, Li Y, Pfeffer MA, et al. Impact of Cardiovascular Events on Change in Quality of Life and Utilities in Patients After Myocardial Infarction. JACC Heart Fail 2014;2(2):159–65.

44. Amin AP, Wang TY, McCoy L, et al. Impact of Bleeding on Quality of Life in Patients on DAPT. J Am Coll Cardiol 2016;67(1):59–65.

45. Yeh RW, Secemsky EA, Kereiakes DJ, et al. Development and Validation of a Prediction Rule for Benefit and Harm of Dual Antiplatelet Therapy Beyond 1 Year After Percutaneous Coronary Intervention. JAMA 2016;315(16):1735.

46. Very High Coronary Artery Calcium (≥1000) and Association With Cardiovascular Disease Events, Non–Cardiovascular Disease Outcomes, and Mortality. doi:10.1161/CIRCULATIONAHA.120.050545.

47. Rosenblit PD. Extreme Atherosclerotic Cardiovascular Disease (ASCVD) Risk Recognition. Curr Diabetes Rep 2019;19(8):61.

48. Briasoulis A, Bakris GL. Chronic Kidney Disease as a Coronary Artery Disease Risk Equivalent. Curr Cardiol Rep 2013;15(3):340.

49. Muntner P, Farkouh ME. Chronic Kidney Disease as a Coronary Heart Disease Risk Equivalent. Curr Cardiovasc Risk Rep 2010;4(2):136–41.

50. Virani SS, Newby LK, Arnold SV, et al. 2023 AHA/ACC/ACCP/ASPC/NLA/PCNA Guideline for the Management of Patients With Chronic Coronary Disease: A Report of the American Heart Association/American College of Cardiology Joint Committee on Clinical Practice Guidelines. Circulation 2023;148(9).

51. McDonagh TA, Metra M, Adamo M, et al. 2021 ESC Guidelines for the diagnosis and treatment of acute and chronic heart failure. Eur Heart J 2021;42(36):3599–726.

Optimal Medical Therapy for Stable Ischemic Heart Disease in 2024

Focus on Exercise and Cardiac Rehabilitation

Sherrie Khadanga, MD[a,b,*], Tanesha Beebe-Peat, MD[c]

KEYWORDS

- Cardiac rehabilitation • Secondary prevention • Lifestyle management
- Behavioral change • Exercise

KEY POINTS

- Secondary prevention plays a pivotal role in the management of chronic coronary disease.
- Cardiac rehabilitation (CR) has been shown to reduce cardiovascular mortality and morbidity as well as improve quality of life, exercise capacity, and functional status, yet it is underutilized.
- Exercise training, a key component of CR, has been shown to reduce symptoms of angina.

INTRODUCTION

Cardiovascular disease (CVD) remains the leading cause of death, with chronic coronary disease affecting more than 20 million individuals in the United States.[1] Numerous randomized controlled trials (RCTs), including COURAGE (Clinical Outcomes Utilizing Revascularization and Aggressive Drug Evaluation), ISCHEMIA (International Study of Comparative Health Effectiveness with Medical and Invasive Approaches), and BARI-2D (Bypass Angioplasty Revascularization Investigation 2 Diabetes) have found no mortality benefit with routine cardiovascular revascularization.[2–4] As such, clinicians should strive for cardiovascular risk factor reduction and optimize guideline-directed medical therapy (GDMT) for these patients. In addition to pharmacotherapy, lifestyle modification plays a pivotal role for prevention and symptom relief.[3–6]

Cardiac rehabilitation (CR) is a comprehensive team-based approach to deliver behavioral, lifestyle, and medical therapies to individuals of CVD. Typically, an outpatient

[a] Division of Cardiology, Department of Medicine, University of Vermont, Burlington, VT, USA;
[b] Vermont Center on Behavior and Health, University of Vermont, Burlington, VT, USA;
[c] Department of Medicine, University of Vermont Medical Center, Burlington, VT, USA
* Correspondig author. University of Vermont Medical Center Cardiac Rehabilitation and Prevention, 62 Tilley Drive, S Burlington, VT 05403.
E-mail address: Sherrie.Khadanga@uvmhealth.org

Med Clin N Am 108 (2024) 509–516
https://doi.org/10.1016/j.mcna.2023.11.005
0025-7125/24/© 2023 Elsevier Inc. All rights reserved.

medical.theclinics.com

program, CR focuses on structured exercise to improve cardiovascular fitness combined with the management of other risk factors such as changes in diet, medication adherence, and smoking cessation.[4,5] Participation in CR has been shown to decrease morbidity and mortality as well as improve quality of life and is therefore a class 1A recommendation by the American Heart Association and the American College of Cardiology.[6] Those with stable symptoms of angina or those who demonstrate ischemia with symptoms would be eligible for CR. Despite the benefits, it remains underutilized, particularly among those with chronic coronary disease. The purpose of this review is to describe the multidisciplinary components of CR and discuss novel ways of implementation (**Fig. 1**).

BENEFITS OF CARDIAC REHABILITATION

Data from various meta-analysis of RCTs have shown that CR participation decreases cardiovascular mortality as well as lead to improvements in physical function, mood, and functional capacity.[7] The effects of CR were recently assessed using meta-analysis in more than 23,000 patients with coronary disease with a median follow-up of 1 year. For those who participated in CR, a 26% reduction in cardiac mortality and 23% reduction in hospitalization was seen compared with those who did not attend CR. In spite of the numerous benefits, CR participation rates remain low. This may be due to barriers such as distance to the program, lack of transportation, scheduling conflicts, cost of copay, or lack of awareness about CR.[4,5] Ritchey and colleagues in 2020 analyzed Centers for Medicare Services data for CR eligible patients in 2016 and noted CR participation to be 24.4%; although it is more than a quarter increase from years 1997 to 2016, better efforts must be made to improve CR engagement.[8,9]

Patients with chronic coronary disease who experience symptoms of stable angina or have evidence of ischemia based on outpatient testing would benefit from a referral to CR as part of optimizing medical management. The referral may be placed by any physician, for example, a primary care physician or cardiologist.

PATIENT ASSESSMENT

Before enrollment in CR, it is recommended to obtain a baseline assessment of functional capacity, ideally with a maximally tolerated exercise tolerance test

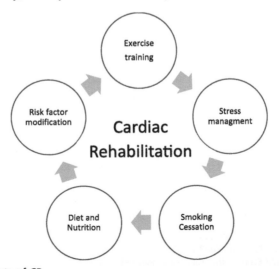

Fig. 1. Components of CR.

(ETT) performed on either a treadmill or bicycle. The ETT can provide both diagnostic and therapeutic information and is a class 2a recommendation for patients with chronic coronary disease who have a change in symptoms or persistent symptoms despite GDMT.[6] The data from the ETT can help provide reassurance to the patient as well as assist staff with tailoring the exercise prescription. Additionally, measures such as body mass index, blood pressure, heart rate, and resting ECG should be obtained and patients should be screened for additional CVD risk factors, for example, diabetes or peripheral arterial disease.[4,5,10] If unable to obtain an ETT, then a submaximal test such as the 6-minute walk test can be used because it can be converted easily to a metabolic equivalent training level and is usually more tolerated than the ETT, especially for elderly patients with arthritis and deconditioning.[11]

EXERCISE TRAINING

Exercise training remains the cornerstone of CR. Exercise has been shown to slow the progression of coronary atherosclerosis as well as positively affect modifiable CVD risk factors such as obesity, diabetes, and hyperlipidemia.[5,6,10] For those with advanced coronary disease and stable symptoms, exercise can improve anginal threshold, meaning it takes more time before symptoms of angina occur. It can therefore be a key component of symptom management along with maximally tolerated GDMT.

Exercise in CR includes both aerobic and resistance training (RT) and is individualized and tailored to the patient's comorbidities as well as the patient's overall goal.[5] In general, aerobic exercise is focused on moderate intensity continuous training with different modalities and walking being a main focus.[5,6] Additionally, RT targeting the major muscle groups is incorporated into the exercise program. This is of critical importance because RT has been found to improve walking endurance and muscle strength thereby increasing overall physical.[12] It is encouraged that patients attend CR 2 to 3 times a week with each session typically lasting 30 to 45 minutes.

During the last 10 to 15 years, the traditional model of CR exercise has evolved, and other alternatives for the appropriate group can further improve outcomes. For example, those who are overweight or obese in CR, exercise should be geared toward maximizing caloric expenditure. In a RCT performed by Ades and colleagues, high-calorie expenditure exercise resulted in double the weight loss (8.2 ± 4 vs 3.7 ± 5 kg; $P < .001$) and a greater waist reduction ($-7 ± 5$ vs $-5 ± 5$ cm; $P = .02$) than standard CR exercise at 5 months.[13]

Although moderate intensity continuous training as led to improvements in fitness, the response is not necessarily consistent. In one study, which consisted of 3925 patients who completed CR, 18% of patients (24% women) failed to demonstrate any improvement, which may be in part due to the type of exercise intensity.[14] Khadanga and colleagues performed an RCT among women participating in CR and found that those randomized to the combination of higher intensity resistance and aerobic interval training improved peak oxygen uptake (peak Vo_2) by 23% compared with standard moderate continuous training. To further improve outcomes, alternatives to traditional CR exercise should be considered.[15]

LIFESTYLE MANAGEMENT AND BEHAVIORAL MODIFICATION

In addition to exercise training, CR is the ideal environment to reduce risk factors and promote secondary prevention through diet, weight management, and smoking cessation. Participants should undergo detailed nutrition counseling to determine areas of nutritional intervention. Both patients and their family members need to be educated on dietary goals and necessary changes in an attempt to ensure dietary compliance.[5] A healthy eating pattern, which includes a variety of fruits and veggies, whole grains, healthy proteins (largely plant based) with limited processed foods, minimal intake of added sugars and foods prepared with little or no salt is generally recommended.[5,6] Specific types of diets such as the Dietary Approaches to Stop Hypertension (DASH) and the Mediterranean diet have demonstrated cardiovascular benefits.[16,17] The DASH diet has been associated with reduced all-cause mortality in adults with hypertension.[16] The diet includes reduced amounts of saturated fat, total fat, and cholesterol with high fiber, protein, and electrolytes from fruits and vegetables.[17]

Similarly, the Mediterranean diet (MedDiet) not only reduces blood pressure but also reduces cardiovascular risk.[16] This diet consists of high amounts of fruits and vegetables, nuts/legumes, whole grains, and seafood with moderate alcohol intake and low amounts of red/processed meat and saturated fats.[18] Some argue the practicality of the MedDiet and whether or not the benefits can be seen for those residing in the United States. To help elucidate this, a large study of 2594 healthy US women were followed over 12 years, and it was noted that for those who consumed a higher amount of the MedDiet, there was an association of a 28% relative risk reduction in CVD events.[19] Additional research is needed to see if there are long-term cardiovascular benefits in US populations.

Weight management is also an important aspect of lifestyle modifications, and with CR, patients should be able to create a plan for diet and exercise with weight management goals in mind (if BMI >25 kg/mg^2, waist >40 inches in men and >35 inches in women) to ensure energy deficit weight loss.[5,20] For those with CVD, when weight loss occurs intentionally due to lifestyle and behavioral changes, there is a cardioprotective effect.[20]

Another goal of CR is to ensure that blood pressure is less than 140/90 mm Hg with isolated hypertension or less than 130/80 in patients with hypertension and additional comorbidities (diabetes, heart failure, or chronic kidney disease).[4] Blood pressure is typically obtained before and following exercise, and if it is elevated, provider is notified to make the necessary adjustments. CR can also be helpful in diabetes management in conjunction with the patient's primary care provider and/or endocrinologist.[4] This can be especially important in patients who are not on cardioprotective antihyperglycemic agents such as sodium-glucose cotransporter-2 (SGLT-2) inhibitors and glucagon-like peptide (GLP-1) receptor agonist that have shown benefits in weight management.[21]

Smoking following a myocardial infarction is associated with higher morbidity and mortality, and these patients are likely to have other unhealthy behavior habits and additional medical comorbidities (stroke, chronic obstructive pulmonary disease (COPD), current asthma, difficulty walking, or climbing stairs).[22] Given that smoking is attributed to 33% of all cardiovascular-related deaths, CR is a great setting to address smoking status and promote cessation.[23]

Participants should be asked about their smoking status or tobacco product use, including those who quit in the last 12 months.[5] Typically, this is obtained through self-report by the patient; however, many patients may not be candid due to fear of judgment or embarrassment.[24] An alternative way to determine smoking status is measuring carbon monoxide (CO) in expired breath. CO can be measured easily with a handheld monitor and CO half-life is approximately 8 hours.[24] Measuring breath CO is not sensitive to the use of nicotine replacement therapies unlike other measures of smoking via nicotine metabolites in saliva, blood, or urine.[22] For those who do smoke, readiness to quit should be assessed and if amenable, treatment options such as nicotine replacement or pharmacotherapy can be discussed. For those who recently quit smoking, positive reinforcement should be given so that they continue to abstain from smoking and tobacco products.[5] Continued education and counseling should be provided for those who are not yet ready. Ideally, the goal is that participants can quit smoking while attending CR. It is imperative to recognize those who smoke given that current smokers are less likely to adhere to CR than their nonsmoking counterparts.[5]

ALTERNATIVE MODALITIES OF CARDIAC REHABILITATION

Hybrid CR model includes both in-person center-based CR (CBCR) and home-based CR (HBCR) in a synchronous way (with real-time audiovisual counseling and education) and asynchronous way (audio only counseling and education).[25] Hybrid CR is an option for certain patients who are "low risk" and can follow the appropriate exercise at home, without having close interactions and monitoring by the CR staff. These programs must still include all the recommended core components that are within the CBCR program. In this model, an initial patient assessment is completed in-person to complete the previously mentioned steps at the start of CR.[25] Heart rate and blood pressure are monitored with at-home devices.[26] Besides exercise recommendations, hybrid CR programs must also address disease-specific self-care (diet, smoking cessation, and treatment of comorbidities such as hyperlipidemia, diabetes, and hypertension). These sessions are allowed to occur in both synchronous and asynchronous ways but there should be follow-up to determine that patients understood the educational concepts of the materials and to allow for question and answer.[25] In a recent review, it seems that hybrid CR provides similar benefits to traditional CR, with improvement in exercise capacity and quality of life and reduced cardiovascular events.[26]

HBCR is not a new type of CR given that patients are expected to participate in home-based exercise training on the days that they are not at the CR facility. Isolated HBCR is fairly new and evolved during the coronavirus disease 2019 (COVID-19) pandemic. A Cochrane review by Dalal and colleagues, compared HBCR versus CBCR and HBCR and found that there was no evidence of different outcomes in patients with stable coronary heart disease both in the short-term (3–12 months) and long-term (up to 24 months) settings.[27] HBCR allows for more flexible and convenient programming and can reduce potential barriers to CR participation, for example, transportation issues or distance. Interestingly, there has been notable improvement in adherence for HBCR (87%) versus CBCR (~49%).[27]

A systematic review by Thomas and colleagues directly compared HBCR and CBCR from January 1980 to January 2017 and could not attribute a single component of CR to be more beneficial in one group over the other.[28] There were no statistically significant differences between HBCR and CBCR among all-cause mortality 12 months after the intervention; exercise capacity and changes in modifiable risk factors were similar between the 2 groups. This may be limited by some of the studies with small sample size and may not be appropriately powered to recognize differences.[28]

Although hybrid or HBCR programs may seem ideal, it is not without limitations. There is less patient accountability and less face-to-face monitoring, and communication.[28] Additionally, there been safety concerns for patients at higher risk, which is why this type of programming is not available to all patients.[28]

CHANGES TO CARDIAC REHABILITATION BECAUSE OF THE CORONAVIRUS DISEASE 2019 PANDEMIC

CR underwent major changes due to the COVID-19 pandemic. Among US Medicare beneficiaries eligible for CR, participation in CR decreased 94% during the start of the pandemic, and although the decline has partially recovered, it has not gone back to prepandemic participation numbers.[29] Additionally, during this time, 220 CR programs closed, which is unfortunate because those that closed were more likely to be affiliated with rural area public hospitals, thereby worsening the gap for vulnerable communities to receive secondary prevention.[29] Although prevalence gained for hybrid and HBCR programs during the pandemic, once the Public Health Emergency expired in May 2023, many programs eliminated virtual or telehealth CR delivery due to lack of reimbursement by Centers for Medicare and Medicaid Services.[30] Future advocacy is needed to ensure adequate delivery of secondary prevention in order to engage as many individuals as possible.

SUMMARY

Medical therapy plays an important role in chronic coronary disease. CR bridges the gap between pharmacologic therapies and lifestyle modification in these patients. CR addresses exercise, weight management, nutrition, psychological conditions, smoking cessation, and multiple medical comorbidities (diabetes, hypertension, and hyperlipidemia). There has been various research determining outcomes for patients who attend CR versus those who do not, and CR participants fair much better in terms of reduction in cardiovascular mortality and hospitalizations. Unfortunately, CR enrollment and adherence remain quite abysmal, and concerted efforts are needed in order to meet the goal of 70% CR participation set by the Million Hearts Cardiac Rehabilitation Collaborative. Given the numerous benefits, cardiac rehabilitation remains a cornerstone for the treatment of chronic coronary disease.[6,31]

CLINICS CARE POINTS

- Nonpharmacologic treatment such as exercise and healthy diet should be recommended for all patients with chronic coronary disease.
- Those with chronic coronary disease should be encouraged to engage in physical activity and limit the amount of sedentary time.
- CR has been shown to reduce cardiovascular mortality and hospitalizations as well as improve quality of life and physical function.
- CR provides tailored exercise prescription consisting of both aerobic exercise as well as strength training.
- For those with chronic coronary disease, exercise can limit symptoms of angina.
- Another key component of CR is lifestyle modification and risk factor reduction all of which can reduce the recurrence of a cardiovascular event.
- Alternative forms of CR, such has hybrid programs or HBCR, have emerged and can be a suitable option for low-risk patients.

FUNDING

This research was supported by National Institutes of Health Center of Biomedical Research Excellence award from the National Institute of General Medical Sciences: P20GM103644 and by the National Heart, Lung, and Blood Institute, United States under Award Number R33HL143305.

DISCLOSURE

All authors have nothing to disclose. There are no relationships with industry for any of the authors.

REFERENCES

1. Tsao CW, Aday AW, Almarzooq ZI, et al. Heart disease and stroke statistics-2022 update: a report from the american heart association [published correction appears in Circulation. 2022 Sep 6;146(10):e141]. Circulation 2022;145(8): e153–639.
2. Boden WE, O'Rourke RA, Teo KK, et al. Optimal medical therapy with or without PCI for stable coronary disease. N Engl J Med 2007;356(15):1503–16.
3. BARI 2D Study Group, Frye RL, August P, et al. A randomized trial of therapies for type 2 diabetes and coronary artery disease. N Engl J Med 2009;360(24): 2503–15.
4. Balady GJ, Ades PA, Bittner VA, et al. Referral, enrollment, and delivery of cardiac rehabilitation/secondary prevention programs at clinical centers and beyond: a presidential advisory from the American Heart Association. Circulation 2011; 124(25):2951–60.
5. Balady GJ, Williams MA, Ades PA, et al. Core components of cardiac rehabilitation/secondary prevention programs: 2007 update: a scientific statement from the American Heart Association Exercise, Cardiac Rehabilitation, and Prevention Committee, the Council on Clinical Cardiology; the Councils on Cardiovascular Nursing, Epidemiology and Prevention, and Nutrition, Physical Activity, and Metabolism; and the American Association of Cardiovascular and Pulmonary Rehabilitation. Circulation 2007;115(20):2675–82.
6. Virani SS, Newby LK, Arnold SV, et al. 2023 AHA/ACC/ACCP/ASPC/NLA/PCNA guideline for the management of patients with chronic coronary disease: a report of the american heart association/american college of cardiology joint committee on clinical practice guidelines. Circulation 2023;148(9):e9–119.
7. Heran BS, Chen JM, Ebrahim S, et al. Exercise-based cardiac rehabilitation for coronary heart disease. Cochrane Database Syst Rev 2011;7:CD001800.
8. Ritchey MD, Maresh S, McNeely J, et al. Tracking cardiac rehabilitation participation and completion among medicare beneficiaries to inform the efforts of a national initiative. Circ Cardiovascular Quality Outcomes 2020;13(1):e005902.
9. Suaya JA, Shepard DS, Normand SL, et al. Use of cardiac rehabilitation by Medicare beneficiaries after myocardial infarction or coronary bypass surgery. Circulation 2007;116(15):1653–62.
10. Jolliffe JA, Rees K, Taylor RS, et al. Exercise-based rehabilitation for coronary heart disease. Cochrane Database Syst Rev 2001;1:CD001800.
11. Saba MA, Goharpey S, Moghadam BA, et al. Correlation between the 6-min walk test and exercise tolerance test in cardiac rehabilitation after coronary artery bypass grafting: a cross-sectional study. Cardiology and Therapy 2021;10: 201–9.
12. Khadanga S, Savage PD, Ades PA. Resistance training for older adults in cardiac rehabilitation. Clinical Geriatric Medicine 2019;35(4):459–68.
13. Ades PA, Savage PD, Toth MJ, et al. High-caloric expenditure exercise: a new approach to cardiac rehabilitation for overweight coronary patients. Circulation 2009;119:2671–8.
14. Rengo JL, Khadanga S, Savage PD, et al. Response to exercise training during cardiac rehabilitation differs by sex. J Cardpulm Rehabil Prev 2020;40(5):319–24.

15. Khadanga S, Savage PD, Pecha A, et al. Optimizing training response for women in cardiac rehabilitation: a randomized clinical trial. JAMA Cardiol 2022;7(2): 215–8.

16. Wang JS, Liu WJ, Lee CL. Associations of ADHERENCE to the DASH diet and the mediterranean diet with all-cause mortality in subjects with various glucose regulation states. Front Nutr 2022;9:828792.

17. Appel LJ, Moore TJ, Obarzanek E, et al. A clinical trial of the effects of dietary patterns on blood pressure. DASH Collaborative Research Group. N Engl J Med 1997;336(16):1117–24.

18. Davis C, Bryan J, Hodgson J, et al. Definition of the mediterranean diet; a literature review. Nutrients 2015;5:9139–53.

19. Ahmad S, Moorthy MV, Demler OV, et al. Assessment of risk factors and biomarkers associated with risk of cardiovascular disease among women consuming a mediterranean diet. JAMA Netw Open 2018;1(8):e185708.

20. Pack QR, Rodriguez-Escudero JP, Thomas RJ, et al. The prognostic importance of weight loss in coronary artery disease: a systematic review and meta-analysis. Mayo Clin Proc 2014;89(10):1368–77.

21. Khadanga S, Barrett K, Sheahan KH, et al. Novel Therapeutics for Type 2 Diabetes, Obesity, and Heart Failure: a review and practical recommendations for cardiac rehabilitation. J Cardiopulm Rehabil Prev 2023;43(1):1–7.

22. Gaalema DE, Bolívar HA, Khadanga S, et al. Current smoking as a marker of a high-risk behavioral profile after myocardial infarction. Prev Med 2020;140: 106245.

23. Centers for Disease Control and Prevention (CDC). Smoking-attributable mortality, years of potential life lost, and productivity losses–United States, 2000-2004. MMWR Morb Mortal Wkly Rep 2008;57(45):1226–8.

24. Khadanga S, Yant B, Savage PD, et al. Objective measure of smoking status highlights disparities by sex. Am Heart J 2022;17:100171.

25. Keteyian SJ, Ades PA, Beatty AL, et al. A review of the design and implementation of a hybrid cardiac rehabilitation program: an expanding opportunity for optimizing cardiovascular care. J Cardiopulm Rehabil Prev 2022;42(1):1–9.

26. Heindl B, Ramirez L, Joseph L, et al. Hybrid cardiac rehabilitation - The state of the science and the way forward. Prog Cardiovasc Dis 2022;70:175–82.

27. Dalal HM, Zawada A, Jolly K, et al. Home based versus centre based cardiac rehabilitation: Cochrane systematic review and meta-analysis [published correction appears in BMJ. 2010;340:c1133]. BMJ 2010;340:b5631.

28. Thomas RJ, Beatty AL, Beckie TM, et al. Home-based cardiac rehabilitation: a scientific statement from the american association of cardiovascular and pulmonary rehabilitation, the american heart association, and the american college of cardiology. Circulation 2019;140(1):e69–89.

29. Varghese MS, Beatty AL, Song Y, et al. Cardiac REHABILITATION and the COVID-19 pandemic: persistent declines in cardiac rehabilitation participation and access among us medicare beneficiaries. Circ Cardiovasc Qual Outcomes 2022;15(12):e009618.

30. Kuehn BM. Pandemic intensifies push for home-based cardiac rehabilitation options. Circulation 2020;142(18):1781–2.

31. Cardiac Rehabilitation, Million Hearts® (hhs.gov), Available at: https://millionhearts.hhs.gov/about-million-hearts/optimizing-care/cardiac-rehabilitation-CRC.html. Accessed Oct 1, 2023.

When to Consider Coronary Revascularization for Stable Coronary Artery Disease

Andrew M. Cheng, MD[a,b], Jacob A. Doll, MD[a,b],*

KEYWORDS

- Revascularization • Coronary artery bypass graft surgery
- Percutaneous coronary intervention • Outcomes • Heart team • Patient preferences

KEY POINTS

- Based on current recommendations, the indications to perform coronary revascularization to improve survival in chronic coronary disease are limited to left main disease and multivessel disease with a reduced left ventricular ejection fraction (LVEF).
- However, revascularization may provide improved quality of life and reduce future adverse cardiovascular events.
- When considering revascularization, these potential benefits should be weighed against procedural risks and costs and often require value-driven discussions with the patient and shared decision-making with a multidisciplinary heart team.

INTRODUCTION

Optimal treatment of chronic coronary disease (CCD) includes lifestyle changes, medical therapy, and revascularization of obstructed coronary vessels for select patients. In comparison to patients with acute coronary syndromes (ACSs) that arise from sudden occlusion of the coronary artery, revascularization of an artery with stable atherosclerotic plaque is less likely to impact overall survival or reduce future cardiovascular events.

Surgical revascularization via coronary artery bypass grafting (CABG) was developed in the 1960s. The first percutaneous coronary intervention (PCI) occurred in 1978 with balloon angioplasty. A decade later bare metal stents were introduced, and ultimately, drug-eluting stents in the early 2000s.[1] Historically, recommendations for revascularization for CCD arose from the early CABG trials in the 1970 and 1980s, comparing surgical revascularization to medical management. These trials predominantly showed that CABG confers a mortality benefit for a subset of high-risk patients, namely those

[a] Division of Cardiology, Department of Medicine, University of Washington, 1959 NE Pacific Street, Seattle, WA 98195, USA; [b] Section of Cardiology, VA Puget Sound Health Care System, 1660 South Columbian Way S111-CARDIO, Seattle, WA 98108, USA
* Corresponding author.
E-mail address: jdoll@uw.edu

Med Clin N Am 108 (2024) 517–538
https://doi.org/10.1016/j.mcna.2023.11.006
0025-7125/24/© 2023 Elsevier Inc. All rights reserved.

with left main (LM) disease ($\geq$50% stenosis) or with three-vessel stenosis ($\geq$70% stenosis in major epicardial vessels).[2] There were no large randomized controlled PCI trials of CCD in the early 1990s, though observational data suggested that PCI conferred a similar survival benefit.[3] These findings led to the paradigm that visual stenosis necessitated intervention ("See one, stent one"), with higher burden of disease increasing the need for revascularization. However, a series of large, randomized trials have challenged this paradigm and emphasize that medical therapy without revascularization is safe and effective for many patients with CCD.

At present, based on the 2023 ACC/AHA recommendations for the management of CCD,[4] the guideline indications to perform coronary revascularization are.

1. To reduce mortality via CABG surgery for:
   a. Patients with LM stenosis
   b. Patients with multivessel coronary artery disease (CAD) and ejection fraction (EF) $\leq$ 35%
2. To reduce future myocardial infarction (MI) or other cardiovascular events for patients with multivessel CAD via CABG and/or PCI.
3. To improve symptoms for patients with refractory angina despite optimal medical therapy (OMT) via CABG and/or PCI.

These recommendations will likely continue to evolve over time. Ongoing advances in surgical and PCI technique, novel medical therapies, and a patient population of increasing age and complexity will continue to shift the balance of risk and benefit for revascularization in CCD. Given this complexity, revascularization decisions require patient-centered and multidisciplinary decision-making.

The following sections will:

1. review the trial data leading to the current guideline recommendations for revascularization
2. review indications for PCI versus CABG treatment decisions
3. highlight remaining controversies and unanswered questions

CASE PRESENTATION

A 77-year-old man with type 2 diabetes had an MI 10 years ago and was successfully revascularized with a right coronary artery (RCA) drug-eluting stent. He now presents with shortness of breath which led to a coronary angiogram showing an 80% proximal left anterior descending artery (LAD) stenosis and a 90% stenosis just distal to his previous mid-RCA stent. An echo was performed which revealed a left ventricular EF of 60%. He is on appropriate secondary prevention medical therapy for stable CAD. His antianginal medication regimen includes metoprolol succinate 25 mg daily only.

In this scenario, our diabetic patient has two-vessel CCD with symptoms that may be anginal in nature. Should this patient undergo revascularization? If so, would PCI or CABG be more appropriate?

DISCUSSION

In 2021, ACC/AHA published coronary revascularization guidelines including indications for revascularization in CCD. In 2023, ACC/AHA published new guidelines for the general management of CCD, also including indications for revascularization. In the following sections, the authors focus primarily on the 2023 guidelines with occasional reference to the 2021 guidelines, as they generally provide complementary recommendations.

REVASCULARIZATION TO REDUCE MORTALITY

Randomized controlled trials have demonstrated a mortality benefit of revascularization for only a relatively small anatomic subset of patients with CCD. A primary goal of the initial assessment and testing of suspected CCD patients is the identification of these high-risk subgroups, with appropriate referral for consideration of CABG or PCI. However, the larger group of patients without high-risk features can be reassured that revascularization is not required urgently, and medical therapy alone may be sufficient to reduce their risk of mortality and MI and manage anginal symptoms.

Left Main Disease

The current 2023 ACC/AHA guidelines recommend revascularization for CCD with significant LM involvement regardless of symptoms. The data for this recommendation comes primarily from two CABG studies (**Table 1**) conducted in the 1970s; the *VA Coop* (VA Cooperative Coronary Surgery Study) and the *European Coronary Surgery Study*. These studies showed a mortality advantage over medical therapy in patients with LM stenosis that received surgical revascularization.[1] At the time, OMT included only aspirin and beta-blockers, and only approximately one-third and one-half of the trial participants were taking these respective medicines.[2] Both medical therapy and surgical technique have advanced markedly since that time, calling into question if these trials are applicable to contemporary practice. Nevertheless, subsequent stable CAD trials have largely excluded LM disease (assuming lack of equipoise) and current guidelines continue to rely on these historic data to guide management for LM stenosis (see **Table 1**).

Multivessel CAD with an Ejection Fraction Less than 35%

Revascularization improves mortality in patients with chronic multivessel CAD with an LVEF less than 35%. There were suggestions of this based on Coronary Artery Surgery Study (CASS), an early CABG versus medical therapy study published in 1983. Although overall a negative study, subgroup analysis showed a survival benefit in CABG participants with an EF less than 50%.[5] The more recent STITCH trial randomized 1212 patients with stable ischemic heart disease, an LVEF less than 35%, and indications for CABG, to OMT alone or CABG + OMT. At a median of 56 months, there was no statistically significant difference in all-cause mortality, though improvements were noted in cardiovascular mortality and heart failure hospitalization.[6] Its extension study, STITCHES, showed that after approximately 10 years patients who underwent CABG had a survival advantage compared with those who received medical therapy alone.[7] Given the late emergence of a mortality benefit of CABG in these studies, the overall benefit must be balanced with consideration of upfront surgical risk.

PCI was not included in the STICH trial, so the REVIVED-BCIS2 trial tested PCI versus medical therapy for a similar patient population. PCI did not confer a benefit for death or heart failure admissions compared with medical therapy alone.[8] Consequently, the class I recommendation for revascularization of chronic multiple-vessel CAD with a low EF is confined to surgical intervention (**Table 2**).

REVASCULARIZATION TO IMPROVE OTHER CARDIOVASCULAR OUTCOMES

Avoiding mortality is the ultimate goal, but reducing the risk of MI or the need for future revascularization procedures are also important objectives. In addition to the studies described above, multiple other landmark randomized controlled trials (RCTs) have tested revascularization versus medical therapy among patients with CCD, most notably *COURAGE, FAME-2,* and *ISCHEMIA*. Although these studies failed to demonstrate a mortality benefit from revascularization, they have added to our understanding

Table 1
Early coronary artery bypass grafting trials versus medical therapy[5,34,35]

Type of Trial	Trial	Study Period	Medical Therapy (n)	CABG (n)	PCI (n)	Enrollment Criteria	Major Outcomes
Early CABG Trials	VA Cooperative Coronary Surgery Study	1972–1974	354	332	N/A	• Angina ≥ 6 mo • At least a 3-mo trial of medical therapy • Angiographic evidence of ≥ 50% stenosis in at least one major coronary artery with a distal by-pass target	Medium follow-up 4 y • Mortality: 14% CABG vs 17% medical therapy (all-comers). P = NS • Mortality: 7% CABG vs 36% medical therapy (subset with LM disease) $P <$ .005. • Mortality: 15% CABG vs 14% medial therapy (subset without LM disease). P = NS
	European Coronary Surgery Study	1973–1976	373	395	N/A	• Men, age <65 y • Angina ≥ 3 mo • Angiographic evidence of ≥ 50% stenosis in at least two major coronary arteries with distal by-pass targets. • LVEF >50%	Medium follow-up 5 y • Mortality: 6.5% CABG vs 15.9% medical therapy (all-comers). $P <$ .001 • Mortality: 7.1% CABG vs 38.3% medical therapy (patients with LM disease) P = .037. • Mortality: 5.1% CABG vs 15.2% medical therapy (pts with three-vessel disease) $P <$ .001
	CASS	1975–1979	390	390	N/A	• Age <65 y • CCS class I or II angina • Angiographic evidence of ≥50% stenosis of left main or ≥70% stenosis of other major coronary artery • LVEF >35%	• Mortality (annual rate): 1.1% CABG vs 1.6% medical therapy (all comers). No significant difference in 1-v, 2-v, 3-v subgroups • Mortality for LVEF < 50% (annual rate): 1.7% CABG vs 3.3% medical therapy. $P <$ .005.

Abbreviations: NS, not significant; 1-v, 2-v, 3-v refer to 1-vessel, 2-vessel, and 3-vessel respectively.

Table 2
Chronic coronary disease: Revascularization versus medical therapy trials for LVEF less than 35%[6–8]

Trial		Study Period	Medical Therapy (n)	CABG (n)	PCI (n)	Enrollment Criteria	Enrollment Characteristics	Major Outcomes
Ischemic Cardiomyopathy	STITCH	2002–2007	602	610	N/A	• Age ≥ 18 • LVEF ≤ 35% • CAD suitable for CABG revascularization	• Mean age = 60 • 12% female • 40% diabetic • 87% CABG group had 2-v or more grafts • NYHA class II (52%) class III (34%) • No angina (37%) CCS class I (16%) class II (43%)	Medium follow-up: 56 mo • All-cause mortality 36% CABG vs 41% medical therapy ($P = .12$) • Death from cardiovascular causes 28% CABG vs 33% medical therapy ($P = .05$) • Death or hospitalization for any cause 58% CABG vs 68% medical therapy ($P = .003$)
	STITCHES	10-year follow-up of STITCH						Medium follow-up: 9.8 y • All-cause mortality 58.9% CABG vs 66.1% medical therapy ($P = .02$) • Death from cardiovascular causes 40.5% CABG vs 49.3% medical therapy ($P = .006$) • Death or hospitalization for any cause 83% CABG vs 89.4% medical therapy ($P = .001$)

(continued on next page)

Table 2
(continued)

Trial	Study Period	Medical Therapy (n)	CABG (n)	PCI (n)	Enrollment Criteria	Enrollment Characteristics	Major Outcomes
REVIVED-BCIS2	2013–2020	353	N/A	347	• Age ≥ 18 • LVEF ≤ 35% • Extensive CAD and viability in at least 4 dysfunctional myocardial segments • CAD suitable for PCI revascularization	• Mean age = 70 • 13% female • 39% diabetic • 71% PCI group with complete revascularization as measured by coronary artery index • NYHA class I-II (74%) class III-IV (26%) • No angina (67%) CCS class I-II (31%) class III (2%)	Medium follow-up: 41 mo • All-cause mortality or heart failure hospitalization 37.2% PCI vs 38% medical therapy (CI, 0.78–1.27; $P = .96$) • All-cause mortality 31.7% PCI vs 32.6% medical therapy (95% CI, 0.75–1.27) • Heart failure hospitalization 14.7% PCI vs 15.3% medical therapy (95% CI, 0.66–1.43) • LVEF change at 1 y: 2% PCI vs 1.1% medical therapy (mean difference, 0.9% point; 95% CI, –1.7–3.4)

of CCD management and indicate a likely reduction in cardiovascular events with contemporary revascularization techniques (**Table 3**).

The summary results of COURAGE—no benefit of PCI compared with OMT with regard to mortality and MI prevention for patients with CCD—changed the treatment paradigm for CAD.[9] However, COURAGE selected and randomized patients after coronary angiography, leading to concern for selection bias and an overall low burden of ischemia among trial participants. There was also concern that revascularization was incomplete in many patients and that targets of PCI were selected by angiography alone without the benefit of invasive functional testing. Critics therefore questioned the validity and applicability of the trial results, particularly to a higher risk population.

In FAME-2, patients with stable angina and at least one epicardial vessel with greater than 50% stenosis were randomized to either fractional flow reserve (FFR)-guided percutaneous intervention + OMT versus OMT alone. FFR is an invasive pressure wire index that can be performed in concert with coronary angiography; it provides a functional assessment that has been well validated to assess the likelihood that a coronary stenosis induces myocardial ischemia. Those without an FFR significant lesion (>0.8) were excluded from the trial as well as those with LM disease or an LVEF less than 30%. In contrast to COURAGE, the difference in combined primary endpoint (death, MI, or urgent revascularization) was statistically significant, and in fact, trial recruitment was halted early due to the major difference between the two treatment arms (4.3% in the PCI group vs 12.7% in the medical-therapy group). However, this difference was driven by urgent revascularization, and there were no differences in the frequency of death or MI.[10] Critics have questioned whether urgent revascularization is an appropriate endpoint for an unblinded trial in which patients in the control arm (and their clinicians) were aware of their untreated ischemic lesion.

Although COURAGE and FAME-2 seemed to have discordant conclusions, COURAGE also revealed an increase in urgent revascularization in the conservative treatment arm. Thus, these trials both support a reduction in unplanned revascularization with PCI, though without reduction in mortality or future MI.

Finally, the ISCHEMIA trial enrolled participants with moderate or severe reversible ischemia based on stress testing, selecting a higher risk patient population with greater potential to benefit from revascularization. Patients with LM disease were excluded, based on coronary CT angiography (CCTA), as well as patients with an EF less than 35%, because these patients had a strong indication for revascularization based on prior evidence. More than 5000 patients were randomized to an immediate invasive strategy (in which patients underwent angiography within 30 days of randomization with the goal of complete revascularization of any ischemic territories) versus conservative therapy (with angiography and revascularization reserved for only those who failed medical therapy). In the invasive arm, 79% of patients were revascularized and of these 74% received PCI and 26% received CABG. There was no difference in the primary composite outcome of death from cardiovascular causes, MI, hospitalization for unstable angina, heart failure, or resuscitated cardiac arrest. There was a late divergence in cardiovascular mortality and MI in favor of the invasive strategy. Spontaneous MIs were less likely in the invasive arm, though this was balanced by more procedural MIs. Of note, 23% of conservatively managed patients crossed over to receive revascularization at 4 years of follow-up.[11]

The ISCHEMIA-EXTEND study published 7-year all-cause, cardiovascular and non-cardiovascular mortality rates for the original cohort. After a median 5.7 years, there was a lower cardiovascular mortality for invasively managed patients, but this was offset by a higher non-cardiovascular mortality, resulting in no overall difference.[12]

Table 3
Chronic coronary disease: Revascularization versus medical therapy trials for LVEF greater than 35%[9–12,23]

	Trial	Study Period	Medical Therapy (n)	CABG (n)	PCI (n)	Enrollment Criteria	Enrollment Characteristics	Major Outcomes
CCS: Clinical Trials	COURAGE	1999–2004	1138	N/A	1149	• Stable CAD • CCS class I, II, III or stabilized class IV angina • ≥70% stenosis in at least one coronary artery • Myocardial ischemia, with ischemic ECG changes at rest, positive stress test, or 80% stenosis with classic angina without provocative testing • Left main (>50%) or LVEF < 30% excluded	• Average age 61.5 y • 15% female • 32% diabetic • No angina 12%, CCS class I (30%), II (36%), III (23%) • 1-v CAD (31%), 2-v (39%), 3-v (30%) Prox LAD (34%) • LVEF 68%	• Medium follow-up 4.6 y • Primary endpoint (PCI vs OMT) • All-cause death and nonfatal MI: 19% vs 18.5% (HR 1.05; 95% CI 0.87–1.27; P = .62) • Secondary endpoint (PCI vs OMT) • Rate of death 7.6% vs 8.3% (P = NS) • Rate of nonfatal MI 13.2% vs 12.3% (P = .33) • Rate of ACS hospitalization 12.4% vs 11.8% (P = .56) • Rate of urgent revascularization 21.1% vs 32.6% (P < .001)
	BARI-2D	2001–2005	1192	1176 378	798	• Diabetic • Angiography with ≥50% stenosis of a major epicardial coronary artery with a positive stress test or ≥70% stenosis and classic angina • Eligible for PCI and/or CABG	• Average age 62 y • 30% female • 100% diabetic • No angina 17.9%, CCS class I–II (42.5%), III–IV (8.6%), unstable angina (9.5%) • 3-v CAD (30.7%) Prox LAD (13.2%) • LVEF 57.2%	• Medium follow-up 5.3 y • Primary endpoint (revascularization vs OMT) • Rates of survival: 88.3% vs 87.8% (P = .97) • Freedom from MACE (death/MI/stroke) 77.2% vs 75.9% (P = .7) • Subanalysis (PCI vs OMT)

Study	Years	N	Inclusion Criteria	Population	Outcomes
			• Left main (>50%) excluded		• Rates of survival: 89.2% vs 89.8% (P = .48) • Freedom from MACE 77% vs 78.9% (P = .15) Subanalysis (CABG vs OMT) • Rates of survival: 86.4% vs 83.6% (P = .33) • Freedom from MACE 77.5% vs 69% (P = .01) • Medium follow-up 213 days
FAME-2	2010–2012	441 N/A 447	• Stable CAD • CCS class I, II, III or stabilized class IV angina • At least one stenosis in a major coronary artery with an FFR ≤ 0.80 • Left main (>50%) or LVEF < 30% excluded	• Average age 63.5 y • 22% female • 27% diabetic • No angina 11%, CCS class I (20%), II (45%), III (16%), IV (7%) • 1-v CAD (75%), 2-v (21%), 3-v (3%) Prox or mid-LAD (64%) • LVEF > 50% (83%)	• Primary endpoint (FFR-guided PCI vs OMT) • All-cause death, nonfatal MI, or urgent revascularization: 4.3% vs 12.7% (P < .001) Secondary endpoint (PCI vs OMT) • Rate of death 0.2% vs 0.7% (P = .31) • Rate of nonfatal MI 3.4% vs 3.2% (P = .89) • Rate of urgent revascularization 1.6% vs 11.1% (P < .001)
ISCHEMIA	2012–2018	2591 2588 534 1520	• Moderate/severe reversible ischemia on stress test • Nuclear perfusion: ≥10% of myocardium ischemic • Echo ≥ 3/16 walls with stress-induced wall motion abnormalities • cMRI ≥12% of myocardium ischemic	• Average age 64 y • 73% CCTA before randomization • 22.6% female • 41% diabetic • No angina 20.1%, CCS class I (26.7%), II (48.8%), III (4.4%) Anatomy based on CCTA (>50% stenosis)	Medium follow-up 3.2 y Primary endpoint (early revascularization vs Med therapy) • CV death, MI, or hospitalization for unstable angina, heart failure, or resuscitated cardiac arrest 16.4% vs 18.2% (P = .34)

(continued on next page)

Table 3
(continued)

Trial	Study Period	Medical Therapy (n)	CABG (n)	PCI (n)	Enrollment Criteria	Enrollment Characteristics	Major Outcomes
ISCHEMIA - EXTEND	7-y Follow-up of the ISCHEMIA Trial				• ETT: exercise-induced ST segment abnormalities • Left main (>50%) or LVEF < 35% excluded	• 1-v CAD (23.3%), 2-v (31.4%), 3-v (45.1%) Prox or mid-LAD (46.8%) • Medium LVEF 60%	Secondary endpoint (PCI vs OMT) • Rate of death 9% vs 8.3% (95% CI, −1.6–3.1) • Rate of nonfatal MI 10.3% vs 11.9% (95% CI, −3.9–0.7) • Rate of CV death or MI 14.2% vs 16.5% (95% CI, −5.0–0.4) Medium follow-up 5.7 y Early revascularization vs Med therapy • All-cause mortality: 12.7% vs 13.4% (HR 1.0: 95% CI, 0.85–1.18) • CV mortality 6.4% vs 8.6% (HR 0.78: 95% CI 0.63–0.96) • Non-CV mortality 5.6% vs 3.3% (HR 1.44: 95% CI 1.08–1.91)

Abbreviations: BARI 2D, Bypass Angioplasty Revascularization Investigation 2 Diabetes; ETT, exercise tolerance test; MACCE, major adverse cardiac and cerebro-vascular events.

In summary, contemporary RCTs show no survival benefit for revascularization (predominantly PCI) in patients with CCD without high-risk features such as LM disease or a low EF. However, some RCTs support a reduction in the frequency of urgent revascularization, spontaneous MIs, and cardiovascular mortality. Therefore, the 2021 and 2023 guidelines provide a class IIa recommendation for revascularization for multivessel CAD to reduce the risk of cardiovascular (CV) events such as spontaneous MI, need for urgent revascularization, or cardiac death.[4] However, given the only modest impact on outcomes, tempered by the uncertainty outlined above, patients should be counseled cautiously regarding their potential benefit balanced with procedural risks.

REVASCULARIZATION TO IMPROVE SYMPTOMS

A more common indication for revascularization in patients with CCD is to provide symptomatic relief from angina. Multiple randomized controlled trials have shown that revascularization provides improvement in quality-of-life measures in the short and intermediate term compared with medical therapy alone. In COURAGE, participants had relatively low levels of angina with more than 40% having no angina or CCS class I symptoms at the inception of the trial. Nevertheless, the rates of angina were significantly lower in the PCI group throughout the study, though there was a "catch-up" in anginal relief within the conservative arm after 3 years of follow-up.[9] Likewise in FAME-2, participants in the invasive arm had a substantial reduction in CCS II–IV symptoms within 1 month of the study compared with the medical therapy cohort and symptomatic relief remained significant until 5-years of follow-up. In the ISCHEMIA trial, there was minimal symptom benefit in revascularizing patients with very low angina burden; however, there was a significant and durable reduction in symptoms among patients with weekly or more episodes of angina, with a pronounced and statistically significant greater likelihood of being angina free within 3 months of revascularization compared with medical therapy alone. There was also significant improvement in quality-of-life scores in the invasive treatment cohort. The differences persisted through at least 3 years of trial follow-up.[13]

Of note, the participants in these studies were not blinded and there were no sham PCI controls, raising the prospect of a significant placebo effect impacting the results. ORBITA was a small, PCI versus sham-PCI trial that randomized 230 patients with stable ischemic symptoms. Patients eligible for the trial had at least one significant lesion with greater than 70% stenosis. Enrollees were blinded to their treatment assignment, and in the sham arm, a coronary angiogram was performed but no stents were placed. There was no difference in the primary outcome of exercise time or patient-reported symptoms on the Seattle Angina Questionnaire, with the exception of a significant improvement in the number of patients with complete freedom from angina.[14] However, the impact of this trial on practice has been limited, with concerns about the small sample size and relatively low burden of angina at baseline.

The quality-of-life improvement associated with revascularization must be weighed against procedural risk. In addition, many patients can achieve satisfactory angina control on medical therapy alone, obviating the need for PCI or CABG. The Appropriate Use Criteria for PCI therefore indicate that a procedure is appropriate for patients with symptoms who are already on at least two antianginal medications,[15] and the current ACC/AHA guidelines suggest revascularization after a failure of "optimal medical therapy."

REVASCULARIZATION STRATEGY: PERCUTANEOUS CORONARY INTERVENTION VERSUS CORONARY ARTERY BYPASS GRAFTING

PCI and CABG are two distinct techniques to revascularize coronary arteries. Determining the most efficacious revascularization technique in select populations has been the focus of numerous trials, and CABG has generally been shown superior, especially for patients with more severe burden of disease.[16] There are several hypotheses to explain this finding. CABG may be more durable and may more frequently achieve complete revascularization. PCI is focused solely on treating flow-limiting lesions, but CABG provides revascularization to the downstream vessel, which may provide more protection from subsequent MIs. However, CABG is associated with increased procedure-related mortality and stroke. A Heart Team discussion, including cardiac surgeons, interventional cardiologists, and general cardiologists, is recommended for each patient with LM or severe multivessel CAD. This will supplement a shared decision-making process with the patient to select an effective and acceptable revascularization strategy.

Three-Vessel CAD

The SYNTAX trial published in 2009 tested the non-inferiority of PCI compared with CABG in treatment of three-vessel CCD or LM disease. Rates of the major composite endpoint (all-cause death, MI, stroke or repeat revascularization) were significantly higher in the PCI group (17.8% vs 12.4%), with the primary contributor being the rate of repeat revascularization (13.5% vs 5.9%). The rate of death or MI was similar between groups and stroke was more likely to occur with CABG (2.2% vs 0.6%). On subgroup analysis, anatomic complexity was a significant mediator of treatment effect. The investigators developed an angiographic scoring system (the SYNTAX score), and SYNTAX score ≤ 22 identified a low-risk group with equivalent outcomes for PCI and CABG treatment. Among those with the most complex disease (SYNTAX score ≥ 33), there was a significant 23.4% increase in the primary composite endpoint with PCI.[17] In the 10-year follow-up (SYNTAXES), investigators found a persistent increase in all-cause mortality among those in the PCI group with three-vessel disease and a high syntax score (≥ 33). These findings support surgical intervention as the preferred technique for complex three-vessel disease.[18]

FAME-3 reopened the PCI versus CABG question using contemporary PCI equipment and invasive functional assessment. In the PCI cohort, only stenotic lesions found to be significant by FFR (≤ 0.8) were treated with second-generation drug-eluting stents. As in SYNTAX, the 1-year primary composite endpoint (all-cause death, MI, stroke, or repeat revascularization) did not meet non-inferiority for PCI compared with CABG. Likewise, the early differences were driven by repeat revascularization, as the incidence of death, MI, or stroke was not significantly different. Incidence of major bleeding, arrhythmia, and acute kidney injury were higher among CABG patients[16] (Table 4).

Based on these studies, current guidelines recommend CABG (class IIa recommendation) in patients requiring revascularization with multivessel disease with diffuse and complex CAD (syntax score > 33).

Left Main Disease

Although evidence of mortality benefit for revascularization of LM stenosis is limited to CABG, PCI has emerged as a potential alternative for low and intermediate disease complexity. A subgroup analysis of the SYNTAX trial showed patients with LM disease did not have worsening mortality compared with CABG at 5 or 10 years but did have increased revascularization; two other smaller trials, the PRECOMBAT trial (600 patients) and LE MANS trial (105 patients), showed relative equipoise in death, MI, and stroke between CABG and PCI in unprotected LM disease, but neither were powered adequately to show differences in the treatment modalities.[19,20] These results led to the NOBLE and EXCEL trials.

Table 4
Chronic coronary disease: Coronary artery bypass grafting versus percutaneous coronary intervention trials[16,17,22,24,36]

Trial	Study Period	Medical Therapy (n)	CABG (n)	PCI (n)	Enrollment Criteria	Enrollment Characteristics	Major Outcomes
Multi-Vessel CAD: CABG vs PCI							
SYNTAX	2005–2007	N/A	897	903	• ≥50% stenosis in ≥3 coronary arteries and/or left main CAD • Anatomy amenable to PCI or CABG	• Average age 65 y • 28% female • 25.1% diabetes • 39% with left main disease	• 12-mo findings CABG vs PCI • MACCE (death, stroke, MI, repeat revascularization) 12.4% vs 17.8% ($P = .002$) • Rate of death, stroke. MI 7.6% vs 7.7% ($P = .99$) • Rate of repeat revascularization 5.9% vs 13.5% ($P < .001$) MACCE: CABG vs PCI Low SYNTAX (<22) 13.6% vs 14.7 ($P = .71$) Intermediate SYNTAX (23–32): 12.0% vs 16.7% ($P = .10$) High SYNTAX (>32): 10.9% vs 23.4%.($P < .001$)
FREEDOM	2005–2010	N/A	894	956	• Diabetic • Multivessel disease (70% stenosis in 2+ major coronary arteries) • Left main disease excluded	• Average age 63 y • 18% female • 100% diabetes • Mean syntax score 26 • 83% 3-v CAD	Medium follow-up 5 y • Mortality, stroke, or myocardial infarction: 18.7% CABG vs 26.6% PCI ($P < .05$) • Mortality: 10.9% CABG vs 16.3% PCI ($P = .049$) (continued on next page)

Table 4
(continued)

Trial	Study Period	Medical Therapy (n)	CABG (n)	PCI (n)	Enrollment Criteria	Enrollment Characteristics	Major Outcomes
					• Anatomy amenable to PCI or CABG		• Stroke: 5.2% CABG vs 2.4% PCI (P = .03). • MI: 6.0% CABG vs 13.9% PCI (P < .001).
FAME-3	2014–2020	N/A	743	757	• Angiographic evidence of ≥ 50% stenosis ≥ three major coronary arteries • Left main excluded • Anatomy amenable to PCI or CABG • Excluded: LM disease/EF < 30%	• Average age 65 y • 18% female • 29% diabetes • Mean syntax score 26 • FFR of ≤ 0.80 were treated with PCI, in the PCI group the mean number of lesions was 4.3, the mean number of drug-eluting stents was 3.7. • CABG had a mean of 4.2 lesions and received a mean of 3.4 distal anastomoses; 97% received a LIMA and 25% received multiple arterial grafts	12-mo findings CABG vs PCI • MACCE (death, stroke, MI, repeat revascularization) 6.9 vs 10.6% (HR, 1.5; 95% CI, 1.1–2.2; P = .35 for noninferiority) • No between-group differences in the incidence of each individual component of the primary end point
LM: CABG vs PCI							
EXCEL	2010–2014	N/A	957	948 (2nd-gen DES)	• Left main disease (≥70% by angiography, or 50%–70% if hemodynamic significance confirmed by FFR) • Syntax score ≤ 32	• Average age 66 y • 23% female • 29% diabetic • LVEF = 57%	Medium follow-up 5 y • Mortality, stroke, or myocardial infarction (5 y): 19.2% CABG vs 22.0% PCI (P = .13). • Mortality: 9.9% CABG vs 12.0% PCI (P = NS).

NOBLE	2008–2015	N/A	603	598	1st-gen DES (12%) 2nd-gen DES (88%)	• Left main disease ≥50% by angiography, or FFR≤0.8 • Syntax score ≤ 32	• Average age 66 y • 22% female • 15% diabetic • Distal LM 81% • LVEF = 60%

• Any myocardial infarction (third universal definition): 4.7% CABG vs 9.6% PCI ($P < .05$)
• Repeated revascularization: 10.0% CABG vs 16.9% PCI ($P < .05$).

Medium follow-up 5 y
Mortality, stroke, myocardial infarction, or repeated revascularization: 19% CABG vs 28% PCI (superiority $P = .0002$)
• Mortality (5 y): 9% CABG vs 9% PCI ($P = .68$).
• Nonprocedural myocardial infarction: 3% CABG vs 8% PCI ($P = .0002$).
Repeated revascularization (5 y): 10% CABG vs 17% PCI ($P = .0009$)

EXCEL and NOBLE were large, randomized control trials comparing PCI to CABG for LM revascularization. Patients with a high SYNTAX score were excluded in EXCEL but not in NOBLE; nevertheless, the mean SYNTAX score was similar in both studies (21 and 23, respectively). Both trials included patients presenting with ACS and CCD. In EXCEL, PCI met the criteria for non-inferiority compared with CABG.[21] However, in NOBLE, the composite endpoint after 5 years was significantly higher for PCI.[22] Importantly, NOBLE included repeat revascularization in its primary endpoint, whereas EXCEL did not and there were also differences in the definitions of periprocedural MI that have prevented a definitive synthesis of these trials. Considering all available data, CABG is the most durable therapy for coronary revascularization in complex LM stenosis and remains the class I recommendation in current guidelines, whereas PCI is a viable alternative for less complex disease and for patients who are unwilling or unable to undergo surgery.

Patients with Diabetes

Patients with diabetes have a higher risk of cardiovascular events and death with potential for greater benefit of CABG therapy. BARI 2D compared prompt revascularization (either PCI or CABG) + OMT versus OMT alone in patients with diabetes with obstructive CAD. The study overall showed no difference in all-cause mortality or adverse cardiovascular events at 5 years. However, in the prespecified subanalysis, the CABG cohort had a reduction in the combined endpoint of death, MI, and stroke. PCI showed no benefit.[23] In the subsequent FREEDOM trial, patients with diabetes and multivessel disease were randomized to PCI with first-generation drug-eluting stents versus CABG. At 5 years, there was a significant reduction in the primary composite endpoint of all-cause death, MI, and stroke for patients receiving CABG (18.7% vs 26.6%). The benefits of CABG were consistent regardless of SYNTAX score, LVEF, or kidney function.[24] Consequently, the 2023 ACC/AHA guidelines recommend CABG over PCI in patients with diabetes with LAD involvement; PCI as an alternative to CABG is relegated to a 2B recommendation.

CONTROVERSIES AND UNANSWERED QUESTIONS
Coronary Artery Bypass Grafting for Mortality Reduction in Multivessel Chronic Coronary Disease Without Left Main Involvement

In the 2014 ACC/AHA guidelines, CABG was recommended to improve survival for patients with CCD having significant LM stenosis, three-vessel disease and two-vessel disease with proximal LAD involvement regardless of LVEF (class I recommendation). As previously described, these recommendations were based on early-CABG trials and a collection of meta-analyses.[25,26] On the heels of ISCHEMA, the 2021 ACC/AHA/SCAI guidelines for revascularization downgraded a survival benefit for CABG from class I to class IIa in patients with multivessel disease with an LVEF 35% to 50% and to class IIb in patients with normal LV function.[27] The 2023 ACC/AHA CCD guidelines provide a class IIa recommendation to revascularize in these situations, but to reduce cardiovascular events rather than for mortality reduction.[4] Critics however argue that ISCHEMIA was not a trial that compared OMT to CABG, and only a minority of patients received CABG in the invasive arm. Consequently, to compare CABG survival outcomes with medical therapy is observational and is subject to confounding by procedural indication.[28] Moreover, ISCHEMIA was not adequately powered to look at mortality alone. Some clinicians and researchers therefore dispute the downgrade to class II and consider CABG strongly indicated in this population.

Percutaneous Coronary Intervention for Patients Who Are Ineligible for Coronary Artery Bypass Grafting

Some patients with indication for CABG may decline or may be deemed ineligible due to comorbidities or frailty. PCI for these patients received a class IIa recommendation from the 2023 ACC/AHA guideline. The OPTIMUM prospective registry enrolled 726 patients who received high-risk PCI after surgical turndown. All-cause mortality at 30 days was high in this group (5.6%), though lower than estimates of surgical mortality.[29] There are no randomized studies of surgical ineligible patients, but extrapolation from other RCTs (REVIVED-BCIS2, SYNTAX, BARI 2D) would imply that PCI confers modestly less long-term benefit than CABG and may not be superior to medical therapy for prevention of mortality. A patient-centered Heart Team discussion is recommended for these complex cases.

Functional Assessments to Guide Revascularization

As noted above, FFR and related invasive techniques can identify ischemic vessels, permitting "functionally-guided" revascularization that may be superior to angiographic assessment alone. Despite early support for this strategy including the FAME 2 trial described above, more recent RCTs have failed to demonstrate a benefit of routine FFR for selection of revascularization targets for PCI or CABG (RIPCORD-2, FARGO, GRAFFITI, FLOWER-MI).[30] As such, these techniques are likely best reserved for assessment of individual lesions of uncertain functional significance, rather than routine use for assessment and treatment of all coronary vessels.

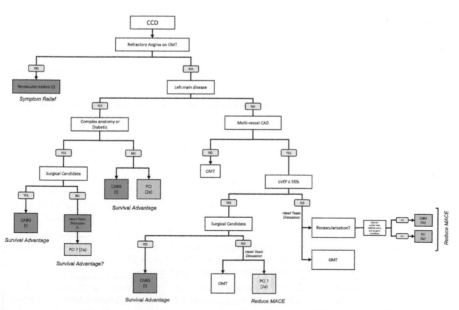

Fig. 1. Proposed pathway to guide revascularization in CCD.[4,27] (*Adapted from* Figure 6: 2021 ACC/AHA/SCAI Guideline for Coronary Artery Revascularization: A Report of the American College of Cardiology/American Heart Association Joint Committee on Clinical Practice Guidelines and modified based on the 2023 American Heart Association (AHA)/American College of Cardiology (ACC) Guideline for the Management of Patients With Chronic Coronary Disease.)

Complete Revascularization

Observational data indicate that patients with residual untreated ischemic vessels after revascularization have worse outcomes than patients who receive complete revascularization.[31] Similarly, complete revascularization has been invoked as an explanation for the superiority of CABG over PCI. It is therefore logical to attempt to optimize revascularization for patients receiving PCI, though similar logic has sometimes failed to translate into successful RCT results for PCI. Achieving complete revascularization may require repeat procedures, more challenging and high-risk techniques, and greater exposure to contrast and radiation. As such, an individualized decision should be made for each patient, considering goals of treatment, risks, and patient preferences.

Table 5
Summary of the 2023 ACC/AHA chronic coronary disease guidelines for revascularization

Chronic Coronary Disease: Indications for Revasculization

COR	LOE	Recommendations
I	A	In patients with CCD and lifestyle-limiting angina despite GDMT and with significant coronary artery stenoses amenable to revascularization, revascularization is recommended to improve symptoms.
I	B-R	In patients with CCD who have significant left main disease or multivessel disease with severe LV dysfunction (LVEF ≤ 35%), CABG in addition to medical therapy is recommended over medical therapy alone to improve survival.
2a	B-NR	In selected patients with CCD and significant left main stenosis for whom PCI can provide equivalent revascularization to that possible with CABG, PCI is reasonable to improve survival.
2a	B-R	In patients with CCD and multivessel CAD appropriate for either CABG or PCI, revascularization in addition to GDMT is reasonable to lower the risk of cardiovascular events such as spontaneous MI, unplanned urgent revascularizations, or cardiac death.

Chronic Coronary Disease: CABG vs PCI

COR	LOE	Recommendations
I	B-R	In patients with CCD who require revascularization for significant left main involvement associated with high-complexity CAD, CABG is recommended in preference to PCI to improve survival.
I	A	In patients with CCD, diabetes, and multivessel CAD with involvement of the LAD who are appropriate candidates for CABG, CABG (with a LIMA) is recommended in preference to PCI to reduce mortality and repeat revascularizations.
2a	B-R	In patients with CCD who require revascularization for multivessel CAD with complex and diffuse CAD (eg, SYNTAX score >33), it is reasonable to choose CABG over PCI to improve survival.
2a	B-NR	In patients with CCD who are appropriate for revascularization but poor candidates for surgery, it is reasonable to choose PCI over CABG to improve symptoms and reduce MACE.

Abbreviations: COR, class of recommendation; LOE, level of evidence.
Adapted from Virani SS, Newby LK, Arnold SV, et al. 2023 AHA/ACC/ACCP/ASPC/NLA/PCNA Guideline for the Management of Patients With Chronic Coronary Disease: A Report of the American Heart Association/American College of Cardiology Joint Committee on Clinical Practice Guidelines. Circulation. 2023;148(9):e9-e119. https://doi.org/10.1161/CIR.0000000000001168

Chronic Total Occlusions

The atherosclerotic process may ultimately progress to complete occlusion of a vessel. There have been substantial advances in PCI for these chronic total occlusions (CTOs) in recent years, resulting in successful revascularization rates of greater than 90% for experienced operators.[32] Improvements in EF and cardiovascular events with CTO intervention are plausible, but the current RCT data are inadequate to assess impact on these clinical outcomes.[33] The 2021 ACC/AHA guideline provides only a class IIb recommendation for CTO intervention for patients with refractory angina.

CASE DECISION-MAKING AND RESOLUTION

Our 77-year-old diabetic patient has two-vessel CCD (including the proximal LAD), normal EF, and shortness of breath that may be an anginal equivalent. Under prior guidelines, CABG would have been a class I indication, but with more recent data, there is not a clear mortality benefit with CABG for this patient. In addition, his advanced age may increase his surgical risk and decrease the likelihood he will benefit from the long-term durability of surgical intervention. Although revascularization may improve his quality of life by reducing his shortness of breath, he has not yet been trialed on an optimal regimen of antianginal medications. Given potential candidacy for CABG, PCI, or a medication-alone strategy, a Heart Team discussion and shared decision-making with the patient are essential. The Heart Team decided both CABG and PCI were technically feasible. Despite having diabetes, his low SYNTAX score and high surgical risk favored PCI. The patient decided for a trial of medical therapy which improved but did not resolve his shortness of breath. PCI was then performed successfully with improvement in symptoms.

The flow diagram (**Fig. 1**) provides a proposed pathway to guide revascularization for CCD.

SUMMARY

Revascularization is an effective adjunct to medical therapy for some patients with CCD. Despite numerous randomized trials, there remains significant uncertainty regarding if and how to revascularize many patients. CABG is a class I indication for patients with significant left main stenosis and multivessel disease with EF $\leq$ 35%. For other patients, clinicians must carefully consider the potential benefits of symptom improvement and reduction of future MI or CV death against the risk and cost of revascularization (**Table 5**). Although guidelines provide a framework for these decisions, each individual patient will have distinct coronary anatomy, clinical factors, and preferences. Decision-making should often involve a multidisciplinary Heart Team discussion and a values-driven discussion with the patient.

DISCLOSURE

Neither author reports any potential financial conflicts of interest.

REFERENCES

1. Mack MJ, Squiers JJ, Lytle BW, et al. Myocardial Revascularization Surgery: JACC Historical Breakthroughs in Perspective. J Am Coll Cardiol 2021;78(4):365–83.
2. Yusuf S, Zucker D, Passamani E, et al. Effect of coronary artery bypass graft surgery on survival: overview of 10-year results from randomised trials by the Coronary Artery Bypass Graft Surgery Trialists Collaboration. Lancet 1994;344(8922):563–70.

3. Jones RH, Kesler K, Phillips HR, et al. Long-term survival benefits of coronary artery bypass grafting and percutaneous transluminal angioplasty in patients with coronary artery disease. J Thorac Cardiovasc Surg 1996;111(5):1013–25.

4. Virani SS, Newby LK, Arnold SV, et al. 2023 AHA/ACC/ACCP/ASPC/NLA/PCNA Guideline for the Management of Patients With Chronic Coronary Disease: A Report of the American Heart Association/American College of Cardiology Joint Committee on Clinical Practice Guidelines. Circulation 2023;148(9):e9–119.

5. Coronary artery surgery study (CASS): a randomized trial of coronary artery bypass surgery. Survival data. Circulation 1983;68(5):939–50.

6. Velazquez EJ, Lee KL, Deja MA, et al. Coronary-Artery Bypass Surgery in Patients with Left Ventricular Dysfunction. N Engl J Med 2011;364(17):1607–16.

7. Velazquez EJ, Lee KL, Jones RH, et al. Coronary-Artery Bypass Surgery in Patients with Ischemic Cardiomyopathy. N Engl J Med 2016;374(16):1511–20.

8. Perera D, Clayton T, O'Kane PD, et al. Percutaneous Revascularization for Ischemic Left Ventricular Dysfunction. N Engl J Med 2022;387(15):1351–60.

9. Boden WE, O'Rourke RA, Teo KK, et al. Optimal Medical Therapy with or without PCI for Stable Coronary Disease. N Engl J Med 2007;356(15):1503–16.

10. De Bruyne B, Pijls NHJ, Kalesan B, et al. Fractional flow reserve-guided PCI versus medical therapy in stable coronary disease. N Engl J Med 2012;367(11):991–1001.

11. Maron DJ, Hochman JS, Reynolds HR, et al. Initial Invasive or Conservative Strategy for Stable Coronary Disease. N Engl J Med 2020;382(15):1395–407.

12. Hochman JS, Anthopolos R, Reynolds HR, et al. Survival After Invasive or Conservative Management of Stable Coronary Disease. Circulation 2023;147(1):8–19.

13. Spertus JA, Jones PG, Maron DJ, et al. Health-Status Outcomes with Invasive or Conservative Care in Coronary Disease. N Engl J Med 2020;382(15):1408–19.

14. Al-Lamee R, Thompson D, Dehbi HM, et al. Percutaneous coronary intervention in stable angina (ORBITA): a double-blind, randomised controlled trial. Lancet 2018;391(10115):31–40.

15. Patel MR, Calhoon JH, Dehmer GJ, et al. ACC/AATS/AHA/ASE/ASNC/SCAI/ SCCT/STS 2017 Appropriate Use Criteria for Coronary Revascularization in Patients With Stable Ischemic Heart Disease: A Report of the American College of Cardiology Appropriate Use Criteria Task Force, American Association for Thoracic Surgery, American Heart Association, American Society of Echocardiography, American Society of Nuclear Cardiology, Society for Cardiovascular Angiography and Interventions, Society of Cardiovascular Computed Tomography, and Society of Thoracic Surgeons. J Am Coll Cardiol 2017;69(17): 2212–41.

16. Fearon WF, Zimmermann FM, De Bruyne B, et al. Fractional Flow Reserve–Guided PCI as Compared with Coronary Bypass Surgery. N Engl J Med 2022; 386(2):128–37.

17. Serruys PW, Morice MC, Kappetein AP, et al. Percutaneous Coronary Intervention versus Coronary-Artery Bypass Grafting for Severe Coronary Artery Disease. N Engl J Med 2009;360(10):961–72.

18. Thuijs DJFM, Kappetein AP, Serruys PW, et al. Percutaneous coronary intervention versus coronary artery bypass grafting in patients with three-vessel or left main coronary artery disease: 10-year follow-up of the multicentre randomised controlled SYNTAX trial. Lancet 2019;394(10206):1325–34.

19. Ahn JM, Roh JH, Kim YH, et al. Randomized Trial of Stents Versus Bypass Surgery for Left Main Coronary Artery Disease: 5-Year Outcomes of the PRECOMBAT Study. J Am Coll Cardiol 2015;65(20):2198–206.

20. Buszman PE, Kiesz SR, Bochenek A, et al. Acute and Late Outcomes of Unprotected Left Main Stenting in Comparison With Surgical Revascularization. J Am Coll Cardiol 2008;51(5):538–45.
21. Stone GW, Sabik JF, Serruys PW, et al. Everolimus-Eluting Stents or Bypass Surgery for Left Main Coronary Artery Disease. N Engl J Med 2016;375(23):2223–35.
22. Mäkikallio T, Holm NR, Lindsay M, et al. Percutaneous coronary angioplasty versus coronary artery bypass grafting in treatment of unprotected left main stenosis (NOBLE): a prospective, randomised, open-label, non-inferiority trial. Lancet 2016;388(10061):2743–52.
23. A Randomized Trial of Therapies for Type 2 Diabetes and Coronary Artery Disease. N Engl J Med 2009;360(24):2503–15.
24. Farkouh ME, Domanski M, Sleeper LA, et al. Strategies for Multivessel Revascularization in Patients with Diabetes. N Engl J Med 2012;367(25):2375–84.
25. Fihn SD, Blankenship JC, Alexander KP, et al. 2014 ACC/AHA/AATS/PCNA/SCAI/STS Focused Update of the Guideline for the Diagnosis and Management of Patients With Stable Ischemic Heart Disease. Circulation 2014;130(19):1749–67.
26. Fihn SD, Gardin JM, Abrams J, et al. 2012 ACCF/AHA/ACP/AATS/PCNA/SCAI/STS Guideline for the Diagnosis and Management of Patients With Stable Ischemic Heart Disease: A Report of the American College of Cardiology Foundation/American Heart Association Task Force on Practice Guidelines, and the American College of Physicians, American Association for Thoracic Surgery, Preventive Cardiovascular Nurses Association, Society for Cardiovascular Angiography and Interventions, and Society of Thoracic Surgeons. J Am Coll Cardiol 2012;60(24):e44–164.
27. 2021 ACC/AHA/SCAI Guideline for Coronary Artery Revascularization: A Report of the American College of Cardiology/American Heart Association Joint Committee on Clinical Practice Guidelines. doi:10.1161/CIR.0000000000001038
28. Bakaeen FG, Ruel M, Calhoon JH, et al. STS/AATS-Endorsed Rebuttal to 2023 ACC/AHA Chronic Coronary Disease Guideline: A Missed Opportunity to Present Accurate and Comprehensive Revascularization Recommendations. Ann Thorac Surg 2023;116(4):675–8.
29. Salisbury AC, Grantham JA, Brown WM, et al. Outcomes of Medical Therapy Plus PCI for Multivessel or Left Main CAD Ineligible for Surgery. JACC Cardiovasc Interv 2023;16(3):261–73.
30. Maznyczka AM, Matthews CJ, Blaxill JM, et al. Fractional Flow Reserve versus Angiography–Guided Management of Coronary Artery Disease: A Meta-Analysis of Contemporary Randomised Controlled Trials. J Clin Med 2022;11(23):7092.
31. Nagaraja V, Ooi S, Nolan J, et al. Impact of Incomplete Percutaneous Revascularization in Patients With Multivessel Coronary Artery Disease: A Systematic Review and Meta-Analysis. J Am Heart Assoc 2016;5(12):e004598.
32. Christopoulos G, Kandzari DE, Yeh RW, et al. Development and Validation of a Novel Scoring System for Predicting Technical Success of Chronic Total Occlusion Percutaneous Coronary Interventions: The PROGRESS CTO (Prospective Global Registry for the Study of Chronic Total Occlusion Intervention) Score. JACC Cardiovasc Interv 2016;9(1):1–9.
33. Megaly M, Buda K, Mashayekhi K, et al. Comparative Analysis of Patient Characteristics in Chronic Total Occlusion Revascularization Studies: Trials vs Real-World Registries. JACC Cardiovasc Interv 2022;15(14):1441–9.

34. Detre K, Murphy MarvinL, Hultgren H. Effect of coronary bypass surgery on longevity in high and low risk patients: Report from the V.A. Cooperative Coronary Surgery Study. Lancet 1977;310(8051):1243–5.
35. Long-term results of prospective randomised study of coronary artery bypass surgery in stable angina pectoris: European Coronary Surgery Study Group. Lancet 1982;320(8309):1173–80.
36. Stone GW, Kappetein AP, Sabik JF, et al. Five-Year Outcomes after PCI or CABG for Left Main Coronary Disease. N Engl J Med 2019;381(19):1820–30.

Antiplatelet Therapy for Patients Who Have Undergone Revascularization Within the Past Year

Which Agents and for How Long?

Khawaja Hassan Akhtar, MD, Usman Baber, MD, MS*

KEYWORDS

- Antiplatelet therapy • Stable ischemic heart disease • P2Y$_{12}$ inhibitors
- Percutaneous coronary intervention • Coronary artery bypass grafting

KEY POINTS

- Clinical guidelines recommend a minimum dual antiplatelet therapy (DAPT) duration of at least 6 months following drug-eluting stent implantation in patients with stable ischemic heart disease undergoing percutaneous coronary intervention, whereas 12 months is mandatory after acute coronary syndrome.
- The use of potent antiplatelet pharmacotherapy reduces ischemic events, albeit with excess bleeding.
- Decisions about duration of antiplatelet therapy after revascularization should include clinical judgment and assessment of the risk of bleeding and ischemic events. To facilitate such decisions, clinicians may rely on validated tools that enable appropriate calibration between patient-level risk and therapeutic intensity.
- Although a minimum duration of DAPT is necessary to prevent early stent-related events, clinical trials have examined continuing antithrombotic therapy with DAPT, dual pathway inhibition comprising aspirin and a low-dose direct oral anticoagulant, and P2Y$_{12}$ inhibitor monotherapy.

INTRODUCTION

The principal goals of myocardial revascularization with either percutaneous coronary intervention (PCI) or coronary artery bypass grafting (CABG) in patients with stable ischemic heart disease (SIHD) or acute coronary syndrome (ACS) are to provide relief of symptoms, prevent future ischemic events, and improve survival.[1,2] Dual antiplatelet therapy (DAPT) with aspirin and a platelet P2Y$_{12}$ inhibitor is universally recommended in

Department of Medicine, Section of Cardiovascular Medicine, University of Oklahoma Health Sciences Center, Oklahoma City, OK 73104, USA
* Corresponding author. Cardiovascular Section, University of Oklahoma Health Sciences Center, 800 Stanton L. Young Boulevard, AAT 5400, Oklahoma City, OK 73104.
E-mail address: usman-baber@ouhsc.edu

Med Clin N Am 108 (2024) 539–551
https://doi.org/10.1016/j.mcna.2023.12.003
0025-7125/24/© 2024 Elsevier Inc. All rights reserved.

all patients after PCI to prevent thrombotic events and reduce ischemic events in patients undergoing CABG.[3–5] However, these salutary benefits are realized at the expense of increased bleeding risk.[5,6] Determining the optimal duration of DAPT that yields the optimal net clinical benefit with respect to lowering thrombosis yet incurring minimal bleeding harm remains an evolving clinical challenge.[6]

Salient factors that inform the intensity and duration of DAPT include clinical presentation (stable vs acute), procedural complexity, time from revascularization, and thrombotic or bleeding risk. At present, clinical practice guidelines (CPGs) recommend a minimum DAPT duration of at least 6 months following drug-eluting stent (DES) implantation in patients with SIHD undergoing PCI. By contrast, ACS patients treated with either PCI or CABG should receive at least 1 year of DAPT.[3,4] Beyond 1 year, patients at high thrombotic risk who have tolerated an initial course of DAPT may be treated with a prolonged duration of antithrombotic pharmacotherapy.[3,4,7] Herein, the authors provide a summary of clinical guidelines and therapeutic strategies focused on identifying the optimal balance between bleeding and thrombotic risk among patients undergoing revascularization.

DUAL ANTIPLATELET THERAPY: CURRENT AGENTS AND RATIONALE OF USE AFTER REVASCULARIZATION

The rationale for DAPT after PCI is to mitigate thrombotic events, the etiology of which varies in relation to time after PCI.[8] Specifically, early events are usually related to procedural and/or technical factors, whereas determinants of later events include systemic factors, such as diabetes mellitus (DM). Risks for stent thrombosis, the most morbid post-PCI event, are highest early after revascularization and attenuate over time.[9] Accordingly, although the clinical imperative for DAPT early after PCI is to prevent culprit lesion and/or stent-related events, the rationale for continued DAPT is to prevent largely non-culprit events that gradually accrue over time.

In this context, the established role of aspirin as the foundation of antiplatelet pharmacotherapy is predicated on its benefits in the secondary prevention of thrombotic events, as compared with placebo.[10] Clopidogrel is an irreversible $P2Y_{12}$ inhibitor and remains the antiplatelet agent of choice as an adjunct to aspirin in patients undergoing revascularization for SIHD.[4,11] The superiority of DAPT over alternative antithrombotic regimens following PCI was established in the Stent Anticoagulation Restenosis Study.[12] In this randomized trial, the safety and efficacy of aspirin alone, aspirin plus warfarin and aspirin plus ticlopidine (a precursor to clopidogrel) was examined in 1965 patients undergoing PCI. The rates of stent thrombosis and composite ischemic events at 30 days were lowest with DAPT, thereby establishing DAPT as the standard-of-care antithrombotic therapy for patients undergoing PCI.[12]

Notwithstanding the established benefits of clopidogrel in the setting of SIHD, variability in pharmacodynamic response and slow onset of action has led to the development of more effective antiplatelet agents.[7,13,14] Potent oral $P2Y_{12}$ inhibitors including prasugrel and ticagrelor are characterized by a much stronger platelet inhibitory effect, yielding significant reductions in thrombotic events as compared with clopidogrel in the setting of ACS.[15–17] In a large randomized trial ($n = 13,608$), prasugrel was superior to clopidogrel with respect to ischemic events among ACS patients undergoing PCI. These benefits were realized at the expense of greater bleeding, including fatal hemorrhage, among those allocated to prasugrel.[18] In a separate trial, ticagrelor-reduced ischemic events as compared with clopidogrel among ACS patients treated medically or with revascularization (CABG or PCI). Although major bleeding was also higher with ticagrelor, rates of fatal bleeding were comparable between groups.[19] Hence, CPGs recommend preferential use of prasugrel or ticagrelor among ACS patients undergoing PCI, whereas ticagrelor or clopidogrel may be used in patients treated medically.[4]

CLINICAL PRACTICE GUIDELINES ON ANTIPLATELET THERAPY AFTER REVASCULARIZATION

The American College of Cardiology (ACC)/American Heart Association (AHA) and the European Society of Cardiology (ESC) Guideline recommendations on DAPT after PCI vary based on the clinical presentation (ACS or SIHD).[3,4] In patient with SIHD undergoing PCI, a loading dose of aspirin (162–325 mg) followed by a maintenance dose of 75 to 100 mg daily is recommended. Initiation of $P2Y_{12}$ inhibitor is usually delayed until coronary anatomy is defined. Clopidogrel is the $P2Y_{12}$ inhibitor of choice in patients with SIHD undergoing PCI. A loading dose of 600 mg followed by a maintenance dose of 75 mg daily is recommended.[3,4,20] In regard to the duration of DAPT after PCI, at least 6 months of DAPT (aspirin and clopidogrel) is the default recommendation (**Table 1**). Among non-high bleeding risk (non-HBR) patients, prolonging DAPT beyond

Table 1
Clinical practice guidelines on antithrombotic therapy among patients with stable ischemic heart disease

Recommendations on Antithrombotic Therapy After Percutaneous Coronary Intervention			
ACC/AHA[4]	COR	ESC[3]	COR
Antiplatelet Agents			
Aspirin (75–100 mg daily) is recommended after PCI in patients with SIHD	I	Aspirin (75–100 mg daily) is recommended after PCI in patients with SIHD	I
Clopidogrel (75 mg daily) is recommended after PCI in patients with SIHD	I	Clopidogrel (75 mg daily) is recommended after PCI in patients with SIHD	I
-	-	Prasugrel or Ticagrelor can be considered as an initial therapy after PCI among patients with a high future thrombotic risk	IIb
Duration of Dual Antiplatelet Therapy			
DAPT (aspirin and clopidogrel) for a duration of 6 mo after PCI	I	DAPT (Aspirin and Clopidogrel) for a duration of 6 mo after PCI	I
Among patients at a high bleeding risk, short duration of DAPT (1–3 mo) followed by monotherapy (preferably aspirin) is recommended	IIb	Among patients at a high bleeding risk, short duration of DAPT (3 mo) followed by monotherapy (preferably aspirin) is recommended	IIa
-	-	Among patients at a very high bleeding risk, short duration of DAPT (1 mo) followed by monotherapy (preferably aspirin) is recommended	IIb
Prolonging DAPT beyond 6 mo may be reasonable to reduce ischemic events among non-HBR patients	IIb	-	-

Abbreviations: ACC, American College of Cardiology; AHA, American Heart Association, COR, class of recommendation; DAPT, dual antiplatelet therapy; ESC, European Society of Cardiology; non-HBR, non-high bleeding risk; PCI, percutaneous coronary intervention; SIHD, stable ischemic heart disease.

6 months may be reasonable to reduce ischemic events, whereas a shorter duration is acceptable for those at HBR.

Among ACS patients treated with PCI, at least 1 year of DAPT is recommended with ticagrelor or prasugrel preferred over clopidogrel.[4] Ticagrelor should be administered as a 180 mg loading dose followed by 90 mg twice daily thereafter. Prasugrel is given as a 60 mg load with a maintenance dose of 10 mg daily. ACS patients with concomitant HBR may be treated with a shorter course of DAPT, whereas non-HBR ACS patients may receive a longer course of antithrombotic therapy.[4,20]

Among patients undergoing CABG, CPGs recommend lifelong use of aspirin (100–325 mg daily) to reduce the risk of adverse cardiovascular events and saphenous vein graft (SVG) closure. Furthermore, in selected patients at low bleeding risk, DAPT with aspirin and $P2Y_{12}$ inhibitor (clopidogrel or ticagrelor) for 1 year can be considered to improve SVG patency.[4,20] A DAPT duration of 1 year is recommended for ACS patients treated with CABG.[4]

BLEEDING AND ISCHEMIC RISK ASSESSMENT

Notwithstanding guideline recommendations, clinical scenarios often require a more nuanced approach to inform therapeutic decisions, particularly with respect to antithrombotic therapy. To facilitate such decisions, clinicians may rely on validated tools to estimate both thrombotic and bleeding risk that enable appropriate calibration between patient-level risk and therapeutic intensity (**Fig. 1**). Indeed, both the US and European guidelines explicitly endorse the concept of formally evaluating the risk benefit calculus *vis-a-vis* antithrombotic therapy using validated scales or established determinants of post-PCI risk.[4,21]

The DAPT trial examined the safety and efficacy of prolonging DAPT beyond 12 months, as compared with aspirin alone, among patients who had undergone PCI and remained event free in the first year after revascularization.[22] Most patients in the experimental arm were treated with clopidogrel-based DAPT. In the overall

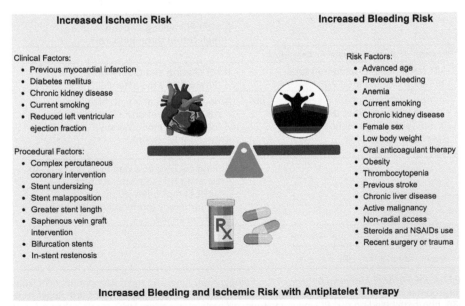

Fig. 1. Risk factors associated with increased ischemic and bleeding risk with antiplatelet therapy. (Created with BioRender.com.)

cohort extending DAPT significantly reduced the co-primary efficacy endpoints of major adverse cardiovascular and cerebrovascular events (MACCE) (4.3% and 5.9%, respectively, $P <$ .001) and definite/probable stent thrombosis (0.4% and 1.4%, respectively, $P <$ .001), whereas major bleeding was increased (2.5% and 1.6%, respectively, $P =$ .001).[22] Yeh and colleagues derived and validated a prediction rule from the study cohort to identify those patients who realized a net clinical benefit (ie, less thrombosis without excess bleeding) with extending DAPT beyond 1 year.[23] Factors associated with greater benefit included DM, prior myocardial infarction (MI) or prior PCI, current cigarette use, congestive heart failure or left ventricular ejection fraction less than 30%, SVG PCI, and stent diameter less than 3 mm, whereas age more than 65 years attenuated the treatment effect of extended DAPT (**Table 2**). Patients with a DAPT score of 2 or higher, which comprised approximately 51% of the trial cohort, realized the greatest benefit with prolonging DAPT compared with their counterparts with a lower DAPT score.[23]

Another useful scoring system to predict the risk of thrombotic and bleeding events is the Patterns of Non-Adherence to Anti-Platelet Regimen in Stented Patients (PARIS) score, derived from the eponymous study.[24] In contrast to the DAPT prediction rule, the PARIS score was constructed from a usual care PCI registry with a 2-year follow-up. Given differences in study design and derivation cohorts, it is not surprising that correlates of thrombosis and bleeding vary somewhat between the DAPT trial and PARIS registry. Specifically, unique correlates of bleeding that emerged from the PARIS study included anemia, use of oral anticoagulation, and body mass index (BMI) (see **Table 2**). However, as a non-randomized study, the effect of different DAPT durations on thrombotic and bleeding risk could not be estimated from the PARIS registry.[24]

Alternative approaches to inform decisions surrounding the duration and/or intensity of antiplatelet therapy consider bleeding or ischemic risk exclusively. With respect to the former, the Predicting Bleeding Complications in Patients Undergoing Stent Implantation and Subsequent Dual Anti-Platelet Therapy (PRECISE-DAPT) score was derived from a patient-level pooled analysis of eight clinical trials ($n = 14,963$) examining the effect of long (12–24 months) versus short (3–6 months) DAPT durations.[25] Constructed to predict the risk of out of hospital bleeding, the PRECISE-DAPT score considers the following five variables: age, creatinine clearance, hemoglobin, white blood cell count, and prior spontaneous bleeding (see **Table 2**). Among patients at elevated bleeding risk (score $\geq$ 25), a prolonged DAPT duration resulted in excess bleeding without ischemic benefit. whereas in those at lower bleeding risk, an ischemic benefit was observed (p interaction [p_{int}] = 0.007).[25]

In regard to the latter, several studies have identified correlates of anatomic or PCI complexity that independently associate with excess ischemic risk. In a pooled analysis of six randomized trials ($n = 9577$), the effect of different DAPT durations was examined in relation to PCI complexity.[26] In this analysis, PCI complexity was defined as PCI involving at least one of the following: 3 vessels treated, $\geq$ 3 stents implanted, $\geq$ 3 lesions treated, bifurcation with 2 stents implanted, total stent length > 60 mm, or chronic total occlusion. PCI complexity was associated with excess thrombotic, but not bleeding, risk in the overall cohort. Moreover, extending DAPT beyond 12 months resulted in an accentuated reduction in major adverse cardiovascular events (MACE) among those with versus without PCI complexity ($p_{int} = 0.01$).[26]

ANTITHROMBOTIC STRATEGIES

Despite the availability of multiple scales to estimate bleeding and thrombotic risk, clinicians must couple a patient's unique risk profile to an individualized therapeutic

Table 2
Risk scoring systems for bleeding and ischemic risk assessment

| Scale | Factors | | Discrimination (C-Statistics) | | Cohorts | |
	Thrombosis	Bleeding	Derivation	Validation	Derivation	Validation
DAPT	Current smoking Diabetes mellitus MI at presentation Prior PCI/prior MI Stent diameter <3 mm Paclitaxel-eluting stent CHF/LVEF <30% SVG PCI	Advanced age	Ischemia: 0.70 Bleeding: 0.68	Ischemia: 0.64 Bleeding: 0.64	RCT	RCT
PARIS	Diabetes mellitus ACS Current smoking CrCl <60 mL/min Prior PCI Prior CABG	Advanced age BMI (<25 or >35) Current smoking Anemia CrCl <60 mL/min Triple therapy on discharge	Ischemia: 0.70 Bleeding: 0.72	Ischemia: 0.65 Bleeding: 0.64	Registry	Registry
PRECISE-DAPT	N/A	Advanced age CrCl Hemoglobin WBC count Prior spontaneous bleeding	Bleeding: 0.73	Bleeding (RCT): 0.70 Bleeding (Registry): 0.66	Meta-analysis of RCTs	RCT and registry

The DAPT Score: Patients with a high DAPT score (DAPT score ≥2) may benefit from a prolonged course of DAPT up to 30 mo after PCI.
 The PARIS Score: For prediction of coronary thrombotic events, the score ranges from 0 to 10 (low risk: 0–2; intermediate risk: 3–4; high risk ≥ 5). For prediction of major bleeding, the score ranges from 0 to 14 (low risk: 0–3; intermediate risk: 4–7; high risk: ≥ 8).
 The PRECISE-DAPT Score: Among patients at elevated bleeding risk (score ≥ 25), prolonged DAPT may result in excess bleeding without ischemic benefit.
 Abbreviations: ACS, acute coronary syndrome; BMI, body mass index; CABG, coronary artery bypass grafting; CHF, congestive heart failure; CrCl, creatinine clearance; LVEF, left ventricular ejection fraction; MI, myocardial infarction; ml, milliliters; mm, millimeters; PCI, percutaneous coronary intervention; RCT, randomized controlled trial; SVG, saphenous vein graft; WBC, white blood cell count.

treatment. In this regard, although a minimum duration of DAPT is necessary to pre-vent early stent-related events, thrombotic risk continues to accrue in many patients after PCI.[7,22] Although aspirin was traditionally considered sufficient for long-term sec-ondary prevention after PCI, emerging evidence has challenged this paradigm. Spe-cifically, clinical trials have tested the following strategies for long-term secondary prevention: prolonged DAPT, dual pathway inhibition (DPI) comprising aspirin and a low-dose direct oral anticoagulant (DOAC), and P2Y$_{12}$ inhibitor monotherapy (**Fig. 2**).

DUAL ANTIPLATELET THERAPY

The benefits of clopidogrel or ticagrelor-based DAPT with respect to preventing thrombotic events seem most pronounced among those with a history of MI or DM. For example, absolute reductions in stent thrombosis (1.4% vs 0.7%) and MACCE (2.9% vs 0.9%) with extended DAPT were larger in magnitude among those with versus without MI randomized in the DAPT trial.[22] In contrast, the incremental absolute increase in bleeding risk with continued DAPT was comparable between groups (1.1% vs 0.9%), suggesting a greater net clinical benefit with extending DAPT in the setting of prior MI and PCI.[22]

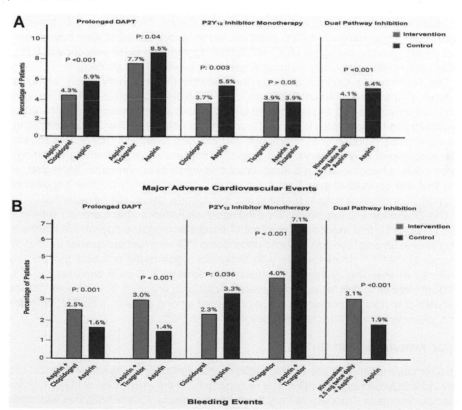

Fig. 2. Effect of different strategies of antithrombotic therapy on ischemic and bleeding events. Bar graphs display the observed rates of major adverse cardiovascular events (A) and major bleeding events (B) with different strategies of antithrombotic therapy. Rates of adverse events for prolonged DAPT based on DAPT and THEMIS trials; P2Y$_{12}$ inhibitor monotherapy from the HOST-EXAM and TWILIGHT trials and for DPI the COMPASS trial. (Created with BioRender.com.)

These findings were extended to ticagrelor-based DAPT in the Prevention of Cardio-vascular Events in Patients with Prior Heart Attack Using Ticagrelor Compared to Placebo on a Background of Aspirin–Thrombolysis in Myocardial Infarction 54 trial.[27] In this randomized study ($n = 21,162$), stable patients with a prior history of MI receiving aspirin were randomized to ticagrelor 90 mg twice daily, ticagrelor 60 mg twice daily, or placebo, respectively. Both doses of ticagrelor were superior to placebo with respect to the primary endpoint of cardiovascular death, MI, or stroke. Although major bleeding was increased with ticagrelor, the absolute increase was slightly lower with the 60 mg bid dosing. Importantly, fatal bleeding or intracranial hemorrhage (ICH) was not increased with ticagrelor.[27]

The effect of ticagrelor versus placebo among patients with DM and SIHD without a prior history of stroke or MI was examined in the THEMIS (A Study Comparing Cardio-vascular Effects of Ticagrelor vs Placebo in Patients with Type 2 Diabetes Mellitus) trial.[28] Among the trial cohort, approximately 58% presented with a prior history of PCI. In the PCI subgroup, ticagrelor resulted in a net clinical benefit, whereas the treatment effect was neutral in the absence of prior PCI ($p_{int} = 0.012$).[29]

MONOTHERAPY WITH P2Y$_{12}$ INHIBITORS

An evolving framework for post-PCI antiplatelet therapy involves the withdrawal of aspirin with continuation of a P2Y$_{12}$ inhibitor alone. Experimental studies have shown that aspirin exerts a negligible effect on platelet aggregation in the presence of P2Y$_{12}$ inhibitor blockade, providing a strong physiologic basis for this strategy.[30]

The Harmonizing Optimal Strategy for Treatment of coronary artery stenosis-Extended Antiplatelet Monotherapy (HOST-EXAM) trial randomized 5438 patients who had undergone PCI and maintained DAPT without any major ischemic or bleeding events for 6 to 18 months to clopidogrel or aspirin monotherapy. Over 2 years, clopidog-rel significantly reduced both thrombotic and bleeding events.[31] This result suggests that clopidogrel may preserve physiologic hemostasis while preventing pathologic thrombosis, a hypothesis that is speculative and warrants confirmation. Moreover, as this trial was conducted in an East Asian cohort, generalizability to other populations with different baseline risks in bleeding and thrombosis should not be assumed.

The Ticagrelor with Aspirin or Alone in High-Risk Patients after Coronary Intervention (TWILIGHT) trial examined the effect of ticagrelor monotherapy versus ticagrelor plus aspirin among high-risk patients undergoing PCI who had completed a 3-month course of DAPT.[32] Monotherapy with ticagrelor significantly reduced the primary endpoint of Bleeding Academic Research Consortium 2, 3 or 5 bleeding by 44% without increasing risk for ischemic events. Additional analyses have shown that the benefits of ticagrelor monotherapy are preserved among patients with DM, complex PCI, or undergoing PCI for non-ST elevation ACSs.[33–35]

DUAL PATHWAY INHIBITION

An alternative antithrombotic strategy after revascularization involves the addition of a low-dose DOAC to aspirin or DPI. The Rivaroxaban for the Prevention of Major Cardio-vascular Events in Coronary or Peripheral Artery Disease (COMPASS) trial examined the effect of adding rivaroxaban 2.5 mg twice daily to aspirin among patients with stable CAD, peripheral artery disease, or both.[36] The trial cohort was enriched with ischemic risk as approximately 20% presented with polyvascular disease and prior MI was present in more than 60%. Over 23 months, rivaroxaban plus aspirin reduced MACE and all-cause mortality by 26% and 23%, respectively. Although major bleeding was increased with rivaroxaban, fatal bleeding or ICH was comparable between groups.

Findings from the overall trial were consistent among those COMPASS participants with a history of PCI ($p_{int} = 0.85$).[36,37]

HIGH BLEEDING RISK PATIENT

The Academic Research Consortium defines HBR based on fulfilling at least one major or two minor criteria with an estimated annualized risk of major bleeding of at least 4%.[38] The HBR phenotype is prevalent among PCI cohorts and its presence confers increased risk for both thrombotic and bleeding events, rendering decisions surrounding duration and intensity of DAPT very difficult.[39] Prior studies suggest that increased exposure to DAPT among HBR patients, even those with elevated thrombotic risk, incurs bleeding harm without ischemic benefit.[40] To formally test this hypothesis, the Management of High Bleeding Risk Patients Post Bioresorbable Polymer Coated Stent Implantation with an Abbreviated Versus Prolonged DAPT Regimen trial randomized HBR patients undergoing PCI treated with 1 month of DAPT to an abbreviated antiplatelet strategy consisting of antiplatelet monotherapy versus continued DAPT for at least two additional months.[41] Over 1 year, the abbreviated strategy resulted in significantly less bleeding (6.5% vs 9.4%; *P*<.001) while maintaining noninferiority for ischemic events (6.1% vs 5.9%; $p_{NI} = 0.001$).[41]

ANTITHROMBOTIC FRAMEWORK

As shown in **Fig. 3**, decisions surrounding the duration and intensity of antithrombotic therapy following PCI may be approached by considering clinical presentation and evaluating thrombotic and bleeding risk (see **Fig. 3**). Among ACS patients deemed HBR, a short (1–3) month course of DAPT is reasonable followed by aspirin or clopidogrel monotherapy. This approach is endorsed by studies showing that longer durations of DAPT in the setting of HBR yield net clinical harm (ie, more bleeding without ischemic reduction). In the absence of HBR, ACS patients may be treated with a default strategy of ticagrelor or prasugrel-based DAPT for 1 year. An alternative bleeding reduction strategy is 3 months of DAPT followed by P2Y$_{12}$ inhibitor monotherapy. The evidence for the latter is most evident with use of ticagrelor monotherapy.

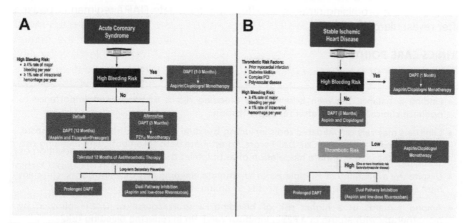

Fig. 3. Clinical algorithm for choice of antiplatelet therapy after percutaneous coronary intervention. (*A*) Clinical algorithm among patients with acute coronary syndrome and (*B*) clinical algorithm among patients with stable ischemic heart disease. (Created with BioRender.com.)

ACS patients who have tolerated at least 1 year of antithrombotic therapy may then be considered for long-term secondary prevention with either continued DAPT or DPI.

Analogously, patients with SIHD undergoing PCI should be evaluated by first considering bleeding risk. Among those with HBR, a 1-month course of DAPT followed by single antiplatelet therapy is reasonable. In the absence of HBR, a default DAPT strategy of clopidogrel-based DAPT for 6 months is appropriate. After 6 months of DAPT, patients may be considered candidates for more intense antithrombotic therapy according to thrombotic risk. For those patients with at least one additional thrombotic risk factor, continued DAPT or DPI is appropriate. In the absence of additional thrombotic risk factors, monotherapy with either aspirin or clopidogrel seems reasonable.

An unanswered and important clinical question relates to the optimal duration of long-term antithrombotic therapy for secondary prevention. Based on existing trials, the relative benefits of prolonged DAPT, DPI, or $P2Y_{12}$ inhibitor monotherapy persist for up to 3 years. However, the durability of this benefit is unknown as the absolute risk for recurrent ischemic events tends to attenuate over time. By contrast, the absolute risk for bleeding tends to accrue in a monotonic fashion with ongoing exposure to antiplatelet therapy.

Another important consideration that remains unanswered is the relative merits of different antithrombotic strategies. At present, existing trials have generally compared antithrombotic strategies to either aspirin monotherapy or DAPT. Direct comparative trials examining the safety and efficacy of different strategies to one another remain an ongoing area of clinical investigation.

SUMMARY

Finding a balance between ischemic and bleeding risk is of paramount importance to optimize future outcomes. Among patients at a higher risk of future bleeding, a short course of DAPT followed by monotherapy with aspirin or a $P2Y_{12}$ inhibitor can help in reducing bleeding risk while minimizing the risk of ischemic events. In the absence of a high bleeding risk, patients at an increased ischemic risk may benefit from prolonging the course of DAPT or by using DPI strategy. An integrated approach using risk scoring systems and individualized assessment of clinical and procedural factors provides the most promising strategy to effectively modulate DAPT regimen in patients after revascularization.

CLINICS CARE POINTS

- Finding a balance between ischemic and bleeding risk is of paramount importance to optimize clinical outcomes after revascularization.
- Clinicians may rely on validated tools including the dual antiplatelet therapy (DAPT) score, the PARIS score, or the PRECISE-DAPT score, to estimate both thrombotic and bleeding risk that can assist in appropriate modulation of antiplatelet therapy.
- Despite the availability of multiple scales to estimate bleeding and thrombotic risk, clinicians must couple a patient's unique risk profile to an individualized therapeutic treatment.
- Among patients at a higher risk of bleeding, a short course of DAPT followed by monotherapy with aspirin or a $P2Y_{12}$ inhibitor can help in reducing bleeding risk.
- Patients at an increased ischemic risk may benefit from prolonging the course of DAPT or by using dual pathway inhibition strategy.

DISCLOSURE

U. Baber: Honoraria/Consulting fees from Amgen, AstraZeneca, Boston Scientific, and Abbott. This research did not receive any funding from agencies in the public, commercial, or not-for-profit sectors.

REFERENCES

1. Virani SS, Newby LK, Arnold SV, et al. 2023 AHA/ACC/ACCP/ASPC/NLA/PCNA Guideline for the Management of Patients With Chronic Coronary Disease: A Report of the American Heart Association/American College of Cardiology Joint Committee on Clinical Practice Guidelines. Circulation 2023;148(9):e9–119.
2. Doenst T, Haverich A, Serruys P, et al. PCI and CABG for Treating Stable Coronary Artery Disease: JACC Review Topic of the Week. J Am Coll Cardiol 2019; 73(8):964–76.
3. Knuuti J, Wijns W, Saraste A, et al. 2019 ESC Guidelines for the diagnosis and management of chronic coronary syndromes. Eur Heart J 2020;41(3):407–77.
4. Levine GN, Bates ER, Bittl JA, et al. 2016 ACC/AHA Guideline Focused Update on Duration of Dual Antiplatelet Therapy in Patients With Coronary Artery Disease: A Report of the American College of Cardiology/American Heart Association Task Force on Clinical Practice Guidelines: An Update of the 2011 ACCF/AHA/SCAI Guideline for Percutaneous Coronary Intervention, 2011 ACCF/AHA Guideline for Coronary Artery Bypass Graft Surgery, 2012 ACC/AHA/ACP/AATS/PCNA/ SCAI/STS Guideline for the Diagnosis and Management of Patients With Stable Ischemic Heart Disease, 2013 ACCF/AHA Guideline for the Management of ST-Elevation Myocardial Infarction, 2014 AHA/ACC Guideline for the Management of Patients With Non-ST-Elevation Acute Coronary Syndromes, and 2014 ACC/ AHA Guideline on Perioperative Cardiovascular Evaluation and Management of Patients Undergoing Noncardiac Surgery. Circulation 2016;134(10):e123–55.
5. Warren J, Baber U, Mehran R. Antiplatelet therapy after drug-eluting stent implantation. J Cardiol 2015;65(2):98–104.
6. Capodanno D, Mehran R, Krucoff MW, et al. Defining strategies of modulation of antiplatelet therapy in patients with coronary artery disease: a consensus document from the academic research consortium. Circulation 2023;147(25):1933–44.
7. Angiolillo DJ, Galli M, Collet JP, et al. Antiplatelet therapy after percutaneous coronary intervention. EuroIntervention 2022;17(17):e1371–96.
8. Dangas GD, Claessen BE, Mehran R, et al. Development and validation of a stent thrombosis risk score in patients with acute coronary syndromes. JACC Cardiovasc Interv 2012;5(11):1097–105.
9. Waksman R, Kirtane AJ, Torguson R, et al. Correlates and outcomes of late and very late drug-eluting stent thrombosis: results from DESERT (International Drug-Eluting Stent Event Registry of Thrombosis). JACC Cardiovasc Interv 2014;7(10): 1093–102.
10. Antithrombotic Trialists' Collaboration. Collaborative meta-analysis of randomised trials of antiplatelet therapy for prevention of death, myocardial infarction, and stroke in high risk patients. BMJ 2002;324(7329):71–86. https://doi.org/10.1136/ bmj.324.7329.71.
11. Colombo A, Chieffo A, Frasheri A, et al. Second-generation drug-eluting stent implantation followed by 6- versus 12-month dual antiplatelet therapy: the SECURITY randomized clinical trial. J Am Coll Cardiol 2014;64(20):2086–97.

12. Leon MB, Baim DS, Popma JJ, et al. A clinical trial comparing three antithrombotic-drug regimens after coronary-artery stenting. Stent Anticoagulation Restenosis Study Investigators. N Engl J Med 1998;339(23):1665–71.
13. Gurbel PA, Bliden KP, Hiatt BL, et al. Clopidogrel for coronary stenting: response variability, drug resistance, and the effect of pretreatment platelet reactivity. Circulation 2003;107(23):2908–13.
14. Sibbing D, Aradi D, Alexopoulos D, et al. Updated Expert Consensus Statement on Platelet Function and Genetic Testing for Guiding P2Y12 Receptor Inhibitor Treatment in Percutaneous Coronary Intervention. JACC Cardiovasc Interv 2019;12(16):1521–37.
15. Franchi F, Angiolillo DJ. Novel antiplatelet agents in acute coronary syndrome. Nat Rev Cardiol 2015;12(1):30–47.
16. Wiviott SD, Trenk D, Frelinger AL, et al. Prasugrel compared with high loading- and maintenance-dose clopidogrel in patients with planned percutaneous coronary intervention: the Prasugrel in Comparison to Clopidogrel for Inhibition of Platelet Activation and Aggregation-Thrombolysis in Myocardial Infarction 44 trial. Circulation 2007;116(25):2923–32.
17. Gurbel PA, Bliden KP, Butler K, et al. Randomized double-blind assessment of the ONSET and OFFSET of the antiplatelet effects of ticagrelor versus clopidogrel in patients with stable coronary artery disease: the ONSET/OFFSET study. Circulation 2009;120(25):2577–85.
18. Wiviott SD, Braunwald E, McCabe CH, et al. Prasugrel versus clopidogrel in patients with acute coronary syndromes. N Engl J Med 2007;357(20):2001–15.
19. Wallentin L, Becker RC, Budaj A, et al. Ticagrelor versus clopidogrel in patients with acute coronary syndromes. N Engl J Med 2009;361(11):1045–57.
20. Lawton JS, Tamis-Holland JE, Bangalore S, et al. 2021 ACC/AHA/SCAI Guideline for Coronary Artery Revascularization: Executive Summary: A Report of the American College of Cardiology/American Heart Association Joint Committee on Clinical Practice Guidelines. Circulation 2022;145(3):e4–17.
21. Valgimigli M, Bueno H, Byrne RA, et al. 2017 ESC focused update on dual antiplatelet therapy in coronary artery disease developed in collaboration with EACTS: The Task Force for dual antiplatelet therapy in coronary artery disease of the European Society of Cardiology (ESC) and of the European Association for Cardio-Thoracic Surgery (EACTS). Eur Heart J 2018;39(3):213–60.
22. Mauri L, Kereiakes DJ, Yeh RW, et al. Twelve or 30 months of dual antiplatelet therapy after drug-eluting stents. N Engl J Med 2014;371(23):2155–66.
23. Yeh RW, Secemsky EA, Kereiakes DJ, et al. Development and Validation of a Prediction Rule for Benefit and Harm of Dual Antiplatelet Therapy Beyond 1 Year After Percutaneous Coronary Intervention. JAMA 2016;315(16):1735–49.
24. Baber U, Mehran R, Giustino G, et al. Coronary Thrombosis and Major Bleeding After PCI With Drug-Eluting Stents: Risk Scores From PARIS. J Am Coll Cardiol 2016;67(19):2224–34.
25. Costa F, van Klaveren D, James S, et al. Derivation and validation of the predicting bleeding complications in patients undergoing stent implantation and subsequent dual antiplatelet therapy (PRECISE-DAPT) score: a pooled analysis of individual-patient datasets from clinical trials. Lancet 2017;389(10073):1025–34.
26. Giustino G, Chieffo A, Palmerini T, et al. Efficacy and Safety of Dual Antiplatelet Therapy After Complex PCI. J Am Coll Cardiol 2016;68(17):1851–64.
27. Bonaca MP, Bhatt DL, Cohen M, et al. Long-term use of ticagrelor in patients with prior myocardial infarction. N Engl J Med 2015;372(19):1791–800.

28. Steg PG, Bhatt DL, Simon T, et al. Ticagrelor in Patients with Stable Coronary Disease and Diabetes. N Engl J Med 2019;381(14):1309–20.
29. Bhatt DL, Steg PG, Mehta SR, et al. Ticagrelor in patients with diabetes and stable coronary artery disease with a history of previous percutaneous coronary intervention (THEMIS-PCI): a phase 3, placebo-controlled, randomised trial. Lancet 2019;394(10204):1169–80.
30. Capodanno D, Mehran R, Valgimigli M, et al. Aspirin-free strategies in cardiovascular disease and cardioembolic stroke prevention. Nat Rev Cardiol 2018;15(8): 480–96.
31. Koo BK, Kang J, Park KW, et al. Aspirin versus clopidogrel for chronic maintenance monotherapy after percutaneous coronary intervention (HOST-EXAM): an investigator-initiated, prospective, randomised, open-label, multicentre trial. Lancet 2021;397(10293):2487–96.
32. Mehran R, Baber U, Sharma SK, et al. Ticagrelor with or without Aspirin in High-Risk Patients after PCI. N Engl J Med 2019;381(21):2032–42.
33. Angiolillo DJ, Baber U, Mehran R. Ticagrelor monotherapy in patients with diabetes mellitus undergoing percutaneous coronary interventions: insights from the TWILIGHT trial. Cardiovasc Res 2020;116(7):e70–2.
34. Dangas G, Baber U, Sharma S, et al. Ticagrelor With or Without Aspirin After Complex PCI. J Am Coll Cardiol 2020;75(19):2414–24.
35. Baber U, Dangas G, Angiolillo DJ, et al. Ticagrelor alone vs. ticagrelor plus aspirin following percutaneous coronary intervention in patients with non-ST-segment elevation acute coronary syndromes: TWILIGHT-ACS. Eur Heart J 2020;41(37):3533–45.
36. Eikelboom JW, Connolly SJ, Bosch J, et al. Rivaroxaban with or without Aspirin in Stable Cardiovascular Disease. N Engl J Med 2017;377(14):1319–30.
37. Connolly SJ, Eikelboom JW, Bosch J, et al. Rivaroxaban with or without aspirin in patients with stable coronary artery disease: an international, randomised, double-blind, placebo-controlled trial. Lancet 2018;391(10117):205–18.
38. Urban P, Mehran R, Colleran R, et al. Defining High Bleeding Risk in Patients Undergoing Percutaneous Coronary Intervention. Circulation 2019;140(3):240–61.
39. Cao D, Mehran R, Dangas G, et al. Validation of the Academic Research Consortium High Bleeding Risk Definition in Contemporary PCI Patients. J Am Coll Cardiol 2020;75(21):2711–22.
40. Costa F, Van Klaveren D, Feres F, et al. Dual Antiplatelet Therapy Duration Based on Ischemic and Bleeding Risks After Coronary Stenting. J Am Coll Cardiol 2019; 73(7):741–54.
41. Valgimigli M, Frigoli E, Heg D, et al. Dual Antiplatelet Therapy after PCI in Patients at High Bleeding Risk. N Engl J Med 2021;385(18):1643–55.

Medical Decision-Making and Revascularization in Ischemic Cardiomyopathy

Alex J. Chang, MD[a], Yilin Liang, MD, MPH[a],
Steven A. Hamilton, MD[b], Andrew P. Ambrosy, MD[b,c],*

KEYWORDS

- Ischemic cardiomyopathy • Coronary artery disease • Heart failure
- Revascularization • Percutaneous coronary intervention
- Coronary artery bypass grafting • Myocardial viability

KEY POINTS

- Ischemic cardiomyopathy (ICM) remains a complex and prevalent form of heart disease, and early diagnosis and comprehensive management strategies are essential in improving outcomes.
- Treatment modalities for patients with heart failure and ICM have significantly advanced.
- While robust and compelling evidence supports optimal medical therapy (OMT) and surgical revascularization in this high-risk patient population, the role of percutaneous coronary intervention (PCI) and routinely assessing viability to guide patient selection remains controversial.

INTRODUCTION

Ischemic cardiomyopathy (ICM) is the most common cause of heart failure (HF) in the United States and presents a significant burden on health care systems and patient quality of life.[1] It is a well-recognized and well-studied clinical entity, as there have been significant advances in the evaluation and management of ICM over the past 2 decades. However, despite this growing body of evidence, several areas remain controversial and uncertain. This review aims to provide a comprehensive overview

[a] Department of Medicine, Kaiser Permanente San Francisco Medical Center, 2425 Geary Boulevard, San Francisco, CA 94115, USA; [b] Department of Cardiology, Kaiser Permanente San Francisco Medical Center, 2425 Geary Boulevard, San Francisco, CA 94115, USA; [c] Clinical Trials Program, Division of Research, Kaiser Permanente Northern California, 2000 Broadway, Oakland, CA 94612, USA
* Corresponding author. Clinical Trials Program, Division of Research, Kaiser Permanente Northern California, 2000 Broadway, Oakland, CA 94612.
E-mail address: andrew.p.ambrosy@kp.org
Twitter: @KPHeartDoc (A.P.A.)

Med Clin N Am 108 (2024) 553–566
https://doi.org/10.1016/j.mcna.2023.11.007
0025-7125/24/© 2023 Elsevier Inc. All rights reserved.

medical.theclinics.com

of the current understanding of ICM, encompassing its epidemiology, diagnostic approaches, and management strategies with a focus on coronary revascularization.

DEFINITION OF ISCHEMIC CARDIOMYOPATHY

The traditional definition of ICM was the presence of any epicardial coronary vessels with ≥75% stenosis or any history of myocardial infarction (MI) or coronary revascularization, either via percutaneous coronary intervention (PCI) or coronary artery bypass grafting (CABG).[2] While simple, this definition did not consider the wide spectrum of coronary artery disease (CAD) and how outcomes can change based on the number of vessels affected and the anatomic distribution of CAD (ie, left main CAD). A widely cited observational study in 2002 aimed to establish a more comprehensive definition of ICM by examining the prognostic power associated with varying degrees of CAD.[2] They found that more extensive CAD was independently associated with reduced survival. Furthermore, they found that reclassifying certain CAD distributions (ie, 1-vessel vs 2-vessel vs 3-vessel CAD) into ICM versus nonischemic cardiomyopathy (NICM) improved prognostic power. Thus, the authors propose the following definition of ICM as a comprehensive consensus definition that should be standardized and utilized for both patient care and research purposes (**Box 1**).

EPIDEMIOLOGY, CLINICAL CHARACTERISTICS, AND OUTCOMES

HF continues to represent a significant burden to the health care system and society. In the United States, the prevalence of HF is 6.7 million, and the incidence is 1 million new cases per year. It has been previously estimated that by 2030, the prevalence of HF in the US will be >8 million.[3,4] In 2019, greater than 1 million hospital discharges were attributed to a principal diagnosis of HF.[5] The medical cost of HF is expected to increase from $20.9 billion to $53.1 billion in 2030, with the largest proportion of cost attributed to inpatient hospitalizations.[6] Overall, HF survival has increased due to improvements in background medical therapy for HF, though recent population data have suggested survival rates have begun to plateau.[4]

HF etiologies are divided into 2 general categories: ICM and NICM. ICM has been found to account for approximately 60% to 70% of patients with HF and left ventricular systolic dysfunction.[1,7] Patients with ICM tend to be older and have more comorbidities commonly associated with CAD, such as diabetes, hypertension, hyperlipidemia, chronic kidney disease, and peripheral artery disease.[8,9] Patients with NICM tend to have lower left ventricular ejection fraction (LVEF) and higher rates of atrial fibrillation.[8,9] When compared to NICM, ICM has been shown to be independently

---

Box 1
Definition of ischemic cardiomyopathy

Left Ventricular Ejection Fraction ≤40% and ≥1 of the following
- ≥75% stenosis of ≥2 coronary arteries
- ≥75% stenosis of:
  ○ Left Main Coronary Artery or Proximal Left Anterior Descending Artery
- History of MI
- History of PCI or CABG

Abbreviations: CABG, coronary artery bypass grafting; MI, myocardial infarction; PCI, percutaneous coronary intervention.

associated with worse outcomes.[8–10] The Global Registry of Acute Coronary Events study found that hospitalized patients with acute coronary syndrome and HF had markedly increased in-hospital and 6-month mortality rates.[10] The Duke database demonstrated ICM was an independent predictor of 5-year mortality with lower 5-year survival rates in patients with ICM compared to NICM.[8] A more recent observational study of the European Society of Cardiology Heart Failure Registries similarly found ICM was an independent predictor of 1-year mortality and HF hospitalization with comparatively higher rates of both endpoints in patients with ICM.[9]

PATHOPHYSIOLOGY OF ISCHEMIC CARDIOMYOPATHY

The fundamental pathophysiological mechanism of ICM involves myocardial ischemia due to atherosclerotic narrowing or occlusion of coronary arteries.[11] Over time, chronic myocardial perfusion abnormalities lead to cardiac remodeling, with the left ventricle (LV) undergoing structural changes to maintain cardiac output. The LV dilates and becomes more spherical, leading to apical displacement of the mitral valve papillary muscles, which manifests as restriction of the mitral valve leaflets and functional mitral regurgitation.[12] This triggers a vicious cycle where regurgitant flow leads to reduced cardiac output and exacerbation of myocardial perfusion abnormalities, leading to further adverse LV remodeling. This adverse remodeling occurs in a background of neurohormonal dysregulation which also contributes to chronic myocardial perfusion abnormalities via systemic vasoconstriction, sodium and fluid retention, and sympathetic activation.[13]

Repetitive ischemic injury leads to adaptive metabolic changes in cardiac myocytes to protect against further ischemia and preserve viable myocardial tissue at the expense of ventricular function.[14] This concept is called "myocardial hibernation" and it is thought that restoring myocardial blood flow (ie, coronary revascularization) leads to partially or completely restored LV function.[15] This theory has been the basis of many historical and recent studies investigating the role of coronary revascularization in patients with ICM.

DIAGNOSTIC EVALUATION OF ISCHEMIA IN HEART FAILURE

The current American Heart Association/American College of Cardiology/Heart Failure Society of America Guidelines on the Management of Heart Failure and European Society of Cardiology (ESC) Guidelines for the Diagnosis and Treatment of Acute and Chronic Heart Failure recommend a multimodal approach when evaluating the etiology of new-onset heart failure with preserved ejection fraction (HFpEF) and reduced ejection fraction (HFrEF).[16,17] The initial diagnostic evaluation involves a complete history and physical examination, laboratory evaluation, 12-lead electrocardiogram, chest x-ray, and transthoracic echocardiography.[16,17] Patients with HFrEF who are likely to have obstructive CAD and are candidates for coronary revascularization should be considered for an ischemic evaluation.[16,17] Of note, the guidelines do not specifically address ischemic evaluation in patients with new-onset HFpEF, likely due to the paucity of available evidence supporting ischemic evaluation and coronary revascularization in HFpEF. As the diagnosis of ischemia in HFpEF is unlikely to yield significant changes in global management that is, coronary revascularization, the authors do not recommend routine ischemic evaluation in this population.

The timing of ischemic evaluation is unclear and there are no clear consensus statements regarding this topic. The authors recommend early ischemic evaluation in patients with new-onset HFrEF given its important downstream effects and the significant differences in treatment strategies between ICM and NICM. A large observational study of patients with new-onset HFrEF found those who received an ischemic evaluation within 90 days of diagnosis had lower 1-year mortality rates and higher treatments rates with guideline-directed medical therapy (GDMT) and coronary revascularization compared to those who did not.[18] Despite this evidence, early ischemic evaluation has yet to be widely embraced and there has been gross under-utilization of CAD testing in new-onset HF. An analysis of the Get With The Guidelines – Heart Failure Registry found that <40% of patients with new-onset HF received CAD testing within 90 days of diagnosis.[19] A subsequent study by Zheng *and colleagues* built on this finding and found that CAD testing rates were lower (<30%) for patients diagnosed as an outpatient.[20] The underutilization of early CAD testing may be related to variability in clinical presentation (ie, some patients are deemed *too sick* to undergo further diagnostic testing), the availability of catheterization laboratories and certain noninvasive modalities, and the level of involvement of local cardiologists. Zheng and colleagues found that patients co-managed by a cardiologist had 5-fold higher adjusted odds for early CAD testing.[20]

There are several guideline-recommended modalities that detect and characterize underlying CAD and myocardial ischemia.[16,17] The selection of modalities should be based on candidacy for coronary revascularization and pre-test probability of CAD, which can be estimated as low, intermediate, or high based on initial diagnostic evaluation. The US and European guidelines have developed several clinical models that can help classify pre-test probability of CAD.[21,22] Invasive coronary angiography (ICA) is the gold standard for assessing and characterizing coronary artery anatomy and stenoses, especially in high-risk patients.[23] However, the procedural risks may make ICA unappealing in certain patient populations. Alternative noninvasive modalities to consider are coronary computed tomography angiography (CCTA) and stress imaging such as stress echocardiography (SE), single-photon emission computed tomography (SPECT), positron emission tomography, and cardiac magnetic resonance (CMR).[16,17,] Stress imaging has been shown to inform long-term prognosis in HF patients with inducible ischemia,[24,25] and has been historically used to guide coronary revascularization decisions.[26] CCTA in particular has increasingly become a viable noninvasive alternative that can provide a more expeditious and possibly more cost-effective means of assessing patients at risk for CAD.[27] Studies evaluating the performance of CCTA in detecting significant coronary stenoses have found it to be comparable to invasive coronary angiography, as well as boast an excellent negative predictive value and the ability to effectively rule out CAD, especially in patients with low to intermediate risk of CAD.[28,29]

Our approach to ischemic evaluation in new-onset HFrEF is based on the current US and European HF guidelines and is presented in **Fig. 1**. The diagnosis of ischemia in HF necessitates a multi-faceted approach that incorporates information from multiple modalities. Clinicians should strive to initiate early ischemic evaluation as this can have downstream effects on clinical outcomes.

MANAGEMENT OF ISCHEMIC CARDIOMYOPATHY
Optimal Medical Therapy

Once ICM and HF have been diagnosed, all patients should be placed on optimal GDMT for CAD and HF. The goals of therapy are to reduce the downstream sequelae of CAD and HF, including cardiovascular (CV) morbidity and mortality.

GDMT consists of the "4 pillars of HF therapy," which include various classes of medications, including evidence-based beta-blockers, renin-angiotensin-aldosterone system inhibitors, mineralocorticoid receptor antagonists (MRAs), and sodium-glucose

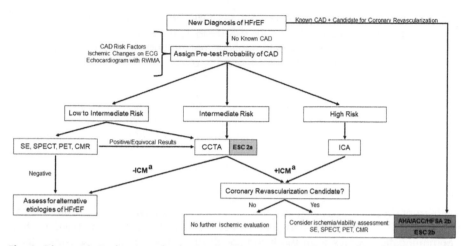

Fig. 1. Diagnostic Evaluation of Ischemic Cardiomyopathy. [a]ICM is angiographically defined by the presence of ≥75% stenosis of ≥2 coronary arteries or ≥75% stenosis of either the left main coronary artery or the proximal left anterior descending artery. ACC, American College of Cardiology; AHA, American Heart Association; CAD, coronary artery disease; CCTA, coronary computed tomography angiography; CMR, cardiac magnetic resonance; ECG, electrocardiogram; ESC, European Society of Cardiology; HFSA, Heart Failure Society of America; HFrEF, heart failure with reduced ejection fraction; ICA, invasive coronary angiography; ICM, ischemic cardiomyopathy; PET, positron emission tomography; SE, stress echocardiography; SPECT, single-photon emission computed tomography, RWMA, regional wall motion abnormality.

co-transporter 2 inhibitors (SGLT2i). Several landmark clinical trials have provided compelling evidence regarding the benefit of pharmacologic therapy in HF and ICM.[16,17] These therapies have been endorsed by both the US and European guidelines.[16,17]

For patients with established atherosclerotic cardiovascular disease (ASCVD), aspirin and statins have clear roles in secondary prevention as they have been proven to reduce the risk of subsequent ASCVD-related events like myocardial infarction and ischemic stroke, as well as incident HF.[30] However, once HF and ICM are established, the role of newly initiating aspirin and statins is less clear. Aspirin has been theorized to antagonize the cardioprotective benefits of GDMT like angiotensin-converting enzyme inhibitors (ACEi), MRAs, and beta-blockers, potentially leading to worse HF outcomes.[31–33] A recent meta-analysis of 14 studies challenged this theory when they found aspirin was associated with lower rates of all-cause mortality in HF patients.[34] Similarly, there is a theoretic concern that cholesterol-lowering agents like statins may have an adverse effect in HF patients, as prior literature has demonstrated an association between low serum cholesterol and worse HF outcomes (ie, often termed the "cholesterol paradox").[35] Two major randomized controlled trials (RCT), Controlled Rosuvastatin Multinational Trial in Heart Failure (CORONA) and Gruppo Italiano per lo Studio della Sopravvivenza nell'Insufficienza Cardiaca (GISSI-HF) tackled this question and found statins had no beneficial or adverse effect on HF outcomes.[36,37] This lack of effect was consistent in patients with ICM and NICM. Overall, whether aspirin and statins improve or worsen HF outcomes remains unclear. This is due to the high competing risks of death due to pump failure and sudden cardiac death versus death due to adverse ASCVD-related events, which ultimately present challenges in demonstrating clear benefits of these therapies in RCTs. Given their established role in ASCVD and the lack of consensus on the risk-benefit profile of aspirin and statin in HF, the authors believe it is reasonable to continue aspirin and statins in these patients, provided there are no clear contraindications.

Coronary Revascularization

While the evidence for optimal medical therapy (OMT) in HF and ICM is ubiquitous and robust, there is more controversy surrounding the ideal timing and approach to coronary revascularization in the setting of ICM. The remainder of this article will discuss the available evidence behind coronary revascularization, the role of myocardial viability studies, and potential areas of future investigation.

Surgical Revascularization

The current US and European guidelines recommend surgical revascularization in patients with HF, LVEF ≤35%, and suitable coronary anatomy.[16,17] The basis for this recommendation comes from the landmark Surgical Treatment for Ischemic Heart Failure (STICH) trial that examined the effect of CABG on HF outcomes in ICM.[38,39] STICH enrolled 1212 patients from 99 clinical sites in 22 countries with HF, LVEF ≤35%, and CAD amenable to CABG. The presence of myocardial viability was not mandated to receive CABG, and 50% of all enrolled patients underwent viability testing as part of a substudy. Patients were randomized in a 1:1 ratio and non-blinded fashion to receive OMT alone or CABG plus OMT. OMT consisted of ACEi/angiotensin receptor blockers (ARBs) and beta-blockers titrated to optimal doses, and device therapy (as appropriate). Patients with cardiogenic shock, recent acute MI, and severe aortic valvular disease were excluded. From 2002 to 2007, patients were enrolled, randomized, and followed every 4 months for the first year and subsequently every 6 months. The primary endpoint was all-cause mortality. Secondary endpoints included all-cause and cause-specific mortality and hospitalizations.

The mean ± standard deviation (SD) age and LVEF of the study cohort was 60 ± 9 years and 30 ± 8%, respectively. The duration of follow-up among all patients ranged between 3.5 years and 13.4 years, with a median of 9.8 years. Initially, CABG plus OMT was associated with a 3-fold higher 30-day mortality rate, but by year 5 a trend toward benefit emerged and subsequently reached statistical significance at year 10. At year 10, CABG was associated with significantly lower risk of all-cause mortality (hazard ratio [HR] = 0.84, 95% confidence interval [CI] 0.73–0.97, P = .02), CV mortality, (HR = 0.79, 95% CI 0.66–0.93, P = .006), the composite of all-cause mortality or CV hospitalization (HR = 0.72, 95% CI 0.64–0.82, P < .001), and the composite of all-cause mortality or HF hospitalization (HR = 0.81, 95% CI 0.71–0.93, P = .002), when compared to OMT alone. Like real-world clinical practice, there was a high rate of cross-over from OMT alone to CABG plus OMT, and on per-protocol analysis, CABG plus OMT was associated with an even greater reduced risk of all-cause mortality (HR = 0.77, 95% CI 0.67–0.90, P = .001). Notably, younger patients experienced a greater reduction in the composite of all-cause mortality or CV hospitalization (HR in age ≤54 years = 0.55, 95% CI 0.43–0.71, HR in age >67 years = 0.73, 95% CI 0.57–0.92, P = .004), and the effect of CABG plus OMT on all-cause mortality diminished with increasing age (HR in age ≤54 years = 0.66, 95% CI 0.49–0.89, HR in age >67 years = 0.82, 95% CI 0.63–1.06, P = .062).[40] Patients with ≥2 out of 3 prognostic factors of 3-vessel CAD, LVEF ≤27%, or LV end-systolic volume index (LVESVI)≥79 mL/m^2, also had a greater reduced risk of all-cause mortality (HR = 0.71, 95% CI 0.56–0.89, P = .004) and CV mortality (HR = 0.72, 95% CI 0.56–0.94, P = .014) with CABG.[41]

Percutaneous Coronary Intervention

Until Revascularisation for Ischaemic Ventricular Dysfunction - British Cardiovascular Intervention Society 2 (REVIVED-BCIS2), there were no RCTs examining the effect of PCI on HF outcomes in ICM.[42] REVIVED-BCIS2 enrolled 700 patients from 40 clinical sites in the United Kingdom with HF, LVEF ≤35%, and extensive CAD (ie, defined as British Cardiovascular Intervention jeopardy score of ≥6, on a scale from 0 to 12, with higher scores indicating greater extent of disease)[43] and demonstrable viability in at least 4 dysfunctional myocardial segments amenable to revascularization with PCI. Patients were randomized in a 1:1 ratio and non-blinded fashion to receive OMT alone or PCI plus OMT, with the aim of revascularizing all diseased proximal coronary vessels supplying areas of viable myocardium. OMT consisted of ACEi/ARBs/angiotensin receptor neprilysin inhibitors (ARNIs), beta-blockers, MRAs, and SGLT2i titrated to optimal doses, and device therapy (as appropriate). Patients with cardiogenic shock, recent acute MI, or sustained ventricular arrhythmias within 72 hours before randomization were excluded. From 2013 to 2020, patients were enrolled, randomized, and followed at 1 month, 6 months, 1 year, 2 years, and annually thereafter. The primary endpoint was the composite of all-cause mortality or HF hospitalization. Secondary endpoints included CV mortality, acute MI, and appropriate automatic implantable cardioverter defibrillator (AICD) therapy.

The mean ± SD age and LVEF of the study cohort was 70 ± 9 years and 27 ± 7%, respectively The duration of follow-up among all patients ranged between 1.9 years and 5 years, with a median of 3.4 years. Compared to OMT alone, PCI plus OMT did not significantly alter the risk of all-cause mortality or HF hospitalization (HR = 0.99, 95% CI 0.78–1.27, P = .96). Similarly, there was no change in risk for CV mortality (HR = 0.88, 95% CI 0.65–1.20) and acute MI (HR = 1.01, 95% CI 0.64–1.60). Additionally, there was no significant difference between groups in the incidence of appropriate AICD therapy at 24 months (RR = 0.42, 95% CI 0.17–1.06) and risk of all-cause mortality or aborted sudden cardiac death (HR = 1.03, 95% CI 0.82–1.30, P = .80), indicating that PCI did not reduce the incidence of potentially fatal ventricular arrhythmias.[44]

Discussion

The key findings in STICH and REVIVED-BCIS2 are summarized in **Table 1**. When analyzing and comparing STICH and REVIVED-BCIS2, several insights merit further mention. First, STICH provides evidence that adding CABG to OMT improves clinical outcomes in patients with ICM and HF. This benefit is more pronounced when patients are younger and have more advanced disease. In contrast, REVIVED-BCIS2 demonstrated adding PCI to OMT had no beneficial or adverse effect. Second, STICH had younger patients (mean age of 60), while REVIVED-BCIS2 had older patients (mean age of 70). The older population in REVIVED-BCIS2 had a higher competing risk of mortality from non-CV causes, which may have masked any treatment effect. This potential effect was demonstrated in the STICH trial when increasing age diminished the magnitude of benefit in all-cause mortality.[40] Third, the beneficial effect of CABG in STICH was not observed until 10-year follow-up. Previous studies have demonstrated that LV recovery occurs months to years after revascularization of hibernating myocardium.[45] REVIVED-BCIS2 only had 3 to 4 years of follow-up, and it very well may take 10 years of restored myocardial perfusion to reverse chronic metabolic and structural changes and manifest as reduced rates of HF and CV-related morbidity and mortality. Finally, STICH and REVIVED-BCIS2 were conducted in different eras of OMT. When STICH occurred, the only Class 1 recommended medical therapies for HF were ACEi/ARBs and beta-blockers. When REVIVED-BCIS2 occurred, GDMT was much more robust with the addition of ARNIs, MRAs, and SGLT2i,

Table 1
Surgical treatment for ischemic heart failure versus REVIVED-BCIS2

Trial Acronym	STICH	REVIVED-BCIS2
Number of Patients	1212	700
Viability Imaging	Not Required	Required
Patients with Viability imaging	50%	100%
Modality Used	CMR 21%, remaining DSE/SPECT	CMR 70%, remaining DSE/SPECT/PET
Patient Demographics		
Mean Age ± SD	60 ± 9 y	70 ± 9 y
Mean LVEF ± SD	30 ± 8%	27 ± 7%
Revascularization Modality	CABG	PCI
Goal-Directed Medical Therapy	Beta-Blocker, ACEi/ARB	Beta-Blocker, ACEi/ARB/ARNI, MRA, SGLT2i
Median Follow-up	9.8 y	3.4 y
Primary Endpoint	All-Cause Mortality	All-Cause Mortality or HF Hospitalization
Outcome	Favors CABG (HR = 0.84, 95% CI 0.73–0.97, $P = .02$)	No Difference (HR = 0.99, 95% CI 0.78–1.27, $P = .96$)

Abbreviations: ACEi, angiotensin-converting enzyme inhibitors; ARB, angiotensin receptor blockers; ARNI, angiotensin receptor neprilysin inhibitors; CABG, coronary artery bypass grafting; CMR, cardiac magnetic resonance; DSE, dobutamine stress echocardiography; HF, heart failure; LVEF, left ventricular ejection fraction; PCI, percutaneous coronary intervention; CV, cardiovascular; MRA, mineralocorticoid receptor antagonists; PET, positron emission tomography; SD, standard deviation; SLGT2i, sodium-glucose co-transporter 2 inhibitors; SPECT, single-photon emission computed tomography.

which likely diluted the potential impact of PCI. The difference in intensity and breadth of OMT can be appreciated between the 2 studies as REVIVED-BCIS2 had much higher utilization rates of various GDMT, as well as device-based therapies like cardiac resynchronization therapy (CRT) and AICDs, which are considered a critical part of OMT. The global nature of STICH likely further contributed to this differential use of GDMT as there are well-known geographic differences in accessibility and affordability of GDMT and device-based therapies.[46] As a result, the differences in OMT led to a narrower gap between the treatment and control arms of REVIVED-BCIS2 compared to STICH, and potentially masked a treatment effect with PCI.

The results of STICH and REVIVED-BCIS2 thrust the topic of CABG versus PCI into the limelight. However, the authors believe the most compelling differences between the 2 trials are population age and competing risk of non-CV mortality, duration of follow-up and anticipated timeframe of benefit, and differential use of GDMT and device-based therapies. If anything, these 2 studies demonstrated the importance of patient selection in coronary revascularization. Younger patients with a life expectancy of at least 10 years are more likely to derive benefit, and if the surgical risk is acceptable, the evidence basis is strongest for CABG.

AREAS OF CONTROVERSY AND TOPICS OF FUTURE INVESTIGATION
Coronary Artery Bypass Grafting Versus Percutaneous Coronary Intervention?

The recent results of REVIVED-BCIS2 question whether PCI is inferior to CABG in ICM. Several studies have investigated this question. An analysis of the Kyoto PCI/CABG

Registry demonstrated an increased risk of all-cause mortality and CV mortality over 5 years in PCI when compared to CABG.[47] Similarly, a study of the Ontario Registry demonstrated higher rates of all-cause mortality, CV mortality, major adverse cardiovascular events (MACE), and hospitalizations for MI and HF over 5 years in PCI compared to CABG.[48] The current available evidence best supports CABG over PCI in ICM, but this is far from a definitive conclusion as the available evidence is limited to these observational studies and comparisons of STICH and REVIVED-BCIS, which had significant variations in study population and protocol. Future research investigating the role of PCI in younger populations, and directly comparing PCI to CABG would provide more conclusive evidence in coronary revascularization strategies in patients with ICM.

When Should We Revascularize? Is Contemporary Medical Therapy Enough?

The lack of effect with PCI in REVIVED-BCIS2 could potentially be explained by the effectiveness of contemporary GDMT, which questions whether STICH would demonstrate the same beneficial effect of CABG if the trial were to be repeated in today's era of GDMT. Furthermore, if indicated, the timing of revascularization is unclear. Should we revascularize soon after diagnosis? Or perhaps only if there is not LV recovery after a trial of GDMT? Future research investigating these questions would help determine coronary revascularization's role and optimal timing in ICM.

The Role of Myocardial Viability Studies

The US and European guidelines provide a Class 2b recommendation for non-invasive stress imaging, such as SE, SPECT, PET, and CMR, to assess myocardial ischemia and viability.[16,17] These tests identify areas of nonviable scarred myocardium and viable hibernating myocardium, which can inform prognosis and guide clinical decisions on whether to revascularize. This approach stems from older observational studies that demonstrated improvement in post-revascularization mortality in patients with viable myocardium compared to patients without viable myocardium.[26] These studies have many limitations as most were retrospective, non-randomized, and had substantial risk for confounding variables. STICH and REVIVED-BCIS2 were the first prospective RCTs that provided evidence for the relationship between viability and revascularization.

STICH and REVIVED-BCIS2 both evaluated whether viability was predictive of HF outcomes. A STICH substudy found that patients with viable myocardium had lower rates of the composite of all-cause mortality and CV hospitalization (HR = 0.59, 95% CI 0.47–0.74, P = .003).[49] REVIVED-BCIS2 found that the magnitude of nonviable scarred myocardium predicted worse outcomes. For each 10% increase in scar volume, there was an 18% higher risk of death or HF hospitalization (HR = 1.18, 95% CI 1.04–1.33, P < .01).[50] While viability was associated with prognosis, it did not modify the treatment effect in STICH and REVIVED-BCIS2. In both studies, there was no significant interaction between the presence or absence of myocardial viability and the treatment effect of CABG/PCI.[42,49,51] Furthermore, patients with viability did not have a significant increase in LVEF after CABG/PCI when compared to those who received OMT.[42,51]

The importance of viability studies remains controversial and recent trials have challenged their role in predicting benefit in coronary revascularization. Conceivably, the value of viability may depend on modality, particularly given the recent emergence of CMR, which has been shown to accurately describe functional and structural consequences of ischemia.[52] Additionally, viable myocardium likely exists on a continuum, including jeopardized, stunned, early hibernation, and advanced hibernation,

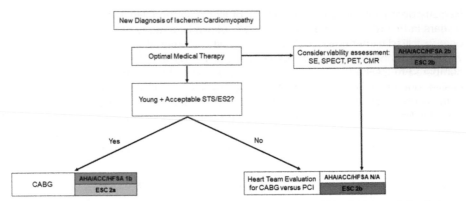

Fig. 2. Management of ischemic cardiomyopathy. ACC, American College of Cardiology; AHA, American Heart Association; CABG, coronary artery bypass grafting; CMR, cardiac magnetic resonance; ESC, European Society of Cardiology; ES2, EuroSCORE-2; HFSA, Heart Failure Society of America; PET, positron emission tomography; PCI, percutaneous coronary intervention; SE, stress echocardiography; SPECT, single-photon emission computed tomography; STS, Society of Thoracic Surgeons.

and this heterogeneity may impact prognostic value and interaction with treatment effect (ie, coronary revascularization). Future research should investigate the role of viability imaging and its various modalities in prognosticating and risk-stratifying those with nonviable and scarred myocardium.

SUMMARY AND INTEGRATING EVIDENCE INTO CLINICAL PRACTICE

ICM remains a complex and prevalent form of heart disease, and early diagnosis and comprehensive management strategies are essential in improving outcomes. Over the past few decades, treatment modalities for patients with HF and ICM have significantly advanced. While robust and compelling evidence supports OMT and surgical revascularization in this high-risk patient population, the role of PCI and routinely assessing viability to guide patient selection remains controversial. Continued research is essential to further unravel the complexities of ICM and lead to more effective therapies, ultimately reducing the attendant risk of morbidity and mortality in patients afflicted with this chronic condition. A summary of our ICM management algorithm is provided in **Fig. 2**, which proposes the sequential steps as follows.

1. Diagnostic Evaluation of ICM in HF (**Fig. 1**): Clinicians should use a multi-faceted approach to assign a pre-test probability of CAD in patients with HF. Those with low-intermediate risk of CAD can first be assessed with CCTA or non-invasive stress imaging.
2. Viability Testing: Per the US and European HF guidelines, consider viability testing in candidates for revascularization. The authors caution clinicians that the current means of assessing viability are limited and have not definitively demonstrated utility in prognosticating treatment response.
3. Optimal Medical Therapy: Once the diagnosis of ICM is made, every patient should be placed on OMT as defined.
4. Method of Coronary Revascularization: If revascularization is pursued, the preferred method is CABG, provided patients are younger with greater than 10-year life expectancy and have acceptable peri-operative risk as defined by the

Society of Thoracic Surgeons risk score and the EuroSCORE-2.[53] In younger patients with $\geq$2 out of 3 prognostic factors of 3-vessel CAD, LVEF $\leq$27%, or LVESVI $\geq$79 mL/m2, the benefit derived with CABG may be even more pronounced.

CLINICS CARE POINTS

The current available evidence best supports surgical revascularization in patients with ischemic cardiomyopathy and amenable coronary anatomy.

- Non-invasive imaging modalities including coronary computed tomography angiography can be useful alternatives to invasive angiography to evaluate for an ischemic etiology of heart failure in patients with low to intermediate risk.

- CABG has been shown to improve cardiovascular outcomes including survival in appropriately selected patients with ICM.

- Percutaneous coronary intervention has not been demonstrated to improve cardiovascular outcomes in patients with underlying ischemic cardiomyopathy.

- The presence of myocardial viability does not modify the anticipated benefit of surgical revascularization in patients with known ischemic cardiomyopathy.

DISCLOSURES

Dr A.P. Ambrosy has received relevant research support through grants to his institution from the National Heart, Lung, and Blood Institute, United States (K23HL150159), the American Heart Association, United States (2nd Century Early Faculty Independence Award), The Permanente Medical Group, Northern California Community Health Program, Garfield Memorial Fund, Abbott Laboratories, Amarin Pharma, Inc., Edwards Lifesciences LLC, Esperion Therapeutics, Inc., and Novartis. All other authors have no relevant financial disclosures.

REFERENCES

1. Bourassa MG, Gurné O, Bangdiwala SI, et al. Natural history and patterns of current practice in heart failure. The Studies of Left Ventricular Dysfunction (SOLVD) Investigators. J Am Coll Cardiol 1993;22(4 Suppl A):14A–9A.
2. Felker GM, Shaw LK, O'Connor CM. A standardized definition of ischemic cardiomyopathy for use in clinical research. J Am Coll Cardiol 2002;39(2):210–8.
3. Ambrosy AP, Fonarow GC, Butler J, et al. The global health and economic burden of hospitalizations for heart failure: lessons learned from hospitalized heart failure registries. J Am Coll Cardiol 2014;63(12):1123–33.
4. Tsao CW, Aday AW, Almarzooq ZI, et al. Heart Disease and Stroke Statistics-2023 Update: A Report From the American Heart Association [published correction appears in Circulation. 2023 Feb 21;147(8):e622] [published correction appears in Circulation. 2023 Jul 25;148(4):e4]. Circulation 2023;147(8):e93–621.
5. Adams KF Jr, Fonarow GC, Emerman CL, et al. Characteristics and outcomes of patients hospitalized for heart failure in the United States: rationale, design, and preliminary observations from the first 100,000 cases in the Acute Decompensated Heart Failure National Registry (ADHERE). Am Heart J 2005;149(2): 209–16.
6. Heidenreich PA, Albert NM, Allen LA, et al. Forecasting the impact of heart failure in the United States: a policy statement from the American Heart Association. Circ Heart Fail 2013;6(3):606–19.

7. Gheorghiade M, Sopko G, De Luca L, et al. Navigating the crossroads of coronary artery disease and heart failure. Circulation 2006;114(11):1202–13.

8. Bart BA, Shaw LK, McCants CB Jr, et al. Clinical determinants of mortality in patients with angiographically diagnosed ischemic or nonischemic cardiomyopathy. J Am Coll Cardiol 1997;30(4):1002–8.

9. Tymińska A, Ozierański K, Balsam P, et al. Ischemic Cardiomyopathy versus Non-Ischemic Dilated Cardiomyopathy in Patients with Reduced Ejection Fraction-Clinical Characteristics and Prognosis Depending on Heart Failure Etiology (Data from European Society of Cardiology Heart Failure Registries). Biology 2022;11(2):341.

10. Steg PG, Dabbous OH, Feldman LJ, et al. Determinants and prognostic impact of heart failure complicating acute coronary syndromes: observations from the Global Registry of Acute Coronary Events (GRACE). Circulation 2004;109(4):494–9.

11. Bhandari B, Quintanilla Rodriguez BS, Masood W. Ischemic cardiomyopathy. StatPearls [Internet]. Treasure Island (FL): StatPearls Publishing; 2023.

12. Bhatt AS, Ambrosy AP, Velazquez EJ. Adverse Remodeling and Reverse Remodeling After Myocardial Infarction. Curr Cardiol Rep 2017;19(8):71.

13. Hartupee J, Mann DL. Neurohormonal activation in heart failure with reduced ejection fraction. Nat Rev Cardiol 2017;14(1):30–8.

14. Bayeva M, Sawicki KT, Butler J, et al. Molecular and cellular basis of viable dysfunctional myocardium. Circ Heart Fail 2014;7(4):680–91.

15. Rahimtoola SH. The hibernating myocardium in ischaemia and congestive heart failure. Eur Heart J 1993;14(Suppl A):22–6.

16. Heidenreich PA, Bozkurt B, Aguilar D, et al. AHA/ACC/HFSA Guideline for the Management of Heart Failure: A Report of the American College of Cardiology/American Heart Association Joint Committee on Clinical Practice Guidelines [published correction appears in J Am Coll Cardiol. 2023 Apr 18;81(15):1551]. J Am Coll Cardiol 2022;79(17):e263–421.

17. McDonagh TA, Metra M, Adamo M, et al. ESC Guidelines for the diagnosis and treatment of acute and chronic heart failure [published correction appears in Eur Heart J. 2021 Oct 14;:]. Eur Heart J 2021;42(36):3599–726.

18. McGuinn E, Warsavage T, Plomondon ME, et al. Association of Ischemic Evaluation and Clinical Outcomes Among Patients Admitted With New-Onset Heart Failure. J Am Heart Assoc 2021;10(5):e019452.

19. O'Connor KD, Brophy T, Fonarow GC, et al. Testing for Coronary Artery Disease in Older Patients With New-Onset Heart Failure: Findings From Get With The Guidelines-Heart Failure. Circ Heart Fail 2020;13(4):e006963.

20. Zheng J, Heidenreich PA, Kohsaka S, et al. Variability in Coronary Artery Disease Testing for Patients With New-Onset Heart Failure. J Am Coll Cardiol 2022;79(9):849–86.

21. Gulati M, Levy PD, Mukherjee D, et al. AHA/ACC/ASE/CHEST/SAEM/SCCT/SCMR Guideline for the Evaluation and Diagnosis of Chest Pain: A Report of the American College of Cardiology/American Heart Association Joint Committee on Clinical Practice Guidelines. Circulation 2021;144(22):e368–454 [published correction appears in Circulation. 2021 Nov 30;144(22):e455].

22. Knuuti J, Wijns W, Saraste A, et al. 2019 ESC Guidelines for the diagnosis and management of chronic coronary syndromes. Eur Heart J 2020;41(3):407–77 [published correction appears in Eur Heart J. 2020 Nov 21;41(44):4242].

23. Ferreira JP, Rossignol P, Demissei B, et al. Coronary angiography in worsening heart failure: determinants, findings and prognostic implications. Heart 2018; 104(7):606–13.
24. Elhendy A, Sozzi F, van Domburg RT, et al. Effect of myocardial ischemia during dobutamine stress echocardiography on cardiac mortality in patients with heart failure secondary to ischemic cardiomyopathy. Am J Cardiol 2005;96(4):469–73.
25. Miller WL, Hodge DO, Tointon SK, et al. Relationship of myocardial perfusion imaging findings to outcome of patients with heart failure and suspected ischemic heart disease. Am Heart J 2004;147(4):714–20.
26. Allman KC, Shaw LJ, Hachamovitch R, et al. Myocardial viability testing and impact of revascularization on prognosis in patients with coronary artery disease and left ventricular dysfunction: a meta-analysis. J Am Coll Cardiol 2002;39(7): 1151–8.
27. Chow BJW, Coyle D, Hossain A, et al. Computed tomography coronary angiography for patients with heart failure (CTA-HF): a randomized controlled trial (IMAGE-HF 1C). Eur Heart J Cardiovasc Imaging 2021;22(9):1083–90.
28. Leschka S, Alkadhi H, Plass A, et al. Accuracy of MSCT coronary angiography with 64-slice technology: first experience. Eur Heart J 2005;26(15):1482–7.
29. Meijboom WB, van Mieghem CA, Mollet NR, et al. 64-slice computed tomography coronary angiography in patients with high, intermediate, or low pretest probability of significant coronary artery disease. J Am Coll Cardiol 2007;50(15):1469–75.
30. Virani SS, Newby LK, Arnold SV, et al. 2023 AHA/ACC/ACCP/ASPC/NLA/PCNA Guideline for the Management of Patients With Chronic Coronary Disease: A Report of the American Heart Association/American College of Cardiology Joint Committee on Clinical Practice Guidelines [published correction appears in Circulation. 2023 Sep 26;148(13):e148. Circulation 2023;148(9):e9–119.
31. Teo KK, Yusuf S, Pfeffer M, et al. Effects of long-term treatment with angiotensin-converting-enzyme inhibitors in the presence or absence of aspirin: a systematic review. Lancet 2002;360(9339):1037–43 [published correction appears in Lancet 2003 Jan 4;361(9351):90].
32. Tweeddale MG, Ogilvie RI. Antagonism of spironolactone-induced natriuresis by aspirin in man. N Engl J Med 1973;289(4):198–200.
33. Lindenfeld J, Robertson AD, Lowes BD, et al. MOCHA (Multicenter Oral Carvedilol Heart failure Assessment) Investigators. Aspirin impairs reverse myocardial remodeling in patients with heart failure treated with beta-blockers. J Am Coll Cardiol 2001;38(7):1950–6.
34. Jiwani S, Mustafa U, Desai S, et al. Survival Benefit of Aspirin in Patients With Congestive Heart Failure: A Meta-Analysis. J Clin Med Res 2021;13(1):38–47.
35. Horwich TB, Hamilton MA, Maclellan WR, et al. Low serum total cholesterol is associated with marked increase in mortality in advanced heart failure. J Card Fail 2002;8(4):216–24.
36. Kjekshus J, Apetrei E, Barrios V, et al. Rosuvastatin in older patients with systolic heart failure. N Engl J Med 2007;357(22):2248–61.
37. Tavazzi L, Maggioni AP, Marchioli R, et al. Effect of rosuvastatin in patients with chronic heart failure (the GISSI-HF trial): a randomised, double-blind, placebo-controlled trial. Lancet 2008;372(9645):1231–9.
38. Velazquez EJ, Lee KL, Deja MA, et al. Coronary-artery bypass surgery in patients with left ventricular dysfunction. N Engl J Med 2011;364(17):1607–16.
39. Velazquez EJ, Lee KL, Jones RH, et al. Coronary-Artery Bypass Surgery in Patients with Ischemic Cardiomyopathy. N Engl J Med 2016;374(16):1511–20.

40. Petrie MC, Jhund PS, She L, et al. Ten-Year Outcomes After Coronary Artery Bypass Grafting According to Age in Patients With Heart Failure and Left Ventricular Systolic Dysfunction: An Analysis of the Extended Follow-Up of the STICH Trial (Surgical Treatment for Ischemic Heart Failure). Circulation 2016;134(18):1314–24.
41. Panza JA, Velazquez EJ, She L, et al. Extent of coronary and myocardial disease and benefit from surgical revascularization in ischemic LV dysfunction [Corrected]. J Am Coll Cardiol 2014;64(6):553–61 [published correction appears in J Am Coll Cardiol. 2014 Oct 7;64(14):1539].
42. Perera D, Clayton T, O'Kane PD, et al. Percutaneous Revascularization for Ischemic Left Ventricular Dysfunction. N Engl J Med 2022;387(15):1351–60.
43. Perera D, Stables R, Booth J, et al. BCIS-1 Investigators. The balloon pump-assisted coronary intervention study (BCIS-1): rationale and design. Am Heart J 2009;158(6):910–6.e2.
44. Perera D, Morgan HP, Ryan M, et al. Arrhythmia and Death Following Percutaneous Revascularization in Ischemic Left Ventricular Dysfunction: Prespecified Analyses From the REVIVED-BCIS2 Trial. Circulation 2023;148(11):862–71.
45. Bax JJ, Visser FC, Poldermans D, et al. Time course of functional recovery of stunned and hibernating segments after surgical revascularization. Circulation 2001;104(12 Suppl 1):I314–8.
46. CHF Investigators G-, Joseph P, Roy A, et al. Global Variations in Heart Failure Etiology, Management, and Outcomes [published correction appears in JAMA. 2023 Sep 5;330(9):880]. JAMA 2023;329(19):1650–61.
47. Watanabe H, Yamamoto K, Shiomi H, et al. Percutaneous coronary intervention using new-generation drug-eluting stents versus coronary arterial bypass grafting in stable patients with multi-vessel coronary artery disease: From the CREDO-Kyoto PCI/CABG registry Cohort-3. PLoS One 2022;17(9):e0267906.
48. Sun LY, Gaudino M, Chen RJ, et al. Long-term Outcomes in Patients With Severely Reduced Left Ventricular Ejection Fraction Undergoing Percutaneous Coronary Intervention vs Coronary Artery Bypass Grafting [published correction appears in JAMA Cardiol. 2020 Jun 1;5(6):732]. JAMA Cardiol 2020;5(6):631–41.
49. Bonow RO, Maurer G, Lee KL, et al. Myocardial viability and survival in ischemic left ventricular dysfunction. N Engl J Med 2011;364(17):1617–25.
50. Perera D. Effect of myocardial viability, functional recovery and PCI on clinical outcomes in the REVIVED-BCIS2 trial. New Orleans, LA, US: Presented at the American College of Cardiology Annual Meeting; 2023.
51. Panza JA, Ellis AM, Al-Khalidi HR, et al. Myocardial Viability and Long-Term Outcomes in Ischemic Cardiomyopathy. N Engl J Med 2019;381(8):739–48.
52. Scatteia A, Dellegrottaglie S. Cardiac magnetic resonance in ischemic cardiomyopathy: present role and future directions. Eur Heart J Suppl 2023;25(Suppl C):C58–62.
53. Bouabdallaoui N, Stevens SR, Doenst T, et al. Society of Thoracic Surgeons Risk Score and EuroSCORE-2 Appropriately Assess 30-Day Postoperative Mortality in the STICH Trial and a Contemporary Cohort of Patients With Left Ventricular Dysfunction Undergoing Surgical Revascularization. Circ Heart Fail 2018;11(11):e005531.

Ischemic Heart Disease in Women

Eleonore Grant, MD[a], Monika Sanghavi, MD[b],*

KEYWORDS

- Ischemic heart disease • women's cardiovascular health
- MI with no obstructive coronary arteries • Spontaneous coronary artery dissection
- acute coronary syndrome

KEY POINTS

- Women have a unique clinical phenotype of ischemic heart disease with higher prevalence of non-occlusive disease, and decreased burden of obstructive atherosclerosis.
- Women share a disproportionate burden of traditional risk-factors for heart disease and have sex-specific risk-factors that are not incorporated into commonly used risk scores.
- Ischemia with non-Obstructive Coronary Arteries (INOCA) is a clinical entity grouping several endotypes including microvascular disease, vasospasm, and myocardial bridging and is more common in women.
- There is a burgeoning understanding of the discordance between angina and ischemia in women, especially in INOCA and this should be carefully considered in treatment strategies.

INTRODUCTION

The landscape of ischemic heart disease in women has expanded significantly with attention to sex-specific differences. The focus has shifted from obstructive epicardial atherosclerosis to a spectrum of ischemic heart disease including nonobstructive etiologies. Better appreciation of the different phenotypes of ischemic heart disease may help reduce disparities between the sexes. Women with ischemic heart disease are reported to have a higher prevalence of angina,[1] lower health-related quality of life,[2] higher emergency room visits,[3] and increased short- and long-term mortality than men.[4] This article reviews the current understanding of ischemic heart disease highlighting sex-specific differences.

---

[a] Department of Internal Medicine, University of Pennsylvania, 3400 Civic Center Boulevard, Philadelphia, PA 19104, USA; [b] Division of Cardiology, University of Pennsylvania, 3400 Civic Center Boulevard, Philadelphia, PA 19104, USA
* Corresponding author.
E-mail address: Monika.Sanghavi@pennmedicine.upenn.edu

Med Clin N Am 108 (2024) 567–579
https://doi.org/10.1016/j.mcna.2023.11.001
0025-7125/24/© 2023 Elsevier Inc. All rights reserved.

BIOLOGIC DIFFERENCES

In addition to differences in hormonal milieu, several sex differences in cardiovascular anatomy and function have been reported, which may contribute to the differences in clinical phenotypes and presentation.[5,6] Women are known to have smaller epicardial arteries compared with men even when matched for body mass index (BMI) and left ventricular mass.[7] They have higher resting blood flow per gram of myocardial mass,[8] which may be due to differences in autonomic function.[9]

RISK FACTORS
Traditional Risk Factors, Differing Burden of Disease

Women share many of the same traditional cardiovascular risk factors as men (hyperlipidemia, hypertension [HTN], diabetes mellitus [DM], abdominal obesity, smoking, and physical inactivity).[10] However, HTN, DM, and smoking are more potent risk factors in women than men (odds ratio of 1.5, 1.6, and 2.0, respectively).[10] Possible reasons for this have been theorized: (1) HTN is often undertreated in women as compared with men;[11] (2) DM may cause heightened impairment of endothelium-dependent vasodilation which may disproportionally affect women[11]; and (3) smoking risk is potentiated by use of combined oral contraceptive pills (tenfold increase in myocardial infarction (MI) and threefold increase in stroke).[12] This underscores the need to target these modifiable risk factors in primary and secondary prevention of Ischemic Heart Disease (IHD) in women.

Sex-Specific Risk Factors

Several sex-specific risk factors have also been reported.[11–16] These include (1) hormonal risk factors, (2) adverse pregnancy outcomes,[17] and (3) inflammation and rheumatologic conditions.[14,18]

Hormonal factors

Endogenous estrogen is cardioprotective due to a myriad of positive effects on the metabolic and vascular system[19] and is theorized to be the reason for the 10-year delay in atherosclerotic events in women compared with men. The loss of endogenous estrogen production during menopause has been associated with increased cardiovascular risk, redistribution of body fat, reduced glucose tolerance, abnormal lipids, and increased blood pressure and arterial stiffening.[19–21] Still, exogenous estrogen replacement has not been proven as a reliable mechanism to reduce cardiovascular risk.[20]

Polycystic ovarian syndrome (PCOS) is associated with adverse cardio-metabolic health and higher incidence of IHD. Although the association is well-established, it is still debated whether PCOS is an independent a risk factor for IHD or if it is due to the adverse metabolic effects (dyslipidemia, insulin resistance, weight gain).[17]

Hypertensive and metabolic disorders of pregnancy

Adverse pregnancy outcomes including hypertensive disorders of pregnancy, gestational diabetes, preterm birth, and small for gestational age infant have all been shown to increase the risk of IHD.[17] This is true for the peripartum period, but also confers a twofold life-time risk of cardiovascular disease (CVD).[17] Preeclampsia is an atherosclerotic CVD (ASCVD) risk enhancer, similar to family history, and should be considered when assessing the risk of ischemic heart disease in women. Timing, severity, and recurrence of preeclampsia are all correlated with future cardiovascular risk and can be gleaned when obtaining a pregnancy history.

Rheumatologic conditions

Women are also disproportionately affected by inflammatory and autoimmune conditions which confer a higher lifetime risk of IHD and are also considered ASCVD risk enhancers. Patients with lupus have a three- to fourfold increased risk of CV events and death.[22] Inflammation is important in the pathogenesis of atherosclerosis and may explain the increased risk in these patients.

Other risk factors affecting women disproportionately include chest wall radiation in patients with breast cancer, psychosocial risk factors,[23] including poor mental health[24] and low socioeconomic status.[25]

PRESENTATION

Ischemic heart disease can present as acute coronary syndrome (ACS) or as chronic disease with stable symptoms of angina pectoris. The definition of "typical" angina pectoris is based on the traditional paradigm of obstructive coronary artery disease that was commonly noted in men. Although chest pain is the most common presentation for both sexes, there are important differences that need to be considered. Highlighted in the following sections are sex differences in the presentation of acute coronary syndrome and chronic ischemic heart disease.

Acute Presentations

The most common symptom of acute ischemic heart disease is chest discomfort; however, women are known to have a broader range of symptoms on presentation. Young women (aged 35–54 years) are 50% more likely than similarly aged men to present without chest pain when they have an ST elevation MI (STEMI).[26,27] Although many women with acute myocardial infarction (AMI) have nonobstructive disease (as discussed below), women with obstructive epicardial disease are more likely to suffer from plaque erosion and embolization compared with plaque rupture in men.[27] Of note, women presenting with AMI are much less likely to receive guideline-recommended therapies than men (lipid-lowering medications, dual antiplatelet therapy, beta-blockers, angiotensin-converting enzyme [ACE]/angiogensin receptor block [ARB]), and less likely to achieve door to balloon time of less than 90 minutes.[2] This discrepancy is likely multifactorial from delayed diagnosis and incomplete understanding of the spectrum of ischemic disease, these discrepancies are even more significant in young women.

MI with no obstructive coronary arteries

Women presenting with ACS are more likely than men to have no evidence of obstructive disease on coronary angiography.[27] MI with no obstructive coronary arteries (MINOCA) is a working diagnosis. It encompasses many possible underlying diagnoses and requires further investigation.[28] In one international, multicenter study, the use of optical coherence tomography and cardiac magnetic resonance (CMR) identified a potential mechanism in 84.5% of women with a diagnosis of MINOCA. Approximately three of four were determined to be of an ischemic cause and the remainder of non-ischemic cause.[29] Ischemic causes of MINOCA can involve the epicardial and/or microvascular circulation. Epicardial causes of MINOCA include plaque disruption, epicardial spasm, spontaneous coronary artery dissection (SCAD), embolism, whereas microvascular causes include microvascular spasm and supply demand mismatch secondary to microvascular disease. Given the heterogeneity of the clinical entity, its treatment is largely dependent on the underlying etiology.

Spontaneous coronary artery dissection

SCAD is defined as a non-iatrogenic and non-atherosclerotic separation of the layers of an epicardial coronary wall by intramural hemorrhage with or without intimal tear. SCAD likely represents less than 4% of all AMIs in women, but up to one-third of MIs in women younger than 50 years. More than 90% of SCAD events occur in women.[30] Diagnosis is made by coronary angiography showing abrupt smooth tapering of the vessel due to intramural hematoma or presence of an intimal flap.[31] Accurate diagnosis is key because management differs significantly from atherosclerotic disease with a preference for conservative management in stable patients.[31] Optimal medical treatment is unknown. The use of antiplatelets is extrapolated from atherosclerotic disease management despite different pathophysiology. Management should target symptom reduction because chest pain is common after the initial event and prevention of recurrence. The use of beta-blockade has been associated with reduced risk of recurrent SCAD in one observational study.[32] Statins are recommended based on atherosclerotic risk.[33] Head-to-pelvis cross-sectional imaging is recommended to evaluate for extracoronary vascular anomalies due to the high prevalence of arteriopathies in this population. In addition, referral to cardiac rehab is recommended for all patients with SCAD.

Stress cardiomyopathy/Takotsubo

Stress cardiomyopathy, an ACS mimicker, presents as sudden and transient left ventricular dysfunction, typically associated with left ventricular apical ballooning and akinesis. Most cases (60%–90%) present after an emotional or physiologic trigger with a predilection for the postmenopausal, elderly female.[34,35] It is thought that microvascular dysfunction may be the pathologic mechanism in Takotsubo, though there is also an overlapping association reported with SCAD and myocardial bridging.[36–39]

Chronic Presentations

Chronic IHD in women most commonly presents as stable angina, independent of underlying etiology.[40] However, compared with men, women report broader symptomology (ie, shortness of breath, nausea, epigastric pain) and are more likely to report atypical symptoms such as fatigue, jaw pain, or dyspnea. Women present later into their symptom onset or will have repeated visits with the medical system before diagnosis. Women with nonobstructive disease will have had a myriad of tests (stress test, invasive angiography, computed tomography angiography [CTA]) and may be falsely reassured or dismissed if they are negative.[41]

PATHOPHYSIOLOGY
Differences in Types of Disease

Although chronic IHD from obstructive epicardial disease is common, women with angina disproportionally suffer from nonobstructive etiologies of ischemic heart disease.[3,18,40,42–44]

Under the umbrella term of open artery ischemia (OAI),[45] several stable clinical phenotypes have emerged.[45]

1. ANOCA (angina with non-obstructive coronary arteries)
2. INOCA (ischemia with non-obstructive coronary arteries)[46]

These clinical phenotypes are manifestations of several endotypes of disease (coronary spasm, myocardial bridge, endothelial dysfunction, coronary microvascular dysfunction [CMD], and microvascular spasm). These endotypes can be divided anatomically into disease of the epicardial and microvascular circulation as discussed below (Fig. 1).

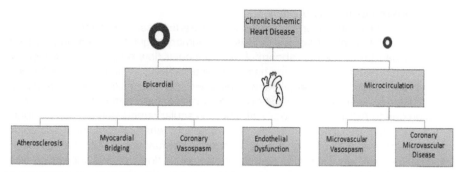

Fig. 1. Etiologies of chronic IHD categorized anatomically.

Epicardial Circulation

Atherosclerosis

Women are more likely to have diffuse and nonobstructive atherosclerosis noted on coronary angiogram. Although focally nonobstructive, diffuse disease can be functionally significant. The WISE study, in women with stable symptomatic CAD, demonstrated that 57% of women with symptoms and signs of ischemia had nonobstructive CAD on angiography.[47] Nonobstructive CAD is defined as less than 50% diameter stenosis of all major epicardial vessels and is at least twice as prevalent in women compared with men.[15] The sex-specific difference in incidence of obstructive atherosclerosis is most notable earlier in life and becomes less significant with age (and menopause).[5]

Epicardial artery vasospasm and endothelial dysfunction

Prinzmetal angina is a clinical syndrome of recurrent angina associated with myocardial ischemia from coronary spasm. Chest pain often occurs at rest or at night; however, exertional symptoms in the morning have also been reported.[46] Smoking is an established risk factor where diabetes and HTN are not. On invasive testing, coronary spasm is defined as severe (>90%) constriction of the coronary artery after administration of acetylcholine with ECG changes indicative of ischemia and associated angina.

Endothelial dysfunction is also diagnosed on invasive testing with administration of acetylcholine and is diagnosed in the setting of constriction of the epicardial vessel (>0% to <90%) with acetylcholine instead of the expected vasodilation in normal vasculature.

Myocardial bridge

This is a congenital anomaly where a segment of epicardial vessel traverses through the myocardium and is thus compressed during systole. The degree of compression is not predictable of the hemodynamic effects. Most commonly, the bridge overlies the left anterior descending artery. Myocardial bridges are common and are reported in 25% of autopsies and CT angiograms. Although most are not hemodynamically or clinically significant, they can been associated with acute and chronic IHD.[37]

Microcirculation

Microvascular spasm

Vasospastic angina can also be due to microvascular spasm. Challenging to diagnose, microvascular spasm is diagnosed by ECG changes and angina in the absence of epicardial constriction with administration of acetylcholine invasively; however, functionally should show decreased coronary blood flow and increased sinus lactate accumulation after administration of acetylcholine.

Coronary microvascular dysfunction

The coronary microcirculation (arterioles and pre-arterioles) represents 90% of the coronary circulating blood volume and is the primary regulator of coronary blood flow. CMD can be defined as abnormal microvascular flow responses or abnormal microvascular resistance[45,48,49] and has multiple underlying etiologies. These include structural and functional abnormalities as well as external causes (myocardial and systemic).[45] Structural etiologies include microvascular luminal obstruction (ie, microembolization during ACS), vascular wall infiltration, vascular remodeling (ie, hypertrophic cardiomyopathy), perivascular fibrosis, or rarefaction, whereas functional etiologies include endothelial, smooth muscle, or autonomic dysfunction.[5] CMD can be diagnosed in the noninvasively with decreased coronary flow reserve (coronary flow reserve [CFR] <2.0–2.5) on PET imaging or invasively with abnormal microvascular resistance (index of microvascualr resistance [IMR] <25 or hyperemic microvascular resistance [hMR]<2.0) on coronary function testing.[40]

Diagnostic Testing in Stable IHD

Evaluation of obstructive disease

Risk stratification of chest pain before test selection helps determine pretest probability of disease. Traditional risk scores (ie, Framingham and Diamond and Forrester) tend to overestimate women's risk for obstructive coronary disease. Young age significantly lowers pretest probability of detecting IHD. Thus, young women with multiple risk factors or risk enhancers (ie, hypertensive disorders of pregnancy, early menopause, diabetes)[50] should have more nuanced risk assessment. Newer risk scores should be considered for more accurate contemporary risk assessment of ischemic heart disease.[51–54] Current risk assessment can help identify low-risk patients not requiring additional diagnostic testing for obstructive CAD.[53]

Choice of initial diagnostic testing

Choosing the appropriate diagnostic test for evaluation of ischemic heart disease in women depends on several factors such as test availability, local expertise, patient's body habitus, and ability to exercise.

The 2021 chest pain guidelines give coronary CTA (CCTA) and stress testing both class I indications in patients with intermediate or high pretest probability and no established coronary disease. Both should be considered and have intrinsic advantages and disadvantages; however, there are some sex differences in noninvasive stress testing that should be considered.

In a sub-study of PROMISE evaluating the association between sex and noninvasive testing results and adverse events (composite of death, myocardial infarction, and unstable angina), women were significantly less likely to have an abnormal CCTA (>70% stenosis) compared with a positive stress test. CCTA was less likely to be positive compared with exercise ECG and nuclear stress (OR: 0.66, $P < .001$) but not compared with stress echocardiography.[55] Women with a positive CCTA were more strongly associated with clinical events than a positive stress test suggesting it is a better predictor of adverse events.[56]

In addition, CCTA can help detect nonobstructive atherosclerotic plaque, which is associated with increased mortality compared with those without CAD. Data from the CAC consortium showed that women with larger and more numerous calcified lesions on CCTA had a 2.2-fold higher CVD mortality compared with men suggesting a higher relative risk in women compared with men.[55,56]

Future guidelines may provide sex-specific recommendations for stress testing as the nuanced differences between men and women are better understood.

Functional coronary assessment

For patients with persistent symptoms, evidence of ischemia, and no obstructive disease on imaging, PET stress testing and stress CMR may provide additional noninvasive imaging options for the evaluation of persistent chest pain symptoms and nonobstructive disease to evaluate for microvascular dysfunction. These are both given a 2a recommendation in the 2021 Chest Pain guidelines.

Coronary function testing is an invasive option to evaluate for microvascular dysfunction but provides the additional opportunity to assess for endothelial dependent dysfunction with the administration of acetylcholine.

Management

Historically, ischemic burden on testing and angina symptoms have thought to be closely linked and targeting ischemia would also treat angina.

However, recent studies have shown that angina symptoms/severity are not directly associated with the presence of ischemia: a discordance not well understood. In the CIAO-ISCHEMIA trial, it was found that among women with INOCA, improvement in ischemia (23%) and angina (43%) were common at 1 year but were not correlated.[57] This highlights the importance of considering both ischemia and angina when managing a patient with ischemic heart disease.

Pharmacotherapy

For traditional atherosclerotic disease, women should be treated aggressively with secondary prevention interventions such aspirin, statins, cardiac rehabilitation.

Pharmacotherapy for OAI should target the underlying endotype (**Fig. 2**). The CorMICA trial tested the use of an invasive diagnostic strategy in angina and nonobstructive coronary artery disease and was able to show an improvement in Seattle Angina Questionnaire and Quality of life.[58]

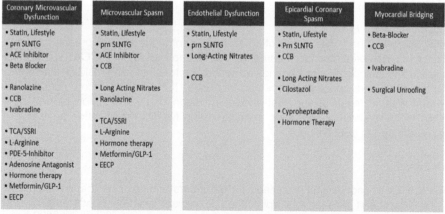

Coronary Microvascular Dysfunction	Microvascular Spasm	Endothelial Dysfunction	Epicardial Coronary Spasm	Myocardial Bridging
• Statin, Lifestyle	• Statin, Lifestyle	• Statin, Lifestyle	• Statin, Lifestyle	• Beta-Blocker
• prn SLNTG	• prn SLNTG	• prn SLNTG	• Prn SLNTG	• CCB
• ACE Inhibitor	• ACE Inhibitor	• Long-Acting Nitrates	• CCB	
• Beta Blocker	• CCB			• Ivabradine
		• CCB	• Long Acting Nitrates	
• Ranolazine	• Long Acting Nitrates		• Cilostazol	• Surgical Unroofing
• CCB	• Ranolazine			
• Ivabradine			• Cyproheptadine	
	• TCA/SSRI		• Hormone Therapy	
• TCA/SSRI	• L-Arginine			
• L-Arginine	• Hormone therapy			
• PDE-5-Inhibitor	• Metformin/GLP-1			
• Adenosine Antagonist	• EECP			
• Hormone therapy				
• Metformin/GLP-1				
• EECP				

Fig. 2. Treatment pathways for patients with ANOCA. This figure includes therapies for patients with ANOCA based on endotype. ACE, angiotensin-converting enzyme; ANOCA, angina with nonobstructive coronary arteries; CCBs, calcium channel blockers; EECP, enhanced external counterpulsation; GLP-1, glucagon-like peptide-1; PDE-5, phosphodiesterase 5 inhibitors; SLNTG, sublingual nitroglycerin; TCA/SSRI, tricyclic antidepressants/selective serotonin reuptake inhibitors. (*Adapted from* Smilowitz NR, Prasad M, Widmer RJ, et al. Comprehensive Management of ANOCA, Part 2—Program Development, Treatment, and Research Initiatives. J Am Coll Cardiol. 2023;82(12):1264-1279. https://doi.org/10.1016/j.jacc.2023.06.044)

The recent JACC State of the Art Review of ANOCA outlines treatment strategies for individual endotypes (see **Fig. 2**). Lifestyle changes and statins are the cornerstone therapy for all endotypes, but additional treatment needs to be individualized.[59]

For coronary microvascular dysfunction, first-line therapy includes nonselective beta blockade, angiotensin converting enzyme inhibitor (ACE-I), and sublingual nitroglycerin. Ranolazine, calcium channel blockers, and ivabradine can also be considered. The second line includes ranolazine, calcium channel blockers, and nitrates.[59]

For vasospasm (both epicardial and microvascular), the mainstay of therapy includes calcium channel blockers and short-acting nitrates.[59] For microvascular spasm, ACE-inhibitors should also be considered.

For myocardial bridging, beta blockade or calcium channel blockers are the treatment of choice and nitrates should be avoided as it is thought to dilate the proximal and distal segments of the compressed artery and can worsen the resulting systolic stenosis. Percutaneous coronary intervention (PCI) or surgical myotomy is the surgical intervention of choice and should be considered on a case-by-case basis.[36,37]

For endothelial dysfunction, nitrates and calcium channel blockers should be considered.

Considerations in Pregnancy

Acute presentation in pregnancy

AMI is uncommon in women of reproductive age. However, pregnancy increases the risk three- to fourfold and is associated with significant morbidity and mortality.[60–62] The recent reported case fatality rate is approximately 5%.[60] There is a higher incidence of myocardial infarction with increasing maternal age.[60] Acute MIs are most common in the third trimester or postpartum period. Approximately 25% of women present with an STEMI and 75% with an non-ST elevation MI (NSTEMI). The anterior wall is most commonly involved (69% of cases). The mechanism of injury is most commonly due to coronary dissection (43%), followed by atherosclerosis (27%) and thrombosis (17%).[63]

Chronic ischemic heart disease

Established coronary disease is not an absolute contraindication to pregnancy. However, it is a risk predictor for maternal cardiac complications in the CARPREG II risk index.[64] The associated risk depends on several factors including residual left ventricular function and ongoing myocardial ischemia. It has been recommended that women wait at least 1-year post-revascularization or postinfarction before pregnancy[65,66] and should undergoing cardiac testing for risk stratification prior as part of preconception counseling.

SUMMARY

Over the last decade, we have gained a better understanding of sex-based differences in ischemic heart disease but application in clinical practice is still limited. With increased testing availability, improved insurance coverage for testing, and development of more targeted treatment options, there is hope that the entire spectrum of ischemic heart disease will be better understood and optimally treated.

CLINICS CARE POINTS

- Review sex-specific risk factors when evaluating a woman's risk for ischemic heart disease.

- Consider the entire spectrum of ischemic heart disease in patients presenting with angina.
- MINOCA is a working diagnosis requiring further investigation.

REFERENCES

1. Hemingway H, Langenberg C, Damant J, et al. Prevalence of Angina in Women Versus Men. Circulation 2008;117(12). https://doi.org/10.1161/circulationaha. 107.720953.
2. Gijsberts CM, Agostoni P, Hoefer IE, et al. Gender differences in health-related quality of life in patients undergoing coronary angiography. Open Heart 2015; 2(1). https://doi.org/10.1136/openhrt-2014-000231.
3. Schmidt KMT, Nan J, Scantlebury DC, et al. Stable Ischemic Heart Disease in Women. Curr Treat Options Cardiovasc Med 2018;20(9). https://doi.org/10. 1007/s11936-018-0665-4.
4. Mehilli J, Presbitero P. Coronary artery disease and acute coronary syndrome in women. Heart 2020;106(7). https://doi.org/10.1136/heartjnl-2019-315555.
5. Reynolds HR, Bairey Merz CN, Berry C, et al. Coronary arterial function and disease in women with no obstructive coronary arteries. Circ Res 2022;130(4). https://doi.org/10.1161/CIRCRESAHA.121.319892.
6. Sanghavi M, Gulati M. Sex differences in the pathophysiology, treatment, and outcomes in IHD. Curr Atheroscler Rep 2015;17(6). https://doi.org/10.1007/s11883-015-0511-z.
7. Hiteshi AK, Li D, Gao Y, et al. Gender differences in coronary artery diameter are not related to body habitus or left ventricular mass. Clin Cardiol 2014;37(10). https://doi.org/10.1002/clc.22310.
8. Taqueti VR. Sex differences in the coronary system. Adv Exp Med Biol 2018;1065. https://doi.org/10.1007/978-3-319-77932-4_17.
9. Aggarwal NR, Patel HN, Mehta LS, et al. Sex differences in ischemic heart disease: advances, obstacles, and next steps. Circ Cardiovasc Qual Outcomes 2018;11(2). https://doi.org/10.1161/CIRCOUTCOMES.117.004437.
10. Yusuf PS, Hawken S, Ôunpuu S, et al. Effect of potentially modifiable risk factors associated with myocardial infarction in 52 countries (the INTERHEART study): Case-control study. Lancet 2004;364(9438). https://doi.org/10.1016/S0140-6736(04)17018-9.
11. Geraghty L, Figtree GA, Schutte AE, et al. Cardiovascular disease in women: from pathophysiology to novel and emerging risk factors. Heart Lung Circ 2021;30(1). https://doi.org/10.1016/j.hlc.2020.05.108.
12. Kaminski P, Szpotanska-Sikorska M, Wielgos M. Cardiovascular risk and the use of oral contraceptives. Neuroendocrinol Lett 2013;34(7).
13. Garovic VD, Dechend R, Easterling T, et al. Hypertension in pregnancy: diagnosis, blood pressure goals, and pharmacotherapy: a scientific statement from the American heart association. Hypertension 2022;79(2). https://doi.org/10. 1161/HYP.0000000000000208.
14. Mulvagh SL, Mullen KA, Nerenberg KA, et al. The Canadian Women's Heart Health Alliance Atlas on the epidemiology, diagnosis, and management of cardiovascular disease in women — chapter 4: sex- and gender-unique disparities: CVD across the lifespan of a woman. CJC Open 2022;4(2). https://doi.org/10. 1016/j.cjco.2021.09.013.

15. Pravda NS, Karny-Rahkovich O, Shiyovich A, et al. Coronary artery disease in women: A comprehensive appraisal. J Clin Med 2021;10(20). https://doi.org/10.3390/jcm10204664.

16. Young L, Cho L. Unique cardiovascular risk factors in women. Heart 2019; 105(21). https://doi.org/10.1136/heartjnl-2018-314268.

17. O'Kelly AC, Michos ED, Shufelt CL, et al. Pregnancy and reproductive risk factors for cardiovascular disease in women. Circ Res 2022;130(4). https://doi.org/10.1161/CIRCRESAHA.121.319895.

18. Samad F, Agarwal A, Samad Z. Stable ischemic heart disease in women: Current perspectives. Int J Womens Health 2017;9. https://doi.org/10.2147/IJWH.S107372.

19. Naftolin F, Friedenthal J, Nachtigall R, et al. Cardiovascular health and the menopausal woman: The role of estrogen and when to begin and end hormone treatment [version 1; peer review: 3 approved]. F1000Res 2019;8. https://doi.org/10.12688/f1000research.15548.1.

20. Cho L, Davis M, Elgendy I, et al. Summary of updated recommendations for primary prevention of cardiovascular disease in women: JACC state-of-the-art review. J Am Coll Cardiol 2020;75(20). https://doi.org/10.1016/j.jacc.2020.03.060.

21. Nappi RE, Chedraui P, Lambrinoudaki I, et al. Menopause: a cardiometabolic transition. Lancet Diabetes Endocrinol 2022;10(6). https://doi.org/10.1016/S2213-8587(22)00076-6.

22. Ajeganova S, Hafström I, Frostegård J. Patients with SLE have higher risk of cardiovascular events and mortality in comparison with controls with the same levels of traditional risk factors and intima-media measures, which is related to accumulated disease damage and antiphospholipid syndrome: A case-control study over 10 years. Lupus Sci Med 2021;8(1). https://doi.org/10.1136/lupus-2020-000454.

23. Vogel B, Acevedo M, Appelman Y, et al. The Lancet women and cardiovascular disease Commission: reducing the global burden by 2030. Lancet 2021;397: 10292. https://doi.org/10.1016/S0140-6736(21)00684-X.

24. Jespersen L, Abildstrøm SZ, Hvelplund A, et al. Persistent angina: Highly prevalent and associated with long-term anxiety, depression, low physical functioning, and quality of life in stable angina pectoris. Clin Res Cardiol 2013;102(8). https://doi.org/10.1007/s00392-013-0568-z.

25. Hamad R, Penko J, Kazi DS, et al. Association of low socioeconomic status with premature coronary heart disease in US adults. JAMA Cardiol 2020;5(8). https://doi.org/10.1001/jamacardio.2020.1458.

26. Minissian MB, Mehta PK, Hayes SN, et al. Ischemic heart disease in young women: JACC review topic of the week. J Am Coll Cardiol 2022;80(10). https://doi.org/10.1016/j.jacc.2022.01.057.

27. Mehta LS, Beckie TM, DeVon HA, et al. Acute myocardial infarction in women : a scientific statement from the american heart association. Circulation 2016;133(9). https://doi.org/10.1161/CIR.0000000000000351.

28. Tamis-Holland JE, Jneid H, Reynolds HR, et al. Contemporary diagnosis and management of patients with myocardial infarction in the absence of obstructive coronary artery disease: a scientific statement from the american heart association. Circulation 2019;139(18). https://doi.org/10.1161/CIR.0000000000000670.

29. Maehara A, Kwong RY, et al. Coronary optical coherence tomography and cardiac magnetic resonance imaging to determine underlying causes of myocardial infarction with nonobstructive coronary arteries in women. Circulation 2021;143: 624–40. Circulation. 2023;147(8). doi:10.1161/CIR.0000000000001132.

30. Mahmoud AN, Taduru SS, Mentias A, et al. Trends of incidence, clinical presentation, and in-hospital mortality among women with acute myocardial infarction with or without spontaneous coronary artery dissection: a population-based analysis. JACC Cardiovasc Interv 2018;11(1). https://doi.org/10.1016/j.jcin.2017.08.016.

31. Kim ESH. Spontaneous coronary-artery dissection. N Engl J Med 2020;383(24):2358–70.

32. Saw J, Humphries K, Aymong E, et al. Spontaneous coronary artery dissection: clinical outcomes and risk of recurrence. J Am Coll Cardiol 2017;70(9). https://doi.org/10.1016/j.jacc.2017.06.053.

33. Hayes SN, Kim CESH, Saw J, et al. Spontaneous coronary artery dissection: current state of the science: a scientific statement from the american heart association. Circulation 2018;137(19). https://doi.org/10.1161/CIR.0000000000000564.

34. Cheema AN, Yanagawa B, Verma S, et al. Myocardial infarction with nonobstructive coronary artery disease (MINOCA): A review of pathophysiology and management. Curr Opin Cardiol 2021;36(5):589–96.

35. Lyon AR, Citro R, Schneider B, et al. Pathophysiology of Takotsubo syndrome: JACC State-of-the-art review. J Am Coll Cardiol 2021;77(7). https://doi.org/10.1016/j.jacc.2020.10.060.

36. Corban MT, Hung OY, Eshtehardi P, et al. Myocardial bridging: Contemporary understanding of pathophysiology with implications for diagnostic and therapeutic strategies. J Am Coll Cardiol 2014;63(22). https://doi.org/10.1016/j.jacc.2014.01.049.

37. Sternheim D, Power DA, Samtani R, et al. Myocardial bridging: diagnosis, functional assessment, and management: JACC state-of-the-art review. J Am Coll Cardiol 2021;78(22). https://doi.org/10.1016/j.jacc.2021.09.859.

38. Kegai S, Sato K, Goto K, et al. Coexistence of spontaneous coronary artery dissection, takotsubo cardiomyopathy, and myocardial bridge. JACC Case Rep 2021;3(2). https://doi.org/10.1016/j.jaccas.2020.11.042.

39. Hausvater A, Smilowitz NR, Saw J, et al. Spontaneous coronary artery dissection in patients with a provisional diagnosis of takotsubo syndrome. J Am Heart Assoc 2019;8(22). https://doi.org/10.1161/JAHA.119.013581.

40. Samuels BA, Shah SM, Widmer RJ, et al. Comprehensive management of ANOCA, part 1—definition, patient population, and diagnosis: JACC state-of-the-art review. J Am Coll Cardiol 2023;82(12):1245–63.

41. Dean J, Cruz SD, Mehta PK, et al. Coronary microvascular dysfunction: Sex-specific risk, diagnosis, and therapy. Nat Rev Cardiol 2015;12(7). https://doi.org/10.1038/nrcardio.2015.72.

42. Kunadian V, Chieffo A, Camici PG, et al. An EAPCI expert consensus document on ischaemia with non-obstructive coronary arteries in collaboration with European society of cardiology working group on coronary pathophysiology & microcirculation endorsed by coronary vasomotor disorders international study group. Eur Heart J 2020;41(37):3504–20.

43. Reeh J, Therming CB, Heitmann M, et al. Prediction of obstructive coronary artery disease and prognosis in patients with suspected stable angina. Eur Heart J 2019;40(18). https://doi.org/10.1093/eurheartj/ehy806.

44. Ford TJ, Corcoran D, Berry C. Stable coronary syndromes: Pathophysiology, diagnostic advances and therapeutic need. Heart 2018;104(4):284–92.

45. Pepine CJ. ANOCA/INOCA/MINOCA: Open artery ischemia. Am Heart J: Cardiol Res Pract 2023;26. https://doi.org/10.1016/j.ahjo.2023.100260.

46. Kenkre TS, Malhotra P, Johnson BD, et al. Ten-year mortality in the wise study (women's ischemia syndrome evaluation). Circ Cardiovasc Qual Outcomes 2017;10(12). https://doi.org/10.1161/CIRCOUTCOMES.116.003863.

47. Beltrame JF, Crea F, Kaski JC, et al. International standardization of diagnostic criteria for vasospastic angina. Eur Heart J 2017;38(33). https://doi.org/10.1093/eurheartj/ehv351.

48. Camici PG, Crea F. Coronary microvascular dysfunction. N Engl J Med 2007; 356(8). https://doi.org/10.1056/nejmra061889.

49. Ford TJ, Ong P, Sechtem U, et al. Assessment of vascular dysfunction in patients without obstructive coronary artery disease: why, how, and when. JACC Cardiovasc Interv 2020;13(16). https://doi.org/10.1016/j.jcin.2020.05.052.

50. Juarez-Orozco LE, Saraste A, Capodanno D, et al. Impact of a decreasing pre-test probability on the performance of diagnostic tests for coronary artery disease. Eur Heart J Cardiovasc Imaging 2019;20(11). https://doi.org/10.1093/ehjci/jez054.

51. Winther S, Schmidt SE, Mayrhofer T, et al. Incorporating coronary calcification into pre-test assessment of the likelihood of coronary artery disease. J Am Coll Cardiol 2020;76(21). https://doi.org/10.1016/j.jacc.2020.09.585.

52. Gulati M, Levy PD, Mukherjee D, et al. 2021 AHA/ACC/ASE/CHEST/SAEM/SCCT/SCMR guideline for the evaluation and diagnosis of chest pain. J Cardiovasc Comput Tomogr 2022;16(1). https://doi.org/10.1016/j.jcct.2021.11.009.

53. Sanghavi M, Parikh NI. Harnessing the power of pregnancy and pregnancy-related events to predict cardiovascular disease in women. Circulation 2017; 135(6). https://doi.org/10.1161/CIRCULATIONAHA.117.026890.

54. Reynolds HR, Hausvater A, Carney K. Test selection for women with suspected stable ischemic heart disease. J Womens Health 2018;27(7). https://doi.org/10.1089/jwh.2017.6587.

55. Pagidipati NJ, Hemal K, Coles A, et al. Sex differences in functional and CT angiography testing in patients with suspected coronary artery disease. J Am Coll Cardiol 2016;67(22). https://doi.org/10.1016/j.jacc.2016.03.523.

56. Rodriguez Lozano PF, Rrapo Kaso E, Bourque JM, et al. Cardiovascular imaging for ischemic heart disease in women: time for a paradigm shift. JACC Cardiovasc Imaging 2022;15(8). https://doi.org/10.1016/j.jcmg.2022.01.006.

57. Reynolds HR, Picard MH, Spertus JA, et al. Natural history of patients with ischemia and no obstructive coronary artery disease: The CIAO-ISCHEMIA study. Circulation 2021;144(13). https://doi.org/10.1161/CIRCULATIONAHA.120.046791.

58. Ford TJ, Stanley B, Good R, et al. Stratified medical therapy using invasive coronary function testing in angina: the CorMicA trial. J Am Coll Cardiol 2018; 72(23). https://doi.org/10.1016/j.jacc.2018.09.006.

59. Smilowitz NR, Prasad M, Widmer RJ, et al. Comprehensive management of ANOCA, part 2—program development, treatment, and research initiatives. J Am Coll Cardiol 2023;82(12):1264–79.

60. James AH, Jamison MG, Biswas MS, et al. Acute myocardial infarction in pregnancy: A United States population-based study. Circulation 2006;113(12). https://doi.org/10.1161/CIRCULATIONAHA.105.576751.

61. Pacheco LD, Saade GR, Hankins GDV. Acute myocardial infarction during pregnancy. Clin Obstet Gynecol 2014;57(4). https://doi.org/10.1097/GRF.0000000000000065.

62. Roth A, Elkayam U. Acute myocardial infarction associated with pregnancy. J Am Coll Cardiol 2008;52(3). https://doi.org/10.1016/j.jacc.2008.03.049.

63. Elkayam U, Jalnapurkar S, Barakkat MN, et al. Pregnancy-associated acute myocardial infarction: a review of contemporary experience in 150 cases between 2006 and 2011. Circulation 2014;129(16). https://doi.org/10.1161/CIRCULATIONAHA.113.002054.
64. Silversides CK, Grewal J, Mason J, et al. Pregnancy outcomes in women with heart disease: the CARPREG II study. J Am Coll Cardiol 2018;71(21). https://doi.org/10.1016/j.jacc.2018.02.076.
65. Regitz-Zagrosek V, Roos-Hesselink JW, Bauersachs J, et al. 2018 ESC Guidelines for the management of cardiovascular diseases during pregnancy. Eur Heart J 2018;39(34). https://doi.org/10.1093/eurheartj/ehy340.
66. Wilson AM, Boyle AJ, Fox P. Management of ischaemic heart disease in women of child-bearing age. Intern Med J 2004;34(12). https://doi.org/10.1111/j.1445-5994.2004.00698.x.

Chronic Coronary Disease in Older Adults

Alexander P. Ambrosini, MD[a,1], Emily S. Fishman, MD[a,1],
Abdulla A. Damluji, MD, PhD[b,c], Michael G. Nanna, MD, MHS[d,*]

KEYWORDS

• Aging • Older adults • Geriatrics • Coronary artery disease • Revascularization

KEY POINTS

- The number of older adults living with chronic coronary disease is on the rise.
- Geriatric syndromes make diagnosing, treating, and managing complications of chronic coronary disease more complex.
- Medical and interventional therapies for chronic coronary disease have similar benefits for both younger and older adults; however, older adults experience more side effects, trade-offs, and complications.
- Medical decision-making should consider patient symptoms, preferences, and goals of care.
- A comprehensive geriatric heart team approach should be implemented when deciding upon treatment option.

INTRODUCTION

Chronic coronary disease (CCD) is a major cause of morbidity and mortality in older adults.[1,2] Despite this, older adults are underrepresented in the current literature supporting treatments in patients living with CCD. This poses a challenge for clinicians attempting to appropriately weigh the risks and benefits of therapeutic options during shared decision-making with patients. This review focuses on CCD in older adults and outlines the current literature, discusses current medical and invasive treatment options, recommends a patient-centered approach to complex decision-making, and suggests areas for future research.

[a] Department of Internal Medicine, Yale School of Medicine, New Haven, CT, USA; [b] Inova Center of Outcomes Research, Inova Heart and Vascular Institute, Falls Church, VA, USA; [c] Johns Hopkins University School of Medicine, Baltimore, MD, USA; [d] Section of Cardiovascular Medicine, Yale School of Medicine, New Haven, CT 06520, USA
[1] These two authors equally contributed to the manuscript.
* Corresponding author.
E-mail address: michael.nanna@yale.edu

Med Clin N Am 108 (2024) 581–594
https://doi.org/10.1016/j.mcna.2023.12.004

What Is an Older Adult?

The traditional definition of older adults in the United States is age ≥ 65 years. As the population of the United States and the world ages, adults are remaining active and healthier for longer. To reflect this change, current cardiovascular literature now classifies the older adult as age ≥ 75 years.[3] This population, however, is heterogeneous in its cognitive and functional status, level of social and financial support, and medical complexity. Therefore, the management of medical conditions in older adults requires a comprehensive and individualistic approach.

Defining Chronic Coronary Disease

CCD, also referred to as stable ischemic heart disease and stable angina, encompasses a variety of cardiac conditions. These can include individuals with obstructive or nonobstructive coronary artery disease (CAD), the presence or absence of prior myocardial infarction, symptoms of chronic angina or anginal equivalents, and coronary artery disease diagnosed with noninvasive testing.[3] The pathophysiology of CAD involves plaque formation and vascular remodeling that is mediated by modifiable and non-modifiable risk factors, including chronologic age.[4] Older adults often have a higher burden of these risk factors and chronic medical conditions that can mimic or mask the symptoms of CCD. On presentation, older adults are more likely to have silent ischemia and experience non-chest pain symptoms compared with younger adults.[3] Anginal equivalents or accompanying symptoms can include fatigue, dyspnea, and epigastric pain, which can be difficult to distinguish from conditions such as anemia, gastroesophageal reflux disease, chronic pulmonary disease, or deconditioning.[5] These complex phenotypic profiles of CCD in older adults can make it difficult to diagnose and identify the need for advancing therapies. This further highlights the importance of taking a thorough clinical history when identifying and managing older patients with suspected CCD.

Prevalence of Chronic Coronary Disease in Older Adults

Roughly 30% of adults aged ≥ 75 years are living with CCD, with similar prevalence observed in men and women.[1,2] The overall prevalence is expected to rise due to multiple factors, including (1) the aging of the population at large (2) the incidence of new CCD is highest in older adults, (3) mortality after acute coronary syndrome (ACS) has improved with modern therapies, and (4) increased performance of existing noninvasive and invasive testing tools to detect more clinically silent disease.[1,2] It is important to note that while the disease burden is greatest in older adults, disease complexity is also increased due to underlying physiologic and anatomic differences. For example, older adults frequently present with more diffuse, calcified, and anatomically complex CAD, increased vessel tortuosity, microvascular disease, and endothelial dysfunction.[1] Additional data suggest that the onset of CCD is a better prognostic marker of future disability than myocardial infarction.[6] Therefore, with an aging population, CCD represents an expanding burden on patients, caregivers, and the health care system at large.

Geriatric Syndromes

Geriatric syndromes are a collection of clinical conditions that occur frequently with aging and influence cardiovascular outcomes.[7,8] Common geriatric syndromes include falls, delirium, frailty, polypharmacy, and functional or cognitive decline. Geriatric syndromes contribute to the complex clinical phenotype of patients with CCD and therefore must influence management strategies and response to treatment. It is important for clinicians to complete a cardiovascular risk assessment alongside a focused geriatric assessment including evaluation of multimorbidity, cognition, frailty, and social support. A recent Expert Panel recommended a minimum geriatric risk assessment that includes functional assessment, activities of daily living (ADLs), instrumental activities of daily living (IADLs), and goals of care, with further targeted comprehensive geriatric assessment of multimorbidity, polypharmacy, cognitive impairment, frailty, and falls **(Fig. 1)**.[9,10]

Diagnosing Chronic Coronary Disease in Older Adults

All patients with CCD are at increased risk for future major adverse cardiovascular events (MACE) and require regular follow-up. Further diagnostic workup is indicated in patients with CCD when there is clinical uncertainty, or a change in symptoms or functional capacity while on guideline-directed medical therapy (GDMT).[3] There are multiple factors that impact the utility of functional and anatomic assessment of CAD in older adults. Barriers to completing exercise stress testing in older adults, even with modified exercise protocols, include decreased muscle mass, reduced

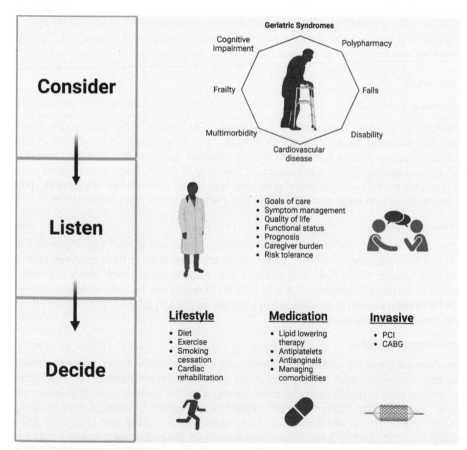

Fig. 1. CCD in Older Adults: "Consider, Listen, Decide" is a framework for approaching shared decision-making in the geriatric population. It highlights the need to consider different geriatric syndromes, listen to patients' goals of care, and decide which treatment options are best. CABG, coronary artery bypass grafting; PCI, percutaneous coronary intervention.

maximal heart rate, musculoskeletal pain, unsteadiness, and baseline electrocardiogram (ECG) abnormalities.[11] Pharmacologic stress tests with accompanying ECG, myocardial perfusion imaging, or echocardiography are feasible alternatives to exercise. Coronary computed tomography angiography (CCTA) presents some challenges in older adults given its increased likelihood of uninterpretable scans, either due to highly calcified plaques or motion artifact.[12] Recent guidelines suggest that CCTA is favored for patient age <65 years, but data are scarce and further dedicated studies are needed to assess generalizability across different ages.[13,14] Diagnostic coronary angiography should be considered within the context of candidacy for percutaneous coronary intervention (PCI) or surgical revascularization and broader goals of care.[3]

Therapeutic Options

The overarching goal of treatment is to prevent disease progression, control symptoms, and maintain patients' level of functioning, independence, and cognition. It is imperative that clinicians understand the risks and benefits of medical therapies and revascularization strategies as they specifically apply to older adults in order to provide the optimal guidance to patients. GDMT is indicated for all patients who have been diagnosed with CAD, regardless of chronologic age. Maximal GDMT for CCD includes preventive measures, optimizing comorbidities, medications aimed at preventing future cardiovascular events, and symptom-directed therapies. Current American and European guidelines recommend an initial medical therapy approach with revascularization reserved for patients with intolerable symptoms despite medical therapy.[3,15]

Lifestyle Modification

Lifestyle modification is essential to managing CCD. Encouraging healthy diet, exercise, and smoking cessation are indicated in all patients. Cardiac rehabilitation can help older adults initiate exercise regimens, improve quality of life, and decrease the risk of hospitalization and cardiovascular mortality.[16] Optimizing comorbidities such as glycemic control, weight, blood pressure, and stress are also key. Importantly, lifestyle modifications have more favorable risk-benefit profiles than medications.

Medical Therapies

Aging causes significant changes to the pharmacokinetics and pharmacodynamics of medical therapies used in CCD.[17] Older adults are more likely to have impaired kidney function, hepatic blood flow, and reduced lean muscle mass which affect the metabolism of certain medications.[17] It is important to recognize that all medical therapies that have been proven to be effective in younger adults can still be used in older adults with additional considerations.

Secondary Prevention

First-line secondary prevention treatment for CAD includes statin and antiplatelet therapy. American Heart Association (AHA) guidelines recommend either moderate-intensity or high-intensity statin for older adults, whereas European guidelines recommend high-intensity statin treatment regardless of age.[3,15] Goals of lipid-lowering therapy are a low-density lipoprotein (LDL) reduction of $\geq 50\%$ and LDL ≤ 70 while on high-intensity statin.[3] Recommendations also include additional lipid-lowering therapies, including ezetimibe and proprotein convertase subtilisin/kexin type 9 (PCSK9) inhibitors if cholesterol goals are not achieved with maximally tolerated statin.[3] Older adults have been underrepresented in trials for novel lipid-lowering therapies, though available data suggest that the benefits of lipid-lowering therapy for preventing secondary atherosclerotic cardiovascular disease events remain consistent across the age spectrum.[18] Additional research supports the use of high-intensity statin over moderate-intensity statin in older adults because of improved survival, however, this is not reflected in current guidelines.[19,20] Furthermore, older adults are less frequently given statins, especially high-intensity statins, for secondary prevention despite having a higher burden of disease and similar tolerability compared to younger adults.[21,22]

Dual antiplatelet therapy (DAPT) with low-dose aspirin and P2Y12 inhibitors have been the cornerstone of medical therapy among those with recent PCI or ACS. DAPT, notably, is not recommended in CCD without recent stent placement or ACS due to higher bleeding risk and absence of reduction in MACE.[3] Clopidogrel and ticagrelor are the preferred P2Y12 inhibitors to use in older adults as prasugrel is associated with increased bleeding risk in those age $\geq$75 years.[23,24] Current guidelines recommend 6 months of DAPT following PCI and potentially shorter durations of DAPT in those with high risk of bleeding.[3] Overall, DAPT is safe to use in older adults but bleeding risk does increase as patients age.[25] Further evidence is required to establish the optimal duration of DAPT in older adults following PCI in the current era of newer generation drug-eluting stents.[26,27] Aspirin monotherapy has historically been preferred as a single antiplatelet agent once transitioned off DAPT; however, recent data suggest that P2Y12 inhibitor monotherapy may reduce the risk of MACE with similar bleeding risk compared to aspirin alone.[28,29] In patients requiring oral anticoagulation following PCI, a short course (less than 30 days duration) of "triple therapy" with a direct oral anticoagulant (DOAC) and DAPT, followed by treatment with a DOAC plus single antiplatelet therapy with clopidogrel is the standard of care based on multiple randomized controlled trials.[3,30] DOAC monotherapy is another potential option for patients with chronic coronary disease (ie, >12 months from PCI) with low ischemic risk and who otherwise require oral anticoagulation.[13,31]

Antianginals

Recommended antianginal therapy includes either a beta-blocker (BB), calcium channel blocker (CCB), or long-acting nitrate for relief of angina and anginal-equivalents.[3] BB and CCB are the current first-line therapies based on US and European guidelines.[3,15] BB work by decreasing myocardial oxygen demand through reduction in heart rate and blood pressure, with the added benefit of disrupting maladaptive ventricular remodeling.[3,32] CCB increase coronary and peripheral vasodilation while also altering myocardial oxygen demand.[33] Use of BB in older adults may be limited by hypotension, bradycardia, dizziness, fatigue, sleep disturbances, sexual dysfunction, and possible cognitive and functional decline.[34] Limitations of CCB vary among dihydropyridine and non-dihydropyridine classes, though they are associated with peripheral edema and constipation. BB should not be initiated in CCD for patients without angina, anginal equivalents, or prior MI or heart failure with reduced ejection fraction.[3] The trials investigating BB and CCB are limited in their inclusion of older adults.[35,36]

Nitrates are just as effective at treating angina as CCB and BB; however, long-acting nitrates are considered second-line antianginals.[37,38] Both short-acting and long-acting nitrates improve exercise tolerance.[39] Common issues faced when using nitrates included headache and tachyphylaxis and they should be avoided in patients with severe aortic stenosis and those taking phosphodiesterase inhibitors.[40]

Refractory angina can be treated with combination therapy of BB, CCB, and nitrates, or with the addition of ranolazine. Ranolazine is an inhibitor of late inward sodium current.[41] Concerns specific to older adults include nausea, constipation, and prolongation of the QTC interval.[15,42]

Additional considerations for further reduction in MACE include sodium-glucose cotransporter-2 (SGLT2) inhibitors, glucagon-like peptide-1 (GLP1) agonists, and angiotensin-converting enzyme (ACE) inhibitors or angiotensin receptor blockers (ARB) in patients with comorbidities such as diabetes, obesity, chronic kidney disease, and systolic dysfunction.[3]

Managing Side Effects

To mitigate the risks of bothersome side effects and polypharmacy, the authors recommend that clinicians routinely screen for adverse events related to cardiovascular medications. If present, consider reducing the dose, switching drug classes, or discontinuing, before re-evaluating at subsequent visits.[43] Other helpful strategies include deliberate dosing schedules and collaboration with primary care providers, pharmacists, nurses, and home health care workers to ensure the maintenance of appropriate medication lists.

Revascularization Strategies

Revascularization in CCD represents a complex clinical scenario with limited data to guide management in older adults. Like medical therapy, the goals of revascularization are to improve symptom burden, prevent secondary events, and improve mortality. Current AHA guidelines recommend revascularization to improve symptoms in patients with CCD and lifestyle-limiting angina despite optimal medical therapy.[3] Mortality benefits have only been demonstrated following coronary artery bypass grafting (CABG) with medical therapy compared with medical therapy alone for either severe left main disease or multivessel disease with left ventricular (LV) systolic dysfunction (ejection fraction ≤35%) or diabetes.[3] A similar survival benefit is also demonstrated with either CABG or PCI for non-complex left main disease with normal LV systolic function.[3,44] When patients are poor surgical candidates, PCI can be used in place of CABG to improve symptoms and reduce MACE.[3] Unfortunately, older adults with complex multimorbid disease and those with geriatric syndromes were underrepresented in these studies.[45–48] Furthermore, current guidelines recommend a heart team approach, including interventionalists, general cardiologists, and surgeons, when there is complex triple vessel disease or when the optimal treatment plan is unclear.[3]

While many of the recommendations in the current guidelines are extrapolated from studies evaluating younger adults, the most compelling data evaluating invasive therapy compared to medical therapy in older adults demonstrate that (1) revascularization can improve angina and quality of life and (2) there is no significant difference in mortality with revascularization versus medical therapy, except in those with severe left main disease, multivessel disease with LV systolic dysfunction, and multivessel disease with diabetes (Table 1).[49–53] These factors must be considered within the context of older adults being at increased risk of in-hospital mortality, periprocedural mortality, and readmission following PCI.[54] With increasing age, patients also have worse outcomes after CABG compared with younger patients.[55] This is at least partially driven by the higher prevalence of frailty in older adults, which is associated with adverse outcomes and mortality following CABG surgery.[56,57] While clinicians may integrate assumptions about known natural life expectancy into therapeutic strategies, survival to older age is a strong predictor of longer life expectancy and many older adults have more than a decade of quality life-years remaining.[58] Furthermore, significant heterogeneity exists in biological aging across patients of similar chronologic ages, which has clear implications for therapeutic decisions.[59] Quantitative pre-procedural risk calculators that incorporate cardiovascular, physiologic, anatomic, and hemodynamic

Table 1
Characteristics and results of randomized trials of revascularization strategies in patients with chronic coronary disease with secondary analyses related to older adults

Trial (Author, Year Published)	Study Population (Sample Size)	Randomized Intervention	Average Age (Years)	Primary Endpoint	Implications for Older Adults
TIME (TIME Investigators, 2001)[49]	Patients ≥75 y with chronic angina classified as CCSC >2 despite ≥2 antianginals (n = 305)	Revascularization vs medical therapy	Mean age = 80	QoL (SF36[a]) at 6 mo: Revascularization = 11.4 vs medical therapy = 3.8; P = .008 MACE at 6 mo: Revascularization 19% vs medical 49% (P < .0001).	Older adults with angina despite medical management have improved QoL with revascularization vs medical therapy alone.
COURAGE (Sedlis et al,[60] 2017)	Patients with chronic stable angina or silent ischemia and angiographic CAD > 70% stenosis (n = 2287)	PCI and medical therapy vs medical therapy alone	Mean age (extended follow up) = 64	Death at 11.9 y: PCI = 25% vs medical therapy = 24%; adjusted HR = 1.03, 95% CI 0.83–1.21, P = .76	In sub-group analysis of age ≥ 65 y, similar clinical events with PCI and medical therapy vs medical therapy alone were observed[52]
BARI-2D (Ikeno et al,[46] 2017)	Patients with type II diabetes and evidence of ischemia (n = 2368)	Prompt revascularization (included CABG and PCI strata) vs medical therapy	Mean age = 62	Death, MI, or stroke at 5 y: low syntax ≤22; CABG 26.1% vs medical therapy 29.9%; P = .41; PCI 17.8% vs medical therapy 19.2%; P = .84; moderate to high syntax ≥23; CABG 15.3% vs medical 30.3%; P = .02; PCI 35.6% vs medical 26.5%; P = .12	Age ≥70 y (n = 514) with no difference in death, MACE, angina, or health status outcomes for revascularization vs medical therapy[53]

(continued on next page)

Table 1
(continued)

Trial (Author, Year Published)	Study Population (Sample Size)	Randomized Intervention	Average Age (Years)	Primary Endpoint	Implications for Older Adults
ISCHEMIA (Maron et al,[61] 2020)	Patients with stable CAD and moderate or severe ischemia (n = 5179)	Invasive vs conservative strategy	Mean age = 64	MACE at median 3.2 y: invasive vs conservative HR 0.93 (95% CI, 0.8–1.08); P = .34. Estimated cumulative event rate 6 mo: invasive = 5.3% vs conservative = 3.4% (95% CI, 0.8–3.0). Estimated cumulative event rate 5 y: invasive 16.4% vs conservative 18.2% (95% CI, −4.7–1.0)	Age ≥75 y (n = 665) had decreased frequency of angina but less improvement in angina-related health status with invasive management compared with younger adults[50]

Abbreviations: BARI-2D, The bypass angioplasty revascularization investigation 2 diabetes trial; CABG, coronary artery bypass grafting; CAD, coronary artery disease; CCSC, canadian cardiac society class; CI, confidence interval; COURAGE, the clinical outcomes utilizing revascularization and aggressive drug evaluation trial; HF, heart failure; HR, hazard ratio; ISCHEMIA, international study of comparative health effectiveness with medical and invasive approaches; MACE, major adverse cardiovascular events; MI, myocardial infarction; PCI, percutaneous coronary intervention; QoL, quality of life; TIME, Trial of Invasive versus Medical Therapy in Elderly Patients With Chronic Symptomatic Coronary-Artery Disease; UA, unstable angina.

a SF36 indicates Short Form 36 Health Survey. SF36 score 0 to 100 with higher scores indicating more favorable status.

risk are improved upon with the addition of a geriatric assessment.[10] These tools can help clinicians provide nuanced risk stratification in this medically complex cohort.

DISCUSSION

In the absence of compelling evidence to recommend medical therapy versus invasive revascularization, it is imperative that clinicians elicit patient preferences regarding treatment of CCD. The authors recommend utilizing the "Consider, Listen, Decide" framework (see **Fig. 1**) that was proposed as a standardized method for approaching treatment decisions in older adults with CCD.[5,43] In this framework, clinicians must first consider a patient's symptoms, comorbidities, and medications to create an impression of the broader clinical context of that individual patient. This can aid in identifying the symptoms that are leading to the greatest functional limitation and allow the clinician to appraise whether therapeutic options are likely to improve those symptoms or, conversely, worsen accompanying symptoms such as fatigue and lightheadedness. Next, clinicians listen to the patient's goals of care, priorities, and preferences. Eliciting a top health goal(s) facilitates the patient-clinician partnership and assists the multidisciplinary heart team in guiding the most appropriate treatment course, weighing the risks and benefits of lifestyle modification, medical therapies, and invasive options to arrive at a person-centered decision.

FUTURE DIRECTIONS

Older adults with CCD are a vulnerable and heterogeneous population with distinct priorities and preferences. To better serve them, there is a significant need for clinical trials enrolling older adults age $\geq$ 75 years with CCD to evaluate the most beneficial medical and revascularization strategies. One ongoing study, LIVEBETTER (A Trial Comparing the Effectiveness and Tolerability of Medications in Older Adults With Stable Angina and Multiple Chronic Conditions, NCT05786417), aims to determine the optimal antianginal approach in older adults with CCD and multiple chronic conditions while also focusing on patient-centered outcomes such as quality of life, symptom control, and mobility. Further evidence, testing of shared decision-making tools, improved risk models, and exploration of patient-centered outcomes that matter most to patients are essential to inform medical decisions and promote the care of older adults.

SUMMARY

The prevalence of CCD is increasing as our population ages and older adults are more likely to experience CCD than younger adults. However, older adults are underrepresented in current CCD literature, and they often present with complex geriatric phenotypes which increase the complexity of shared decisions. A holistic shared decision-making approach considering the broader patient context can assist patients in the delicate balance between treatment benefits, harms, and tradeoffs. Dedicated studies in representative geriatric populations are urgently needed to better inform clinicians and patients in these complex decisions.

CLINICS CARE POINTS

- Incorporating geriatric syndromes is necessary to guide optimal treatment decisions for CCD in older adults.

- Older adults should be optimized on GDMT, albeit with close attention to the potential burden of adverse effects, drug-drug interactions, and polypharmacy.
- Older adults generally derive similar benefits from most medical and invasive treatments compared to younger adults.
- Older adults have increased risk of morbidity and mortality when undergoing invasive treatments for CCD compared with younger adults.
- A geriatric heart team approach is critical to person-centered revascularization decisions in older adults with CCD.

DISCLOSURE

Drs E.S. Fishman and A.P. Ambrosini report no disclosures. A.A. Damluji: Dr A.A. Damluji receives research funding from the Pepper Scholars Program of the Johns Hopkins University Claude D. Pepper Older Americans Independence Center, United States funded by the National Institute on Aging P30-AG021334 and receives mentored patient-oriented research career development award from the National Heart, Lung, and Blood Institute, United States K23-HL153771 to 01. M.G. Nanna: Dr M.G. Nanna reports current research support from the American College of Cardiology Foundation, United States supported by the George F. and Ann Harris Bellows Foundation, the Patient-Centered Outcomes Research Institute, United States (PCORI), the Yale Claude D. Pepper Older Americans Independence Center (P30AG021342), and the National Institute on Aging/National Institutes of Health from R03AG074067 (GEMSSTAR award). Consulting from Heartflow, Inc, Merck.

REFERENCES

1. Dai X, Busby-Whitehead J, Forman DE, et al. Stable ischemic heart disease in the older adults. J Geriatr Cardiol 2016;13(2):109–14.
2. Tsao CW, Aday AW, Almarzooq ZI, et al. Heart Disease and Stroke Statistics-2023 Update: A Report From the American Heart Association. Circulation 2023; 147(8):e93–621.
3. Virani SS, Newby LK, Arnold SV, et al. AHA/ACC/ACCP/ASPC/NLA/PCNA Guideline for the Management of Patients With Chronic Coronary Disease: A Report of the American Heart Association/American College of Cardiology Joint Committee on Clinical Practice Guidelines. Circulation 2023. https://doi.org/10.1161/CIR.0000000000001168.
4. Libby P, Theroux P. Pathophysiology of coronary artery disease. Circulation 2005; 111(25):3481–8.
5. Nanna MG, Wang SY, Damluji AA. Management of Stable Angina in the Older Adult Population. Circulation: Cardiovascular Interventions 2023;16(4):e012438.
6. Pinsky JL, Jette AM, Branch LG, et al. The Framingham Disability Study: relationship of various coronary heart disease manifestations to disability in older persons living in the community. Am J Public Health 1990;80(11):1363–7.
7. Tinetti ME, Inouye SK, Gill TM, et al. Shared risk factors for falls, incontinence, and functional dependence. Unifying the approach to geriatric syndromes. JAMA 1995; 273(17):1348–53.
8. Damluji AA, Chung SE, Xue QL, et al. Frailty and cardiovascular outcomes in the National Health and Aging Trends Study. Eur Heart J 2021;42(37):3856–65.

9. Nanna MG, Sutton NR, Kochar A, et al. A Geriatric Approach to Percutaneous Coronary Interventions in Older Adults, Part II: A JACC: Advances Expert Panel. JACC Adv 2023;2(5). https://doi.org/10.1016/j.jacadv.2023.100421.

10. Nanna MG, Sutton NR, Kochar A, et al. Assessment and Management of Older Adults Undergoing PCI, Part 1: A JACC: Advances Expert Panel. JACC Adv 2023;(4):2. https://doi.org/10.1016/j.jacadv.2023.100389.

11. Goraya TY, Jacobsen SJ, Pellikka PA, et al. Prognostic value of treadmill exercise testing in elderly persons. Ann Intern Med 2000;132(11):862–70.

12. Laggoune J, Nerlekar N, Munnur K, et al. The utility of coronary computed tomography angiography in elderly patients. J Geriatr Cardiol 2019;16(7):507–13.

13. Lowenstern A, Alexander KP, Hill CL, et al. Age-Related Differences in the Noninvasive Evaluation for Possible Coronary Artery Disease: Insights From the Prospective Multicenter Imaging Study for Evaluation of Chest Pain (PROMISE) Trial. JAMA Cardiol 2020;5(2):193–201.

14. Writing Committee M, Gulati M, Levy PD, et al. AHA/ACC/ASE/CHEST/SAEM/SCCT/SCMR Guideline for the Evaluation and Diagnosis of Chest Pain: A Report of the American College of Cardiology/American Heart Association Joint Committee on Clinical Practice Guidelines. J Am Coll Cardiol 2021;78(22):e187–285.

15. Knuuti J, Wijns W, Saraste A, et al. ESC Guidelines for the diagnosis and management of chronic coronary syndromes. Eur Heart J 2020;41(3):407–77.

16. Dibben G, Faulkner J, Oldridge N, et al. Exercise-based cardiac rehabilitation for coronary heart disease. Cochrane Database Syst Rev 2021;11(11):CD001800.

17. Damluji AA, Forman DE, Wang TY, et al. Management of Acute Coronary Syndrome in the Older Adult Population: A Scientific Statement From the American Heart Association. Circulation 2023;147(3):e32–62.

18. Gencer B, Marston NA, Im K, et al. Efficacy and safety of lowering LDL cholesterol in older patients: a systematic review and meta-analysis of randomised controlled trials. Lancet 2020;396(10263):1637–43.

19. Rodriguez F, Maron DJ, Knowles JW, et al. Association Between Intensity of Statin Therapy and Mortality in Patients With Atherosclerotic Cardiovascular Disease. JAMA Cardiol 2017;2(1):47–54.

20. Cholesterol Treatment Trialists C. Efficacy and safety of statin therapy in older people: a meta-analysis of individual participant data from 28 randomised controlled trials. Lancet 2019;393(10170):407–15.

21. Nanna MG, Navar AM, Wang TY, et al. Statin Use and Adverse Effects Among Adults >75 Years of Age: Insights From the Patient and Provider Assessment of Lipid Management (PALM) Registry. J Am Heart Assoc 2018;7(10). https://doi.org/10.1161/jaha.118.008546.

22. Nanna MG, Nelson AJ, Haynes K, et al. Lipid-lowering treatment among older patients with atherosclerotic cardiovascular disease. J Am Geriatr Soc 2023;71(4):1243–9.

23. Husted S, James S, Becker RC, et al. Ticagrelor versus clopidogrel in elderly patients with acute coronary syndromes: a substudy from the prospective randomized PLATelet inhibition and patient Outcomes (PLATO) trial. Circ Cardiovasc Qual Outcomes 2012;5(5):680–8.

24. Wiviott SD, Braunwald E, McCabe CH, et al. Prasugrel versus clopidogrel in patients with acute coronary syndromes. N Engl J Med 2007;357(20):2001–15.

25. Cay S, Cagirci G, Aydogdu S, et al. Safety of clopidogrel in older patients: a non-randomized, parallel-group, controlled, two-centre study. Drugs Aging 2011;28(2):119–29.

26. Gargiulo G. To EncourAGE Individualized Dual Antiplatelet Therapy Duration After Drug-Eluting Stent Implantation: A New pAGE of an Intriguing Book. JACC Cardiovasc Interv 2018;11(5):444–7.
27. Lee SY, Hong MK, Palmerini T, et al. Short-Term Versus Long-Term Dual Antiplatelet Therapy After Drug-Eluting Stent Implantation in Elderly Patients: A Meta-Analysis of Individual Participant Data From 6 Randomized Trials. JACC Cardiovasc Interv 2018;11(5):435–43.
28. Kang J, Park KW, Lee H, et al. Aspirin Versus Clopidogrel for Long-Term Maintenance Monotherapy After Percutaneous Coronary Intervention: The HOST-EXAM Extended Study. Circulation 2023;147(2):108–17.
29. Aggarwal D, Bhatia K, Chunawala ZS, et al. P2Y(12) inhibitor versus aspirin monotherapy for secondary prevention of cardiovascular events: meta-analysis of randomized trials. Eur Heart J Open 2022;2(2):oeac019.
30. Sullivan AE, Nanna MG, Rao SV, et al. A systematic review of randomized trials comparing double versus triple antithrombotic therapy in patients with atrial fibrillation undergoing percutaneous coronary intervention. Catheter Cardiovasc Interv 2020;96(2):E102–9.
31. Yasuda S, Kaikita K, Akao M, et al. Antithrombotic Therapy for Atrial Fibrillation with Stable Coronary Disease. N Engl J Med 2019;381(12):1103–13.
32. Krumholz HM, Radford MJ, Wang Y, et al. National use and effectiveness of beta-blockers for the treatment of elderly patients after acute myocardial infarction: National Cooperative Cardiovascular Project. JAMA 1998;280(7): 623–9.
33. Joyal M, Cremer KF, Pieper JA, et al. Systemic, left ventricular and coronary hemodynamic effects of intravenous diltiazem in coronary artery disease. Am J Cardiol 1985;56(7):413–7.
34. Steinman MA, Zullo AR, Lee Y, et al. Association of beta-Blockers With Functional Outcomes, Death, and Rehospitalization in Older Nursing Home Residents After Acute Myocardial Infarction. JAMA Intern Med 2017;177(2):254–62.
35. Fleg JL, Aronow WS, Frishman WH. Cardiovascular drug therapy in the elderly: benefits and challenges. Nat Rev Cardiol 2011;8(1):13–28.
36. Shanmugasundaram M, Alpert JS. Acute coronary syndrome in the elderly. Clin Cardiol 2009;32(11):608–13.
37. Heidenreich PA, McDonald KM, Hastie T, et al. Meta-analysis of trials comparing beta-blockers, calcium antagonists, and nitrates for stable angina. JAMA 1999; 281(20):1927–36.
38. Fihn SD, Blankenship JC, Alexander KP, et al. ACC/AHA/AATS/PCNA/SCAI/STS focused update of the guideline for the diagnosis and management of patients with stable ischemic heart disease: a report of the American College of Cardiology/American Heart Association Task Force on Practice Guidelines, and the American Association for Thoracic Surgery, Preventive Cardiovascular Nurses Association, Society for Cardiovascular Angiography and Interventions, and Society of Thoracic Surgeons. J Am Coll Cardiol 2014;64(18):1929–49.
39. Wei J, Wu T, Yang Q, et al. Nitrates for stable angina: a systematic review and meta-analysis of randomized clinical trials. Int J Cardiol 2011;146(1):4–12.
40. Thadani U. Challenges with nitrate therapy and nitrate tolerance: prevalence, prevention, and clinical relevance. Am J Cardiovasc Drugs 2014;14(4): 287–301.
41. Hasenfuss G, Maier LS. Mechanism of action of the new anti-ischemia drug ranolazine. Clin Res Cardiol 2008;97(4):222–6.

42. Belsey J, Savelieva I, Mugelli A, et al. Relative efficacy of antianginal drugs used as add-on therapy in patients with stable angina: A systematic review and meta-analysis. Eur J Prev Cardiol 2015;22(7):837–48.

43. Goyal P, Nanna MG. Stable Coronary Artery Disease in the Age of Geriatric Cardiology. J Am Coll Cardiol 2023;81(17):1710–3.

44. Ahmad Y, Howard JP, Arnold AD, et al. Mortality after drug-eluting stents vs. coronary artery bypass grafting for left main coronary artery disease: a meta-analysis of randomized controlled trials. Eur Heart J 2020;41(34):3228–35.

45. Chaitman BR, Hardison RM, Adler D, et al. The Bypass Angioplasty Revascularization Investigation 2 Diabetes randomized trial of different treatment strategies in type 2 diabetes mellitus with stable ischemic heart disease: impact of treatment strategy on cardiac mortality and myocardial infarction. Circulation 2009; 120(25):2529–40.

46. Ikeno F, Brooks MM, Nakagawa K, et al. SYNTAX Score and Long-Term Outcomes: The BARI-2D Trial. J Am Coll Cardiol 2017;69(4):395–403.

47. Farkouh ME, Domanski M, Dangas GD, et al. Long-Term Survival Following Multivessel Revascularization in Patients With Diabetes: The FREEDOM Follow-On Study. J Am Coll Cardiol 2019;73(6):629–38.

48. Stone GW, Kappetein AP, Sabik JF, et al. Five-Year Outcomes after PCI or CABG for Left Main Coronary Disease. N Engl J Med 2019;381(19):1820–30.

49. Investigators T. Trial of invasive versus medical therapy in elderly patients with chronic symptomatic coronary-artery disease (TIME): a randomised trial. Lancet 2001;358(9286):951–7.

50. Nguyen DD, Spertus JA, Alexander KP, et al. Health Status and Clinical Outcomes in Older Adults With Chronic Coronary Disease: The ISCHEMIA Trial. J Am Coll Cardiol 2023;81(17):1697–709.

51. Boden WE, O'Rourke RA, Teo KK, et al. Optimal medical therapy with or without PCI for stable coronary disease. N Engl J Med 2007;356(15):1503–16.

52. Teo KK, Sedlis SP, Boden WE, et al. Optimal medical therapy with or without percutaneous coronary intervention in older patients with stable coronary disease: a pre-specified subset analysis of the COURAGE (Clinical Outcomes Utilizing Revascularization and Aggressive druG Evaluation) trial. J Am Coll Cardiol 2009;54(14):1303–8.

53. Chung SC, Hlatky MA, Faxon D, et al. The effect of age on clinical outcomes and health status BARI 2D (Bypass Angioplasty Revascularization Investigation in Type 2 Diabetes). J Am Coll Cardiol 2011;58(8):810–9.

54. Park DY, Hanna JM, Kadian S, et al. In-hospital outcomes and readmission in older adults treated with percutaneous coronary intervention for stable ischemic heart disease. J Geriatr Cardiol 2022;19(9):631–42.

55. Lemaire A, Soto C, Salgueiro L, et al. The impact of age on outcomes of coronary artery bypass grafting. J Cardiothorac Surg 2020;15(1):158.

56. Solomon J, Moss E, Morin JF, et al. The Essential Frailty Toolset in Older Adults Undergoing Coronary Artery Bypass Surgery. J Am Heart Assoc 2021;10(15): e020219.

57. Lee JA, Yanagawa B, An KR, et al. Frailty and pre-frailty in cardiac surgery: a systematic review and meta-analysis of 66,448 patients. J Cardiothorac Surg 2021; 16(1):184.

58. Centers for Disease Control and Prevention NCfHS. Table 4. Life expectancy at birth, age 65, and age 75, by sex, race, and Hispanic origin: United States, selected years 1900–2018. https://www.cdc.gov/nchs/data/hus/2019/004-508.pdf.

59. Hamczyk MR, Nevado RM, Barettino A, et al. Biological Versus Chronological Aging: JACC Focus Seminar. J Am Coll Cardiol 2020;75(8):919–30.
60. Sedlis SP, Hartigan PM, Teo KK, et al. Effect of PCI on Long-Term Survival in Patients with Stable Ischemic Heart Disease. N Engl J Med 2015;373(20): 1937–46.
61. Maron DJ, Hochman JS, Reynolds HR, et al. Initial Invasive or Conservative Strategy for Stable Coronary Disease. N Engl J Med 2020;382(15):1395–407.

Racial and Ethnic Disparities in the Management of Chronic Coronary Disease

Wilson Lay Tang, MD[a], Fatima Rodriguez, MD, MPH[b],*

KEYWORDS

- Chronic coronary disease • Race • Ethnicity • Disparities • Management

KEY POINTS

- Chronic coronary disease (CCD) is common across diverse patient populations.
- Racial and ethnic representation disparities are pervasive in CCD guideline-informing clinical trials.
- Disparities remain in the multifaceted approach toward CCD management including lifestyle approaches, medical management, and cardiac rehabilitation.

INTRODUCTION

Chronic coronary disease (CCD) comprises a continuum of conditions that include obstructive and non-obstructive coronary artery disease (CAD) with or without prior acute coronary syndrome (ACS).[1] It is estimated that there are 20 million individuals in the United States with CCD, and death from coronary heart disease (CHD) remains the leading cause of death worldwide, with significant disparities by race and ethnicity (**Table 1**). The recent 2023 CCD management guidelines released by the American College of Cardiology/American Heart Association (AHA) highlighted the importance of social determinants of health in the risk and outcomes for CCD.[1]

There is a rising incidence in the disease burden of cardiovascular disease with an estimated global prevalence of 1655 per 100,000 population with the United States having a higher prevalence of 2929 per 100,000.[2] The aging population and increasing prevalence of co-morbidities such as hyperlipidemia, obesity, and diabetes are major factors in the increasing impact of CCD for the future to come.[2]

[a] Department of Medicine, Stanford University, 300 Pasteur Drive, L154, Stanford, CA 94305-5133, USA; [b] Division of Cardiovascular Medicine and Cardiovascular Institute, Department of Medicine, Center for Academic Medicine, Stanford University School of Medicine, Stanford, CA, USA
* Correspondence author. 453 Quarry Road, Palo Alto, CA 94304.
E-mail address: frodrigu@stanford.edu
Twitter: @FaRodriguezMD (F.R.)

Med Clin N Am 108 (2024) 595–607
https://doi.org/10.1016/j.mcna.2023.11.008
0025-7125/24/© 2023 Elsevier Inc. All rights reserved.

Table 1
Prevalence of coronary heart disease, myocardial infarction, angina pectoris

Population Group	Prevalence, CHD, 2017–2020, ≥20 y of Age	Prevalence, MI, 2017–2020, ≥20 y of Age	Prevalence, AP, 2017–2020, ≥20 y of Age
Both sexes	20,500,000 (7.1%) [95% CI, 6.1%–8.3%]	9,300,000 (3.2%) [95% CI, 2.5%–4.0%]	10,800,000 (3.9%) [95% CI, 3.3%–4.5%]
Males	11,700,000 (8.7%)	6,100,000 (4.5%)	5,600,000 (4.3%)
Females	8,800,000 (5.8%)	3,200,000 (2.1%)	5,200,000 (3.6%)
NH White males	9.40%	4.80%	4.70%
NH White females	5.90%	2.20%	3.50%
NH Black males	6.20%	4.00%	2.70%
NH Black females	6.30%	2.30%	4.10%
Hispanic males	6.80%	3.10%	3.60%
Hispanic females	6.10%	1.90%	4.30%
NH Asian males	5.20%	2.80%	2.70%
NH Asian females	3.90%	0.50%	2.70%

Abbreviation: NH, Non-Hispanic.
Prevalence obtained using age-adjusted estimates of self-reported data.
Data from the 2023 heart disease and Stroke Statistics Report (Tsao CW, et al. Circulation. 2023;147(8): e93-e621.) using the National Health and Nutritional Examination Survey (NHANES) dataset.

For most patients with CCD, the primary treatment approaches include intensive lifestyle interventions and optimization of guideline-directed medical therapy (GDMT).[1,3] Invasive interventions are also used in select patient populations with CCD including those with significant left main disease, 3-vessel CAD with diabetes, heart failure with reduced ejection fraction and those with limiting angina despite GDMT. Outside of these population groups, there have been recent studies showing that revascularization does not improve mortality or morbidity on top of GDMT for patients with CCD, even in the presence of significant ischemia on non-invasive testing.[4,5]

With the long history of known racial and ethnic inequalities in procedural utilization, treatment strategies and cardiovascular health outcomes for patients with CCD,[6–8] this review will focus on the racial and ethnic disparities of the multifaceted approach toward CCD management.

TERMINOLOGY
Race and ethnicity

Race and ethnicity are often conflated but they represent separate social constructs. Race refers to a population group of ancestral descent and physical traits whereas ethnicity refers to a population group of similar cultural, linguistic, or religious background.[9] The racial categories in 2020 US Census include White, Black or African American, Asian, American Indian/Alaska Native, and Native Hawaiian/Other Pacific Islander. The term Hispanic or Latino refers to a heterogeneous group of individuals of any race, ancestry, ethnicity, or combination, who have origins in South America, Central America, Mexico, the Caribbean, or any other Spanish-speaking country or culture.[10] Importantly, race and ethnicity are not biological but instead reflect deeply rooted social constructs that have profound effects on cardiovascular risk and outcomes.[11]

Population shift and socioeconomic status

There has been a shift in population size and distribution between the 2010 and 2020 US Census with a notable decrease in non-Hispanic White population size/percentage and an increase in the Hispanic/Latinx, Asian, and 2 or More Race population.[10,12]

There are notable differences by socioeconomic factors by race and ethnicity. On average, non-Hispanic White and Asian populations have higher mean incomes compared to the average American household income of $69,717 per the 2021 American Community Survey.[13] Black and American Indian/Alaska Indian populations had the lowest median household incomes at $46,774 and $53,149 respectively.[13]

Prevalence of chronic coronary disease by race and ethnicity

The 2023 AHA Heart Disease and Stroke Statistics noted that the prevalence rate of CHD was 7.1% with higher rates in males (8.7%) versus females (5.8%) (see **Table 1**).[14] Non-Hispanic White male individuals had the highest rate (9.4%) whereas Asian females had the lowest (3.9%).

DIVERSITY IN CLINICAL TRIALS

There have been numerous landmark trials that have shaped the 2023 AHA CCD Guidelines and prior guidelines to date. This section will highlight the demographics of a few selected trials to better understand the diversity of these randomized controlled trials throughout the years and whether they accurately represented the current population of this country (**Table 2**).

One of the earliest landmark trials, the Coronary Artery Surgery Study (CASS) trial in 1983, found that aggressive initial coronary artery bypass graft treatment does not improve outcomes in CCD.[15] However, 98.3% of their enrolled patients were White. Another trial, the Clinical Outcomes Utilizing Revascularization and Aggressive Drug Evaluation (COURAGE) trial in 2007 that found an initial percutaneous coronary intervention (PCI) strategy for CCD did not improve mortality or major adverse cardiovascular events (MACE), also underrepresented non-White population with 85.9% of patients being White.[16] Even more contemporary trials informing management of CCD have had limited racial and ethnic representation. For example, the 2021 Aspirin Dosing: A Patient-Centric Trial Assessing Benefits and Long-Term Effectiveness (ADAPTABLE) trial which compared dosing of 81 mg versus 325 mg of aspirin in patients with established atherosclerotic cardiovascular disease, nearly 80% of the study population identified as White. Similarly in the 2022 Revascularization for Ischemic Ventricular Dysfunction (REVIVED-BCI2) trials which found revascularization via PCI in patients with ischemic left ventricle ejection fraction less than 35% heart failure does not improve mortality or hospitalization rates for heart failure, 90.6% of their enrolled patients were White.[17,18]

However, there are some trials such as the Bypass Angioplasty Revascularization Investigation 2 Diabetes (BARI-2D) trial in 2009, which investigated whether early revascularization in patients with CCD and type 2 diabetes mellitus (T2DM) improved outcomes and found no significant difference in mortality and MACE, enrolled a population much more representative of the US population, with 16.8% of the study participants identifying as Black and 12.5% identifying as Hispanic.[19] More recently in 2022, the International Study of Comparative Health Effectiveness with Medical and Invasive Approaches (ISCHEMIA) trial in 2022 found no reduction in risk of ischemic cardiovascular events or deaths with an initial invasive strategy in those with stable coronary disease with moderate or severe ischemia.[4] This trial was more representative of races and ethnicities but had an overrepresentation of Asian patients, accounting for

Table 2
List of selected landmark clinical trials in CCD: demographics

	2020 US Census	CASS (1983)		COURAGE (2007)		BARI-2D (2009)[a]		ADAPTABLE (2021)[b]		REVIVED-BCIS2(2022)[c]		ISCHEMIA (2022)[d]		CLEAR-OUTCOMES (2023)	
	%	Total	%	Total	%	Total	%	Total	%	Total	%	Total	%	Total	%
White (non-Hispanic)	57.8%	767	98.3%	1963	85.9%	1561	65.9%	11,990	79.5%	634	90.6%	3403	65.7%	12,732	91.1%
Hispanic or Latino	18.7%			126	5.5%	296	12.5%	481	3.2%			763	14.7%	2333	18.3%
Black	12.1%			114	5.0%	398	16.8%	1311	8.7%	6	0.9%	204	3.9%		
Asian	5.9%					114	4.8%	146	1.0%	49	7.0%	1485	28.7%		
American Indian and Alaska Native	0.7%							114	0.8%						
Native Hawaiian and Other Pacific Islander	0.2%														
Other Race	0.5%			82	3.6%			401	2.7%			37	0.7%		
Two or More Race	4.1%							134	0.9%	11	1.6%				
Total		780		2285		2368		15,076		700		5179		13,975	

[a] Only 63% of enrolled patients were from the US asian population group includes other races.

[b] 6.5% of patients reported "Prefer not to say" regarding race and ethnicity.

[c] Study did not distinguish between non-Hispanic and Hispanic White population group. The 11 in mixed race group includes other or not reported.

[d] 50 patients did not report race.

Abbreviations: ADAPTABLE, aspirin dosing: a patient-centric trial assessing benefits and long-term effectiveness; BARI 2D, bypass angioplasty revascularization investigation 2 diabetes; CASS, coronary artery surgery study; CLEAR, cholesterol lowering via bempedoic acid [ECT1002], an ACL-inhibiting regimen outcomes trial; COURAGE, clinical outcomes utilizing revascularization and aggressive drug evaluation; ISCHEMIA, International Study of Comparative Health Effectiveness with Medical and Invasive Approaches; REVIVED, revascularization for ischemic ventricular dysfunction trial.

28.7% of the trial population, exceeding the US 2020 census estimate of 5.9% for the Asian population.

The recently reported Cholesterol Lowering via Bempedoic Acid [ECT1002], an ACL-Inhibiting Regimen (CLEAR) Outcomes trial in 2023 randomized statin-intolerant patients to bempedoic acid or placebo enrolled 18.3% Hispanic or Latinx individuals but 91.1% of enrollees were White.[20]

Increasing clinical trial diversity in practice-informing CCD trials is a priority and will involve concerted efforts from policy makers, study sponsors, and academic partners.

DISPARITIES IN NON-INVASIVE MANAGEMENT
Lifestyle Changes

Lifestyle modification is one of the main pillars of secondary prevention of CCD, especially in reducing co-morbidities such as hypertension and diabetes mellitus. Dietary change is one effective component of lifestyle changes. One widely known diet, the Dietary Approaches to Stop Hypertension (DASH) diet has been shown to reduce blood pressure substantially.[21] Another diet, the Mediterranean diet, has been shown to be an effective secondary prevention method to reduce incidence of major cardiovascular events.[22] However, there are racial and ethnic disparities present in both utilization and adherence to these diets. In 1 study looking at NHANES data from 2001 to 2002, adherence to the DASH diet was associated with higher socioeconomic status and education, and was lower in disadvantaged groups, with non-Hispanic Black population having the lowest adherence.[23] Another study looked at dietary quality trend from 1999 to 2010, using a health score based on the mean consumption of industrially produced *trans*-fat, and found that lower socioeconomic status was associated with worse dietary quality.[24]

Other studies looking at the impact of food insecurity and food deserts, defined as low-income communities with limited access to healthy food, have found that across a national level, lower income food deserts are associated with increased cardiovascular burden and increased mortality.[25,26] Furthermore, the prevalence of food insecurity continues to persist, especially in non-Hispanic Black and Hispanic populations.[27]

Physical activity is another modifier that has been shown to be vital in secondary prevention of CCD. However, there remain disparities in the amount of physical activity seen. One study looked at self-reported leisure-time physical activity from the 2007 California Health Interview Survey and found that all non-White race and ethnicities engaged in less vigorous physical activity compared with the White population.[28] Another study looking at low-income Black and White population found that Black population had higher odds of self-reported physical inactivity via the National Health Interview Survey.[29]

GUIDELINE-DIRECTED MEDICAL THERAPY FOR CHRONIC CORONARY DISEASE

GDMT is the cornerstone for CCD management. However, there are persistent and pronounced racial and ethnic disparities in access and adherence to evidence-based therapies for secondary prevention.

Antiplatelet therapy is one component of CCD GDMT. One study found that Black and Hispanic populations with CCD are less likely to take aspirin compared with White population, even after accounting for sociodemographic components.[30] This was corroborated with the Multi-Ethnic Study of Atherosclerosis that found that although there has been an increase in aspirin use since the USPSTF recommendation in 2002, there remains underutilization across non-White race and ethnicities.[31] In a study utilizing in-home interviews, Black older adults were less likely to use aspirin or statins compared with White older adults, even after controlling for socioeconomic differences, access to care, and co-morbidities.[32]

After acute myocardial infarction, either managed solely with medical therapy or with revascularization, dual antiplatelet therapy is indicated for a period of time afterward. In recent years, newer P2Y12 inhibitors such as ticagrelor or prasugrel have been shown to be superior in efficacy compared to clopidogrel and have been increasingly prescribed since its introduction.[33–35] However, one retrospective study found that Hispanic ethnicity and lower household income were associated with clopidogrel initiation over these newer agents. Lower adherence rates were also noted in patients of underrepresented races and ethnicities.[36] Notably, socioeconomic predictors for clopidogrel use over these newer agents include no insurance, insurance with Medicare or Medicaid.[35]

Lipid control with medications is another key component of the management of CCD with the aim to achieve reduction in LDL-C levels to reduce risk of MACE. Although historically achieved by statin medications, there has been a rapid development in non-statin agents for LDL-C reduction including ezetimibe, proprotein convertase subtilisin/kexin type 9 (PCSK9) inhibitors such as alirocumab and evolocumab, as well as newer novel agents such as bempedoic acid. These agents are now increasingly used as adjuncts to statin therapy, especially if patients are on maximally tolerated statin therapy or judged to be high risk. However, there are large differences in utilization of lipid-lowering drugs. Black older adults with CCD were found to be less likely to use statins.[31] Another cross-sectional study using the Medical Expenditure Panel Survey found Black and Hispanic men alongside all non-White women were less likely to report statin usage compared to White men.[37] Poor access to care, due to either lack of insurance or routine location for health, were identified as key factors for lower statin use.[38]

There are also racial and ethnic disparities in initiating non-statin medications such as ezetimibe or PCSK9 inhibitors in those who are on maximal statin therapy. One study found that Black patients had lower rates of ezetimibe and PCSK9 inhibitor initiation compared to White patients.[39] PCSK9 inhibitor initiation was also found to be lower among veterans of a race or ethnicity other than non-Hispanic White.[40]

Use of novel and emerging therapies

With the 2023 CCD guidelines, one important new distinction is the rise of sodium-glucose transport protein 2 inhibitors (SGLT2i) and glucagon-like peptide 1 receptor agonist (GLP-1 RA) in GDMT especially in those with diabetes or heart failure.[1] Already, there is mounting evidence of the potential disparities in utilization of these powerful therapies. One study found that Asian, Black, and Hispanic patients with diabetes had lower rates of GLP-1 agonist use compared to White patients.[41] Another study similarly found that Veterans of several different racial groups and Hispanic Veterans with diabetes were less likely to receive prescription for SGLT2i or GLP-1 RA.[42] Early initiation of GLP-1 RA or SGLT2i in adults with diabetes following new diagnosis of CVD was low especially among Black or other races and ethnicity.[43] With new evidence for the role of GLP-1 in CCD patients without diabetes, efforts are needed to ensure that these therapies are accessible to diverse populations to ensure that all patients can benefit.

CARDIAC REHABILITATION

Cardiac rehabilitation has been a known anchor to optimize secondary prevention of CCD. However, it is important to understand the barriers as well as disparities in participation and access to care.

In one retrospective study, participation in cardiac rehab was lower in Asian, Black, and Hispanic patient populations in comparison to White population. Furthermore, time to cardiac rehab attendance was significantly longer for these patient populations in comparison to White population. This was consistent across all different household incomes levels.[44] In another study looking more closely at Los Angeles County, non-Hispanic Black people lived further away from a cardiac rehab facility than non-Hispanic White people.[45]

Referral rates for cardiac rehab were also found to be significantly lower for Black, Hispanic and Asian patients, who are 20%, 36%, and 50% less likely respectively in comparison to White patients at time of discharge.[46] In another observational study looking at cardiac rehab participation rates amongst Medicare patients eligible for cardiac rehab, Black, Hispanic, and Asian patients had participation rates of 13.6%, 13.2%, 16.3%, respectively, compared with 25.8% in non-Hispanic White patients.[47]

DISPARITIES IN INVASIVE MANAGEMENT AND OUTCOMES

There have been numerous studies documenting racial and ethnic disparities in the utilization of revascularization, particularly among Black patients.[6–8,48,49] However, even in more contemporary studies, racial and ethnic disparities in the treatment of patients presenting with ACS remain. One study, using the National Inpatient Sample database from 2009 to 2018, found that Black patients who undergo PCI for STEMI were less likely to receive drug eluting stents (DES) compared to White patients.[50] Furthermore, 1 study found that alongside Black ethnicity, lower median household income, lack of private insurance, as well as non-urban and for-profit hospital status, were also independently associated with not undergoing primary PCI on day of admission for AMI.[51] Even lower neighborhood-level income regardless of race, was associated with a lower likelihood of receiving angiography.[52]

Lower-income patients continue to be less likely to receive an angiogram within a day of admission for STEMI and less likely to be using a DES alongside with slightly worsened mortality rates in STEMI patients.[53] Notably, the proportions of revascularization procedures increased from 2003 to 2016 across all races and ethnicities with no disparities noted in incidence of STEMI-related cardiogenic shock.[54,55] However, differences in management and in-hospital mortality rate in those with AMI complicated by cardiac arrest persists with Black patients and patients of other races and ethnicities having lower use of coronary angiography and PCI, longer time to angiography, and greater use of palliative care consultation compared to white patients.[56] Patient of other races and ethnicities were also noted to have higher in-hospital mortality rate compared to White patients.[56] During the COVID-19 pandemic, Black, Asian, and Hispanic populations also had disproportionate rise in deaths caused by heart disease.[57]

ADDRESSING DISPARITIES AND CONCLUSIONS

CCD is increasingly more prevalent, with growing burden on the healthcare system. Individuals from historically marginalized racial and ethnic backgrounds experience a disproportionate burden of CCD risk factors and adverse outcomes. Identifying disparities in the management of CCD can help inform strategies to mitigate them, and these include solutions involving patients, clinicians, health systems, and communities (**Fig. 1**).

From a clinician's perspective, being cognizant of the additional risk factors and racial and ethnic disparities present in CCD management is a key to guiding patient care. Understanding one's own intrinsic and external biases is also imperative to minimize

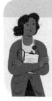
Clinician

- Continual education for CCD treatment updates and advances
- Ensure mandatory implicit bias training and patient-centered approach to CCD
- Bridge language barriers with certified medical interpreters
- Leverage care team models for increased access

Patient

- Personalized patient education that considers health literacy
- Empower patients to establish care goals and provide patient-recorded outcomes
- Care coordination and increasing accessibility
- Document adherence to GDMT at each visit

Community Partnerships

- Improve awareness for healthy dietary habits and lifestyles
- Increase access to fresh, healthy food products
- Expand recreational areas for physical activity and improve the built environment

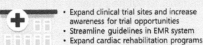
Health System

- Expand clinical trial sites and increase awareness for trial opportunities
- Streamline guidelines in EMR system
- Expand cardiac rehabilitation programs
- Increase accessibility of telehealth services
- Promote diversity in healthcare teams, research investigators, and research staff

Fig. 1. Strategies to reduce disparities in the management of chronic coronary disease.

disparities in care. Addressing disparities in utilization and adherence to GDMT is essential to improving health in diverse populations. Utilizing auxiliary staff to follow up and improving accessibility to telehealth services can allow for better adherence to GDMT. Creating personalized patient education considering varying health literacy and languages can be utilized to empower patient awareness of CCD. Increasing utilization of certified medical interpreters is the key to bridging language barriers.

At a community level, there are potential opportunities that can be taken to improve lifestyle management of CCD. Increasing access to fresh, healthy food products, especially in food deserts, as well as increasing awareness of healthy dietary habits and physical lifestyles can be avenues of approach for further intervention. Promoting awareness of the Supplemental Nutrition Assistance Program (SNAP) to address food insecurity is the key to improving dietary health disparities.[58] Expanding recreational areas for physical activity with continued investments in ongoing infrastructure is important to foster a healthier community and reducing burden of CCD.

Furthermore, there are many aspects that can be improved to reduce disparities across the different aspects of CCD at a health system level. From a clinical trial perspective, expanding enrollment and trial sites to better include underrepresented races and ethnicities in underserved populations is key to reflecting the changing demographics of this nation.[59,60] By doing so provides equity and fairness in opportunities for clinical trials. However, it is important to acknowledge the long-standing history of distrust in the medical system after historical maleficent activities, such as the Tuskegee syphilis study, as well as logistical and socioeconomic barriers to trial sites that may prove to be challenges in bridging the gap in trial enrollment. Additionally, expanding research toward healthier diets that cater toward cultural and dietary habits of Americans could be options toward having accessible and feasible food options for our diverse nation. There have been studies, such as the ¡Viva Bien! that have looked at Mediterranean diet in Hispanic patients but found nonadherence at 12 months due to cultural differences in diet.[61] Promoting diversity in the medical field can help open new perspectives and allow a cultural melting pot of ideas to emerge as a result.

Opportunities are plentiful in streamlining guidelines in the electronic medical records system to encourage prescription and utilization of drugs for secondary prevention of CCD as well as promote automated referrals for cardiac rehab. Further expansion in cardiac rehabilitation programs as well as allocating additional resources to alleviate the socioeconomic burdens that may arise with ongoing participation.

It is noted that there are components not touched upon in this review including focuses on the impact of social support, mental health, sex, and gender biases that play a compounding role in the racial and ethnic disparities seen.

There is more research in CCD management that needs to be done to better understand the complexity and various factors contributing to racial and ethnic healthcare disparities. Equally important is applying this knowledge and to create solutions for addressing these differences in care and moving toward implementation of these solutions throughout health systems.

CLINICS CARE POINT

- CCD is increasingly prevalent and disproportionately affects historically marginalized populations.
- Racial and ethnic disparities are pervasive in the management and outcomes of CCD.
- Solutions to reduce disparities in CCD should include multiprong interventions that address patient, clinician, and health system factors.

FUNDING

Rodriguez was funded by grants from the NIH, United States, National Heart, Lung, and Blood Institute, United States (1K01HL144607), the American Heart Association, United States/Harold Amos Faculty Development program, and the Doris Duke Foundation (Grant #2022051).

ACKNOWLEDGMENTS

We are grateful for the contributions of Summer Ngo for her editorial assistance, without whom this work would not have been possible.

DISCLOSURE STATEMENT

FR reports consulting relationships with Healthpals, Novartis, Amgen, NovoNordisk (CEC), Movano Health, and Kento Health. The remaining authors report no relevant disclosures or competing interests.

REFERENCES

1. Virani SS, Newby LK, Arnold SV, et al. 2023 AHA/ACC/ACCP/ASPC/NLA/PCNA guideline for the management of patients with chronic coronary disease: a report of the american heart association/american college of cardiology joint committee on clinical practice guidelines. Circulation 2023;148(9):e9–119.
2. Khan MA, Hashim MJ, Mustafa H, et al. Global epidemiology of ischemic heart disease: results from the global burden of disease study. Cureus 2020;12(7): e9349.
3. Boden WE, Marzilli M, Crea F, et al. Evolving management paradigm for stable ischemic heart disease patients. J Am Coll Cardiol 2023;81(5):505–14.
4. Maron DJ, Hochman JS, Reynolds HR, et al. Initial invasive or conservative strategy for stable coronary disease. N Engl J Med 2020;382(15):1395–407.

5. Al-Lamee R, Thompson D, Dehbi HM, et al. Percutaneous coronary intervention in stable angina (ORBITA): a double-blind, randomised controlled trial. Lancet 2018;391(10115):31–40.

6. Slater J, Selzer F, Dorbala S, et al. Ethnic differences in the presentation, treatment strategy, and outcomes of percutaneous coronary intervention (a report from the National Heart, Lung, and Blood Institute Dynamic Registry). Am J Cardiol 2003;92(7):773–8.

7. Whittle J, Conigliaro J, Good CB, et al. Racial differences in the use of invasive cardiovascular procedures in the Department of Veterans Affairs medical system. N Engl J Med 1993;329(9):621–7.

8. Wenneker MB, Epstein AM. Racial inequalities in the use of procedures for patients with ischemic heart disease in massachusetts. JAMA 1989;261(2):253–7.

9. Flanagin A, Frey T, Christiansen SL. AMA manual of style committee. updated guidance on the reporting of race and ethnicity in medical and science journals. JAMA 2021;326(7):621–7.

10. Bureau UC. Measuring racial and ethnic diversity for the 2020 census. The United States Census Bureau. Available at: https://www.census.gov/newsroom/blogs/random-samplings/2021/08/measuring-racial-ethnic-diversity-2020-census.html. Accessed August 20, 2023.

11. Roberts D. Dorothy Roberts: The problem with race-based medicine, TED Talk. Available at: https://www.ted.com/talks/dorothy_roberts_the_problem_with_race_based_medicine. Accessed October 10, 2023.

12. Bureau UC. Racial and ethnic diversity in the United States: 2010 census and 2020 census. Census.gov. Available at: https://www.census.gov/library/visualizations/interactive/racial-and-ethnic-diversity-in-the-united-states-2010-and-2020-census.html. Accessed August 20, 2023.

13. S1903: MEDIAN INCOME IN THE PAST 12 ... - Census Bureau Table. Available at: https://data.census.gov/table?q=median+household+income+race&tid=ACSS T1Y2021.S1903. Accessed September 9, 2023

14. Tsao CW, Aday AW, Almarzooq ZI, et al. Heart disease and stroke statistics—2023 update: a report from the American Heart Association. Circulation 2023; 147(8):e93–621.

15. Coronary artery surgery study (CASS): a randomized trial of coronary artery bypass surgery. Survival data. Circulation 1983;68(5):939–50.

16. Boden WE, O'Rourke RA, Teo KK, et al. Optimal medical therapy with or without pci for stable coronary disease. N Engl J Med 2007;356(15):1503–16.

17. Jones WS, Mulder H, Wruck LM, et al. Comparative effectiveness of aspirin dosing in cardiovascular disease. N Engl J Med 2021;384(21):1981–90.

18. Perera D, Clayton T, O'Kane PD, et al. Percutaneous revascularization for ischemic left ventricular dysfunction. N Engl J Med 2022;387(15):1351–60.

19. A randomized trial of therapies for type 2 diabetes and coronary artery disease. N Engl J Med 2009;360(24):2503–15.

20. Nissen SE, Lincoff AM, Brennan D, et al. Bempedoic acid and cardiovascular outcomes in statin-intolerant patients. N Engl J Med 2023;388(15):1353–64.

21. Sacks FM, Svetkey LP, Vollmer WM, et al. Effects on blood pressure of reduced dietary sodium and the dietary approaches to stop hypertension (DASH) Diet. N Engl J Med 2001;344(1):3–10.

22. Delgado-Lista J, Alcala-Diaz JF, Torres-Peña JD, et al. Long-term secondary prevention of cardiovascular disease with a Mediterranean diet and a low-fat diet (CORDIOPREV): a randomised controlled trial. Lancet 2022;399(10338):1876–85.

23. Monsivais P, Rehm CD, Drewnowski A. The DASH diet and diet costs among ethnic and racial groups in the United States. JAMA Intern Med 2013;173(20): 1922–4.

24. Wang DD, Leung CW, Li Y, et al. Trends in dietary quality among adults in the United States, 1999 through 2010. JAMA Intern Med 2014;174(10):1587–95.

25. Kelli HM, Kim JH, Samman Tahhan A, et al. Living in food deserts and adverse cardiovascular outcomes in patients with cardiovascular disease. J Am Heart Assoc 2019;8(4):e010694.

26. Lloyd M, Amos ME, Milfred-Laforest S, et al. Residing in a food desert and adverse cardiovascular events in US veterans with established cardiovascular disease. Am J Cardiol 2023;196:70–6.

27. Brandt EJ, Chang T, Leung C, et al. Food insecurity among individuals with cardiovascular disease and cardiometabolic risk factors across race and ethnicity in 1999-2018. JAMA Cardiology 2022;7(12):1218–26.

28. August KJ, Sorkin DH. Racial/ethnic disparities in exercise and dietary behaviors of middle-aged and older adults. J Gen Intern Med 2011;26(3):245–50.

29. Wilson-Frederick SM, Thorpe RJ, Bell CN, et al. Examination of race disparities in physical inactivity among adults of similar social context. Ethn Dis 2014;24(3): 363–9.

30. Brown DW, Shepard D, Giles WH, et al. Racial differences in the use of aspirin: an important tool for preventing heart disease and stroke. Ethn Dis 2005;15(4): 620–6.

31. Johansen ME, Hefner JL, Foraker RE. Antiplatelet and statin use in US patients with coronary artery disease categorized by race/ethnicity and gender, 2003 to 2012. Am J Cardiol 2015;115(11):1507–12.

32. Qato DM, Lindau ST, Conti RM, et al. Racial and ethnic disparities in cardiovascular medication use among older adults in the United States. Pharmacoepidemiol Drug Saf 2010;19(8):834–42.

33. Wallentin L, Becker RC, Budaj A, et al. Ticagrelor versus clopidogrel in patients with acute coronary syndromes. N Engl J Med 2009;361(11):1045–57.

34. Wiviott SD, Braunwald E, McCabe CH, et al. Prasugrel versus clopidogrel in patients with acute coronary syndromes. N Engl J Med 2007;357(20):2001–15.

35. Faridi KF, Garratt KN, Kennedy KF, et al. Physician and hospital utilization of P2Y12 inhibitors in ST-segment–elevation myocardial infarction in the United States. Circ Cardiovasc Qual Outcomes 2020;13(3):e006275.

36. Nathan AS, Geng Z, Eberly LA, et al. Identifying racial, ethnic, and socioeconomic inequities in the use of novel p2y12 inhibitors after percutaneous coronary intervention. J Invasive Cardiol 2022;34(3):E171–8.

37. Salami JA, Warraich H, Valero-Elizondo J, et al. National trends in statin use and expenditures in the US adult population from 2002 to 2013: insights from the medical expenditure panel survey. JAMA Cardiology 2017;2(1):56–65.

38. Jacobs JA, Addo DK, Zheutlin AR, et al. Prevalence of statin use for primary prevention of atherosclerotic cardiovascular disease by race, ethnicity, and 10-year disease risk in the US: National Health and Nutrition Examination Surveys, 2013 to march 2020. JAMA Cardiology 2023;8(5):443–52.

39. Colvin CL, Poudel B, Bress AP, et al. Race/ethnic and sex differences in the initiation of non-statin lipid-lowering medication following myocardial infarction. J Clin Lipidol 2021;15(5):665–73.

40. Derington CG, Colantonio LD, Herrick JS, et al. Factors associated with PCSK9 inhibitor initiation among US veterans. J Am Heart Assoc 2021;10(8):e019254.

41. Eberly LA, Yang L, Eneanya ND, et al. Association of race/ethnicity, gender, and socioeconomic status with sodium-glucose cotransporter 2 inhibitor use among patients with diabetes in the US. JAMA Netw Open 2021;4(4):e216139.

42. Lamprea-Montealegre JA, Madden E, Tummalapalli SL, et al. Association of race and ethnicity with prescription of SGLT2 inhibitors and GLP1 receptor agonists among patients with type 2 diabetes in the veterans health administration system. JAMA 2022;328(9):861–71.

43. Cromer SJ, Lauffenburger JC, Levin R, et al. Deficits and disparities in early uptake of glucagon-like peptide 1 receptor agonists and SGLT2i among medicare-insured adults following a new diagnosis of cardiovascular disease or heart failure. Diabetes Care 2023;46(1):65–74.

44. Garfein J, Guhl EN, Swabe G, et al. Racial and ethnic differences in cardiac rehabilitation participation: effect modification by household income. J Am Heart Assoc 2022;11(13):e025591.

45. Ebinger JE, Lan R, Driver MP, et al. Disparities in geographic access to cardiac rehabilitation in los angeles county. J Am Heart Assoc 2022;11(18):e026472.

46. Li S, Fonarow GC, Mukamal K, et al. Sex and racial disparities in cardiac rehabilitation referral at hospital discharge and gaps in long-term mortality. J Am Heart Assoc 2018;7(8):e008088.

47. Ritchey MD, Maresh S, McNeely J, et al. Tracking cardiac rehabilitation participation and completion among medicare beneficiaries to inform the efforts of a national initiative. Circ Cardiovasc Qual Outcomes 2020;13(1):e005902.

48. Ayanian JZ, Udvarhelyi IS, Gatsonis CA, et al. Racial differences in the use of revascularization procedures after coronary angiography. JAMA 1993;269(20):2642–6.

49. Bradley EH, Herrin J, Wang Y, et al. Racial and ethnic differences in time to acute reperfusion therapy for patients hospitalized with myocardial infarction. JAMA 2004;292(13):1563–72.

50. Bhasin V, Hiltner E, Singh A, et al. Disparities in drug-eluting stent utilization in patients with acute st-elevation myocardial infarction: an analysis of the national inpatient sample. Angiology 2023;74(8):774–82.

51. Casale SN, Auster CJ, Wolf F, et al. Ethnicity and socioeconomic status influence use of primary angioplasty in patients presenting with acute myocardial infarction. Am Heart J 2007;154(5):989–93.

52. Rose KM, Foraker RE, Heiss G, et al. Neighborhood Socioeconomic and racial disparities in angiography and coronary revascularization: the ARIC surveillance study. Ann Epidemiol 2012;22(9):623–9.

53. Yong CM, Abnousi F, Asch SM, et al. Socioeconomic inequalities in quality of care and outcomes among patients with acute coronary syndrome in the modern era of drug eluting stents. J Am Heart Assoc 2014;3(6):e001029.

54. Alkhouli M, Alqahtani F, Kalra A, et al. Trends in characteristics and outcomes of hospital inpatients undergoing coronary revascularization in the United States, 2003-2016. JAMA Netw Open 2020;3(2):e1921326.

55. Movahed MR, Khan MF, Hashemzadeh M, et al. Age adjusted nationwide trends in the incidence of all cause and ST elevation myocardial infarction associated cardiogenic shock based on gender and race in the United States. Cardiovasc Revasc Med 2015;16(1):2–5.

56. Subramaniam AV, Patlolla SH, Cheungpasitporn W, et al. Racial and ethnic disparities in management and outcomes of cardiac arrest complicating acute myocardial infarction. J Am Heart Assoc 2021;10(11):e019907.

57. Wadhera RK, Figueroa JF, Rodriguez F, et al. Racial and ethnic disparities in heart and cerebrovascular disease deaths during the COVID-19 pandemic in the United States. Circulation 2021;143(24):2346–54.
58. Samuel LJ, Crews DC, Swenor BK, et al. Supplemental nutrition assistance program access and racial disparities in food insecurity. JAMA Netw Open 2023; 6(6):e2320196.
59. Schwartz AL, Alsan M, Morris AA, et al. Why diverse clinical trial participation matters. N Engl J Med 2023;388(14):1252–4.
60. Improving Representation in clinical trials and research: building research equity for women and underrepresented groups at NAP. Edu. doi:10.17226/26479. Accessed September 15, 2013
61. Toobert DJ, Strycker LA, Barrera M, et al. Outcomes from a multiple risk factor diabetes self-management trial for latinas: ¡Viva Bien. Ann Behav Med 2011; 41(3):310–23.

Moving?

Make sure your subscription moves with you!

To notify us of your new address, find your **Clinics Account Number** (located on your mailing label above your name), and contact customer service at:

Email: journalscustomerservice-usa@elsevier.com

800-654-2452 (subscribers in the U.S. & Canada)
314-447-8871 (subscribers outside of the U.S. & Canada)

Fax number: 314-447-8029

Elsevier Health Sciences Division
Subscription Customer Service
3251 Riverport Lane
Maryland Heights, MO 63043

*To ensure uninterrupted delivery of your subscription, please notify us at least 4 weeks in advance of move.

Printed and bound by CPI Group (UK) Ltd, Croydon, CR0 4YY

03/10/2024

01040466-0001